Cognitive Analytic Therapy for Offenders

Cognitive Analytic Therapy (CAT) is an established form of integrated psychotherapy, which has been applied in a variety of clinical settings to a diversity of disorders with promising outcomes. In *Cognitive Analytic Therapy for Offenders*, the authors describe the application of CAT to forensic settings, illustrating the use of this type of therapy with a range of offence types and clinical disorders.

CAT is presented as a new form of forensic psychotherapy which can enhance the understanding, conceptualisation, treatment and management of offenders. The book offers a novel description of clinical practice and describes the innovative application of CAT to forensic work in a variety of contexts and settings for numerous offence types and clinical disorders, including:

- CAT in the treatment of child sex offenders in secure forensic settings
- The use of CAT with women in secure settings
- CAT for parents within prisons
- CAT for borderline and psychopathic personality disorder
- CAT for a stalking offender
- Community-based CAT with perpetrators of domestic violence
- CAT for homicide perpetrators (rage-type, serial sexual, dissociative homicides)
- The application of CAT for court reporting and managing boundary violations.

This book provides an account of a fresh, new approach to conceptualisation and treatment in forensic psychotherapy, and offers the first description of CAT presented in the form of a compilation of illustrations of practice. It will be essential reading for clinical psychologists and psychiatrists, occupational therapists, and anyone who works within services for offenders.

Philip H. Pollock is the Clinical Director of M. V. Psychology Consultancy, a private practice based in Belfast, Northern Ireland, providing forensic psychological services worldwide to government agencies, prisons, secure hospitals and private organisations. He is a consultant forensic clinical psychologist, and author of two previous books on CAT.

Mark Stowell-Smith is a senior psychotherapist in the Wirral and West Cheshire Partnership NHS Trust and has previously worked in a high-security hospital. He is a CAT psychotherapist and trainer, having been involved with CAT from the late 1980s.

Michael Göpfert trained as a child psychiatrist at the Royal London Hospital and at the Clarke Institute of Psychiatry in Toronto. He is presently helping to develop therapeutic community services with Webb House in Crewe. One constant focus of his work for over 20 years has been the area of mental illness and its effect on parenting, resulting in two books and several other publications.

Cognitive Analytic Therapy for Offenders

A new approach to forensic psychotherapy

Edited by Philip H. Pollock,
Mark Stowell-Smith and
Michael Göpfert

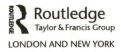
Routledge
Taylor & Francis Group

LONDON AND NEW YORK

First published 2006
by Routledge
27 Church Road, Hove, East Sussex BN3 2FA

Simultaneously published in the USA and Canada
by Routledge
270 Madison Avenue, New York, NY 10016

Routledge is an imprint of the Taylor & Francis Group, an informa business

Typeset in Times by RefineCatch Limited, Bungay, Suffolk
Printed and bound in Great Britain by
MPG Books Ltd, Bodmin, Cornwall
Cover design by Hybert Design

British Library Cataloguing in Publication Data
A catalogue record for this book is available from the British Library

Library of Congress Cataloging-in-Publication Data
Cognitive analytic therapy for offenders : a new approach to forensic
psychotherapy / [edited by] Philip H. Pollock, Mark Stowell-Smith
and Michael Göpfert.
   p. cm.
Includes bibliographical references and index.
ISBN 1–58391–924–4
  1. Prisoners—Mental health. 2. Criminals—Mental health. 3.
Prisoners—Mental health services. 4. Criminals—Mental health
services. 5. Cognitive-analytic therapy. 6. Forensic psychiatry.
  [DNLM: 1. Forensic Psychiatry—methods. 2. Cognitive
Therapy—methods. W 740 C676 2006] I. Pollock, Philip, 1968–
II. Stowell-Smith, Mark. III. Göpfert, Michael, 1947–
  RC451.4.P68C64 2006
  365′.66—dc22   2005015516

ISBN13: 978-1-58391-924-8 ISBN10: 1-58391-924-4

Contents

List of figures

About the editors

Dr Philip H. Pollock is the author of *Cognitive Analytic Therapy for adult survivors of childhood abuse: Approaches to case management and treatment* (Wiley, 2001), joint author of *Cognitive Analytic Therapy for borderline personality disorder: The model and the method* (Ryle, Leighton & Pollock, 1997; Wiley) and the Clinical Director of M. V. Psychology Consultancy, a forensic private practice based in Belfast, Northern Ireland, providing forensic psychological services worldwide to government agencies, prisons, secure hospitals and private organisations. He is a consultant forensic clinical psychologist who also manages the Adult Mental Health Department of Down Lisburn Trust, Northern Ireland.

Dr Mark Stowell-Smith is a senior psychotherapist in the Wirral and West Cheshire Partnership NHS Trust and has previously worked in a high-security hospital. He is a Cognitive Analytic Therapy (CAT) psychotherapist and trainer, having been involved with CAT from the late 1980s.

Dr Michael Göpfert qualified in medicine at Munich University, trained in neurology at the University of Ulm, and pursued general psychiatric training at Guy's and St George's Hospitals in London. He then trained as a child psychiatrist at the Royal London Hospital and at the Clarke Institute of Psychiatry in Toronto. He set up a residential psychotherapy service in Constance, Germany, and then became the first full-time NHS psychotherapist in Liverpool, where he established a truly integrative team. He is presently helping to develop therapeutic community services with Webb House in Crewe. One constant focus of his work for over 20 years has been the area of mental illness and its effect on parenting, resulting in two books and several other publications.

About the contributors

Gill Aitken has a long-standing commitment to social justice and social inclusion. After gaining a DPhil at the University of York (1989) and lecturing in social psychology, she trained as a clinical psychologist and CAT practitioner. For the last 9 years, she has worked mainly with women in community, medium- and high-security psychiatric and prison settings. She is currently employed as Lead Consultant Clinical Psychologist at the National High Secure Services for Women based at Rampton Hospital, and is seconded to CSIP-NIMHE Northwest as the Women's Programme Lead. In 2005, she received the British Psychological Society Distinguished Contributions to Professional Psychology award.

Calvin Bell is a CAT practitioner and is founder and director of Ahimsa and has extensive experience of working in the domestic violence field, particularly with men (both individually and in groups) with histories of violence, including those on life licence. His clinical work has also involved supporting both male and female victims of domestic abuse, and he has worked in a women's refuge, where he gained experience of working with children exposed to domestic violence against their mothers. He has acted as an expert witness in disputed contact and care proceedings since 1996. He is an international consultant and has received numerous commissions to design and deliver training in various aspects of domestic violence from numerous UK and overseas organisations, having just completed a commission to establish Guyana's first intervention programme for domestic violence perpetrators.

Philip Clayton is a Senior Nurse Therapist at Calderstones NHS Trust, Lancashire, England. He is a CAT practitioner and is currently in the final stages of CAT psychotherapy training. He has worked in secure environments for 25 years, making the transition from nursing in ward environments to working as a therapist. He became interested in CAT while working as manager of a therapeutic unit in high-secure provision. Current interests include the use of CAT tools in shared case formulations and adapting the CAT approach for use with the learning disabled population, having also published works on the subject.

Arthur Fairbanks is a Cognitive-Behavioural Therapist with a career background in Forensic Psychiatric Nursing. He has experience of providing care for child sexual offenders within secure settings and of engaging that group in structured treatment focused on their offending.

Justin Hamill holds a Certificate and Diploma in counselling and is an accredited CAT practitioner. He has worked and delivered training in mental health and has experience of working with both female and male clients with a wide range of mental health problems and relationship difficulties, and he has also worked as a counselling supervisor. Justin has 10 years' experience of working with perpetrators of domestic violence and has been actively involved with the development and delivery of services at Ahimsa since its inception.

Ian B. Kerr qualified in medicine at Edinburgh University. After junior hospital posts, he worked for several years in cancer research. He subsequently underwent dual training in psychiatry and psychotherapy at Guy's, the Maudsley and St George's Hospitals in London. He is currently Consultant Psychiatrist and Psychotherapist in Sheffield Care Trust and Honorary Senior Lecturer at the School of Health and Related Research (ScHARR) in the University of Sheffield.

Kirsten McDonnell is a Clinical Psychologist working in Ashworth Hospital for Merseycare NHS Trust. She is currently in the process of completing the Association of Cognitive Analytic Therapy North Practitioner Level training. She has experience of using CAT-informed approaches in work with women in different settings, including prison and high-security care.

James McGuire is Professor of Forensic Clinical Psychology and Director of Studies on the DClinPsychol Programme at the University of Liverpool. He has written extensively on the applications of psychology to criminal justice, the treatment of offenders, adolescent aggression, social problem solving and cognitive-behavioural therapies.

Aisling O'Kane is a Consultant Clinical Psychologist at Wirral and West Cheshire Partnership NHS Trust. Previously, she has worked in high-security hospitals, in medium-secure settings and at the University of Liverpool as Course Director of the MSc in Forensic Behavioural Science. Her research and clinical interests include personality disorders, sexual offending and risk assessment.

Steve Potter is a UKCP-accredited psychotherapist and a supervisor and trainer in CAT. He is part of the CAT North Training Group and co-directs the Inter-Regional Psychotherapy Training in Cognitive Analytic

Therapy. He was Chair of the Association for Cognitive Analytic Therapy for 6 years, until 2003. He is Director of the University of Manchester Counselling Service.

Karen Shannon is a Chartered Clinical Psychologist and deputy head of Mersey Forensic Psychology Service. She has completed her Cognitive Analytic Therapy Practitioner Level Training.

Mark Westacott is Course Director of the CAT course at the University of East Anglia and is also a Consultant Clinical Psychologist in the Forensic Psychiatry Service in Huntingdon, Cambridgeshire. He has extensive experience in the application of CAT in various forensic settings and has a particular interest in the use of CAT with personality-disordered offenders. He trained in Clinical Psychology in Cambridge and the University of East Anglia and became interested in CAT during forensic psychotherapy training at the Portman Clinic, London. He has directed the University of East Anglia CAT course for the past 2 years and is currently working toward the further development of CAT therapy and research in the East Anglia region.

Abigail Willis is a Chartered Clinical Psychologist employed at Mersey Forensic Psychology Service. She has completed her Cognitive Analytic Therapy Practitioner Level Training.

Ruth Wyner originally trained and worked as a journalist. She then spent 20 years in the homelessness sector, initially on the front line and subsequently developing and managing a range of projects in East and Mid-Anglia. Her career in homelessness abruptly came to an end when she was convicted of allowing the supply of heroin at an open-door day centre, one of several projects run by Wintercomfort in Cambridge. Ruth was director of the Charity and was sentenced to 5 years in prison, but she was released after 7 months following a successful appeal against sentence. She wrote about her prison experience in *From the inside* (Aurum Press, 2003). Ruth is now Coordinator of a new charity she helped set up, the Dialogue Trust, which runs applied median groups for offenders in prisons and on probation. She started her professional training as a group analyst 3 months after leaving prison, co-conducts some of the Trust's prison groups and develops research on these groups.

Preface

> To name something gives us a certain amount of power over it. Knowing its name, I know something of the dimensions of that force. Because I have that much of safe ground on which to stand, I can afford to be curious as to its nature. I can afford to move toward it.
>
> (Scott-Peck, 'Healing human evil', 1991; p. 176)

It could be argued that every crime is a window onto the offender's internal world and represents the relational, interpersonal expression of these inner processes as external manifestations. To act destructively, to damage or to abuse is to induce another person, forced to assume the role of victim, into a specific position. Something inside the offender is translated into relational actions in the external world, impacting on the states of mind and consciousness of the victim. This 'relational' analysis is relatively simplistic, yet it accentuates the need to incorporate intrapersonal and interpersonal perspectives in a way that facilitates an accurate conceptualisation of the relationship between the offender's personality and the crime. Exploring and understanding the internal and external facets of crime are core tasks for forensic psychotherapists, who, most often, encounter offenders who cannot name, identify, decipher or think about their own states of mind that have generated the crime or its effects on the victim. As cited by Scott-Peck above, offenders are rarely capable of spontaneously explaining their actions and their ramifications without relying upon a therapeutic relationship and process which promote self-knowledge and provide mental space for conjecture and contemplation. Forensic psychotherapy offers a means to generate this space for reflective analysis and learning.

The offender-to-victim relationships that are created through crimes range across a vast spectrum of impact. The designer of a devastating computer virus that causes mayhem across the cyberworld does so with the intent of achieving certain psychological rewards and expresses an inner narrative through action from a distance. The killer who intimately tortures a victim generates very different states of mind and expresses an idiosyncratic narrative that forces the chosen victim to assume a given role as the perpetrator acts out an internal fantasy. As clinicians, we try to derive a formulated impression from the crime and the criminal by making informed inferences about internal processes such as intentions, motivation and rewards. When we attempt to define those worst components of criminal behaviours considered 'heinous', 'evil' or 'depraved', we concentrate, in part, on making inferences regarding the offender's internally created intent (e.g. intent to traumatise emotionally either through humiliation, maximising terror, or creating an indelible emotional memory of the event; intent to carry out a crime for the excitement of the act alone; or intent to carry out a crime to terrorise others; e.g. the Depravity Scale (Welner, 1998). To help define the quality of the criminal act, we consider elements of the crime which focus upon the relational roles between perpetrator and victim, the respective and reciprocally related states of mind induced and the gratifications derived by the offender. The internal workings of offenders are inferred through their attitudes, intentions and behaviours, and are fundamental considerations when conceptualising the basis for an understanding of the criminal act. Psychological models of the offender's crimes should account for the intrapsychic and relational facets of the act.

The task of helping the criminal to become an improved person within society is a laudable and challenging endeavour. Forensic psychotherapy, as a specialism of psychotherapy established to achieve this virtuous goal, has advanced in terms of the theory, clinical models and therapeutic techniques used to understand the 'criminal mind'. Much of the progress in this arena must be attributed to the pioneering work of Cordess & Cox (1995) and Welldon & Van Velson (1997). These practitioners' ardour for developing and expanding forensic psychotherapy as an enterprise cannot be underestimated.

Within this book, we hope to describe the application of a particular psychological theory and therapy, known as Cognitive Analytic Therapy (CAT), to facilitate an understanding and conceptualisation of the internal–external and relational facets of crimes. CAT lends itself explicitly to this level of analysis. CAT is an integrative psychotherapy which has been applied in a variety of clinical settings and to a diversity of disorders with promising outcomes. We here describe the innovative application of the CAT model and therapy for offenders to illustrate the utility of CAT as a new approach to forensic psychotherapy. Psychotherapy can achieve much with offenders, and we are, with realism, declaring the value of a new form of forensic psychotherapy for offenders and attempting to illustrate its practice.

As a foundation for the application of CAT, it could be argued that a valid forensic psychotherapy should demonstrate a number of attributes. These attributes should include the following:

1   An explicit emphasis is placed on the link between the offender's *personality functioning* and *idiosyncratic actions* during the crime itself. The psychotherapeutic process should make graphic and definite formulation of the pathological relating which underlies the commission of the

offence. This is achieved through a collaborative therapeutic relationship which helps exploration and identification of the offender's unique life experiences, internal structures and processes, and patterns of relating to promote the development of portable 'tools' for self-knowledge and self-reflection. The internal–external and relational facets of the personality–offence link are made explicit.

2   Consideration should be given to the nature of the relationship between *offender and victims*. The manner in which the victim is treated is a central aspect of the analysis of the offender's relating, which ranges in pathology. How the victim is perceived, approached, controlled, treated and left are important idiosyncratic features of the offender's relating. When multiple victims are involved, the generic, nuclear pattern of relating can be extracted and identified. Often, defining and conceptualising the offender-to-victim relationship are the most difficult tasks for the offender.

3   Therapy constructs an internal model of self that equips the offender with the capacity to *self-monitor*, *self-regulate* and *self-manage* as independently as possible. Development of such self-knowledge and self-reflection is a vital component of the rehabilitation of offenders, who are charged with the task of taking ownership and responsibility for their risk potential. Making the therapy 'portable' should be a critical component of forensic psychotherapy.

4   *Risk potential* should be viewed as being, essentially, located within the offender's personality and can be defined as a sequence or pattern of internal events, often catalysed and impelled by external influences (substance abuse, relationship context, etc.), that culminate in the offence itself as a pinnacle event. In this conceptualisation, the sequence of events can be self-initiated through intentional action or through premeditation, and instigated through fantasy, or it can represent a combined accumulation of internal and external events that influence actions. Fantasy is thought of as a vehicle for generating offender-to-victim scenarios and planning the crime, escalating the risk propensity and catalysing the offender's underlying potential to commit crime. The offence is perceived as a point of crescendo and the ultimate climax of expression of the offender's personality. The predictions about when, under what circumstances and how a future offence is likely to occur can be analysed within the psychological reformulation and plans made with the offender to forecast these conditions.

We propose that CAT incorporates the aforementioned components of a well-founded forensic psychotherapy that aims to do the following:

1   consider the internal processes of the offender that culminate in the crime's occurrence, and address the contribution of both internal and external processes and events and their interaction involved in the offending

2   explicitly identify patterns of relating which are evident during the com-
     mission of the offences, particularly the offender-to-victim relationship
3   provide a method that develops insight and self-knowledge through
     provision of a mental model of self
4   encourage offenders to take ownership of their risk potential; improve
     self-awareness, monitoring and self-management, permitting both ther-
     apist and offender to examine the location and pinnacle of risk potential
     and design plans for its regulation. This permits forecasting of crime
     scenarios by the offender and supervising professionals.

At this juncture, the aim is not to overstate the merits of CAT or to parade an
evidence base for CAT as a therapy of choice for offenders; the substance of
our approach relies on case studies to demonstrate the processes of CAT. It is
acknowledged that CAT is an innovative, unproven approach, yet it is hoped
that the examples offered here will stimulate clinicians to apply CAT to
accumulate an evidence base. Given the gravity of the types of problems dealt
with in forensic settings, the responsibilities borne by professionals for the
interventions and decisions they make, and the human consequences of 'failures', it is vital that data are gathered to support or refute the viability of
CAT as a method for offenders.

This book is composed of an account of CAT theory specifically designed for
forensic work, using examples of the application of these methods and tools in
different settings with differing offence categories and offender groups. The contributors received the remit of describing and illustrating their own, perhaps
unique, utilisation of CAT, and of deliberating its value and limitations. We
hope that the illustrations can be viewed as a collection of 'essays' expressing
our collective thoughts about this therapeutic model's uses, that they will
stimulate clinicians and professionals to consider CAT as a fresh way of
thinking about their work, and that they will provide an additional conceptualisation and therapy for achieving effective changes in forensic practice.

Many details have been altered in case materials to safeguard the anonymity
of persons described throughout the book.

Philip H. Pollock
Hong Kong, May 2004

References

Cordess, C. & Cox, M. (1995). *Forensic psychotherapy: Crime, psychodynamics and the
    offender patient*. London: Jessica Kingsley.
Scott-Peck, M. (1991). Healing human evil. Chapter 37. In J. Abrams & C. Zweig
    (Eds), *Meeting the shadow: The hidden power of the dark side of human nature*. New
    York: Penguin.
Welldon, E. & Van Velson, C. (1997). *A practical guide to forensic psychotherapy*.
    London: Jessica Kingsley.
Welner, M. (1998). Defining evil: The Depravity Scale for today's courts. *Forensic
    Echo, 2*, 4–12.

Acknowledgements and dedications

The editors would like to take the opportunity to thank several people who have encouraged and facilitated this endeavour. All of our thanks to the publishers, who have been patient when patience has been in short supply.

I would like to thank Tony Ryle for his 'un-guru-like' pioneering of psychotherapy, willingness to listen to others' ideas, and encouragement of innovative thinking and practice. 'Till Amie an Conor: sin A hae ye in aboot me, ma gates is mair sonsie gat' (P. H. P.).

Many thanks to Michael Guilfoyle and Mick McKeown for help with one of my chapters (M. S.-S.).

Families invariably suffer when a parent engages in the narcissistic endeavour of enriching the world with his writing. It is therefore important to acknowledge the plight of Julia, Anya, Max and Leo, who end up short-changed because of this. The support of all my colleagues, but especially Jenny Davenport in difficult times at work, is gratefully acknowledged (M. J. G.).

Chapter I

Cognitive Analytic Therapy applied to offending

Theory, tools and practice

Philip H. Pollock & Mark Stowell-Smith

Forensic psychotherapy as a specialism

Forensic psychotherapy is the offspring of forensic psychiatry and psycho-analytic psychotherapy, and aims to provide a psychodynamic perspective to the understanding, management and treatment of the offender. The over-arching aim of forensic psychotherapy is to help offenders understand, and take responsibility for, their actions in order to reduce the likelihood of reoffending (Cordess, Riley & Welldon, 1994). In this respect, a central focus is maintained on the criminal act, the psychoanalytic understanding of which can be traced at least back to Freud's (1957) hypothesis that certain criminal acts may have an unconscious meaning and motivation, representing, for example, a means of expressing and discharging unresolved guilt. Within the discipline of forensic psychotherapy, a useful differentiation can be made between careerist criminals, for whom the cost-benefits of the offence may be carefully calculated, and the offender for whom the offence may be the equivalent of a neurotic symptom, the expression of a severe, underlying psychopathology or a defence against underlying depression. Conceptualised in this way, the therapist may address the offence with the offender as, for example, an attempt to gain 'symptom relief' or as an attempt to resolve an internal conflict.

Away from direct clinical work, McGauley & Humphreys (2003) also note how forensic psychodynamic psychotherapy has a role in providing psycho-dynamically informed consultation which enables a dynamic understanding of, for example, the offender in the context of the ward or the institution as a whole. The application of some of these concepts under the heading 'forensic psychotherapy' has been comprehensively detailed by Cordess & Cox (1996) and Welldon & Van Velsen (1998). Other forms of psychological therapy, such as cognitive-behavioural therapy (CBT) in particular, have proved beneficial for offenders, Maden, Williams, Wong & Leis (2004) claiming, 'the evidence shows that, on the balance of probabilities, completion of a suitable CBT programme will decrease the risk of recidivism' (p. 379). The 'what works' debate (McGuire, 1995), which considers the effectiveness of programmes and psychotherapies for offenders, continues to flourish, and it is into this forum that we introduce Cognitive Analytic Therapy (CAT) as a new form of forensic psychotherapy.

The origins of CAT

From the early theoretical developments of the late 1970s, CAT has matured into a form of time-limited psychotherapy that draws together a range of ideas from psychoanalytic, cognitive and personal construct theory. More recently, ideas from Vygotsky (1978) and Bakhtin (1984) have been increasingly emphasised. Both in spirit and in practice, CAT is best represented as a form of integrative, relational psychotherapy. The theme of integration is expressed in Ryle's early attempts to utilise cognitive concepts as the basis for a 'common language' for psychotherapy (Ryle, 1978) and persists in the idea of CAT as a 'comprehensive theory which aims to integrate the more robust and valid findings of different schools of psychotherapy as well as developmental psychology and observational research' (Ryle & Kerr, 2002; p. 2).

The emergence of CAT owes much to the zeal and innovation of its creator, Anthony Ryle, whose exposition of CAT as a form of generic psychotherapy can be traced through various texts (Ryle, 1990; 1995; Ryle & Kerr, 2002). While the popularisation of CAT clearly has much to do with the conceptual and practical innovations which Ryle and his co-workers have contributed to psychotherapy, its evolution has also been stimulated by a variety of economic and cultural influences (such as the growing movement in the public mental health sector toward the implementation of differing forms of brief psychotherapy, and financial accountability). Van Schoor (1996) has also noted the way in which technique-oriented forms of brief therapy appear to have taken precedence in the technologically saturated culture of the late twentieth century. According to Van Schoor, this culture involves 'regimentation, specialisation and standardisation', qualities that are reflected in brief psychotherapy's use of standardised procedure, its manipulation of time and its use of technical procedure. CAT is a brief, time-limited and focused integrative psychotherapy which has found its place within this evolving culture.

CAT for offenders: The history so far

The application of CAT to offenders can be traced to the initial work by Brockman & Smith in Ryle's first book in 1990. Very little work was reported until 1994, with the publication of an article titled 'Women who stab: A personal construct analysis of sexual victimization and offending behaviour' by Pollock & Kear-Colwell (1994). This paper described a combination of repertory grid analysis and CAT for two female offenders who had histories of severe childhood sexual abuse, and who had stabbed their male partners.

In a follow-up paper, Pollock (1996a) reported the changes achieved through the use of CAT for an additional seven women who had similarly sexually abusive histories and interpersonal, intimate offences, with improvements noted for dissociation, psychological symptoms and abuse resolution. An explicit link between personality disorder and interpersonal crime was made within these works. In 1997, Pollock further reported the relevance of CAT in an illustrative case study of a male sexual offender who was diagnosed with borderline personality disorder, incorporating the use of diagrams into the reformulation process and highlighting the importance of deciphering the underlying roles of the offender-to-victim relationships. Pollock & Belshaw (1998) described two cases of offenders who completed CAT with good outcomes, this paper considering the significance of locating risk potential within the offender's personality. A paper which described the benefits of CAT for a female stalker, deemed to exhibit an obsessional form of pathological relating (borderline erotomania), who attempted to kill her therapist was also published (Pollock, 2001a & b); it presented the management of a destructive therapeutic relationship.

Although this series of case studies cannot be displayed as a significant evidence base within forensic psychotherapy practice, CAT for offenders has produced interesting advances in terms of psychological formulation as a means of scaffolding the therapy process, the changes achievable and enhancement of the prediction of risk potential. The works described in the following chapters further illustrate the applications of CAT to a variety of offence categories (e.g. homicide), clinical disorders (e.g. psychopathic personality disorder), settings (e.g. community-based domestic violence services) and contexts (e.g. gender issues).

What follows is a description of CAT theory and therapy and its essential components and facets. The reader is directed to the work of Ryle & Kerr (2002) for a comprehensive review of the evolution in theory and practice of CAT with a diversity of disorders, populations and settings.

The theoretical basis: The language of CAT

For clients, it is necessary that their problems are described to them in a clear, simple and portable form. If we acknowledge that clients enter therapy with a lack of personal insight, and unformulated ideas about their thoughts, feelings, behaviours and tendencies, the importance of providing tools to think about and reflect on internal and external processes can be considered of paramount importance. As a theoretical model and psychotherapy modality, it has been refined over a 20-year period to date and offers the client a clear, succinct set of methods to enhance insight (i.e. through letters, diagrams, etc.) and improve self-knowledge, self-monitoring and self-control.

As an integrative model of psychopathology and therapy, CAT blends and revises several concepts from, in particular, psychoanalytic and object relations thinking. The theory synthesises features from personal construct theory (Kelly, 1955), cognitive-behavioural practice and object-relations perspectives. A thorough account of the origins, history and features of CAT is provided by Ryle (1995; 1997).

Basic concepts in CAT

In developmental terms, the core premise of CAT theory is the assertion that the child acquires and learns to convert interpersonal experiences into intrapsychological processes and structures. Learning is achieved through the internalisation of higher-order language and goal-directed action units, referred to as *procedures* in CAT. The fundamental process in CAT is that *interpsychological* processes occurring between parent (or others) and child become *intrapsychological* experience, evident within structures forming the substance of the child's personality. This occurs during play, when learning skills and even during a parent's explanation of events in terms of logic and cause–effect relationships in the real world.

Differences between psychotherapies can be traced to the level of inference and 'structures', which represent this internalisation. CAT is founded on this specific model of learning that describes how the client internalises portable, psychological 'tools' to understand, reflect upon and negotiate the developmental tasks of life and relationships. In CAT, the basic structures of the self and relationships (relationships with others, ways of relating to oneself) are referred to as *reciprocal role procedures* (RRPs). The model suggests that the transition from inter- to intrapsychological learning occurs between parent and child and similarly between therapist and client in 'tool-mediated, goal-directed' action (Ryle, 1990). Ryle describes how a child learns to internalise a parent's actions as a sign-mediated tool (a Vygotskian idea).

The proposal in CAT is that, through internalisation of our interactions with others, particularly our parents, a range of RRPs structure the self and guide our repertoire of actions toward others and toward ourselves. For example, the soothing, comforting, nurturing role provided by a caring parent is internalised and will guide the client's actions toward, perhaps, a family pet and also toward him/herself when emotionally upset. The 'voice' of the parent may be 'heard' in an inner dialogue such as, 'There there, everything will be OK, you will be all right. I'm here for you.' The nature of the roles of self and other (and the inner dialogue experienced) reflects the child's encounters with others and the repertoire of RRPs internalised. Of course, unhealthy and negative RRPs are internalised similarly, and a unique repertoire of relating can be observed with a spectrum of harmful (to self and others) and healthy RRPs.

The sequence enacted between parent/teacher/significant other and child is, in substance, a blueprint for the interaction sequence between therapist and client during CAT. The process of learning is sequenced through a range of factors and processes (the parent-to-child and therapist-to-client parallels). The sequence includes the consideration of the child's cognitive readiness (i.e. the client is orientated to focus on the tasks of therapy), the parent transfers agentic responsibility to the child (the therapist explicitly shares and facilitates the client's use of the tools of therapy), the adult helps the child to reflect on the task (the therapist focuses attention on the processes and work of therapy), the adult prescriptively directs the child about what to do (the therapist scaffolds the process of therapy and directs the client), the child incorporates and masters the relational, dyadic sequence in dialogical structure from outside to inside (the offender internalises the new learning and the internal image and 'voice' of the therapist as an introject), and emphasis is given to the shared, collaborative internalisation of learning, self-understanding and acquisition of language-based tools or skills. The capacity to reflect and observe oneself in relation to others (and oneself) is developed through external, real-life learning's becoming an internalised 'dialogue', which influences thinking, affects feeling and guides acting.

Therefore, as the parent encourages and guides the child, the therapist uses similar processes and actions in the relationship to scaffold the client's changes. Both scenarios facilitate change through *internalisation* of portable knowledge and skills in the form of procedures promoting growth and change.

Reciprocal role procedures (RRPs)

A rudimentary description of this process of internalisation is here described (readers interested in the theoretical underpinnings of these concepts should refer to Ryle, 1990; Leiman, 2004).

The concept of a *procedure* was introduced as a fundamental unit of analysis and level of inference within CAT (Ryle, 1982) to describe intentional acts or enactment of roles in relationships, similar to yet also different from object-relations thinking. These procedures are sustained by repetitive sequences of mental, behavioural and environmental processes. The procedural sequence occurs as follows: (1) mental processes (perception, appraisal of knowledge, action planning, prediction); (2) the effective enactment of an action or role; (3) evaluation of the consequences of the action or enactment, particularly the response of others; and (4) confirmation or revision of the aim or the means attempted to achieve this aim. The central procedures underlying the client's difficulties are termed RRPs, which represent, theoretically, a direct incorporation of object-relations concepts into CAT theory. RRPs are the core, relational units within the theory.

RRPs are derived from early care-taking and care-receiving relationships. Gradually and by repeated experiences, the child acquires a *repertoire* of RRPs, forming the structures of the self. During human development, the sequence whereby a child learns about possible options for relating to another person and himself are evident in the unique repertoire of RRPs. Learning occurs through socially derived meaning (e.g. language, symbols, signs) (Leiman, 2004), and, once acquired, this repertoire of RRPs is often, because of its procedural qualities, difficult to alter and revise (Crittenden, 1985). RRPs are enacted in relationships on two levels; *self–other* transactions and *self–self* management, defined in terms of Ryle's procedural sequence object relations model (PSORM) (Ryle, 1995). In this model, RRPs form the most basic units of mental development, organising interactions with others and representing repertoires of joint action sequences (Leiman, 2004). self–other (and, vice versa, other–self) relations are organised with the inherent prediction of the other person's response being of paramount consideration. A person may enact or choose to act a certain *role* (which combines action, affect, expectation and communication) with an implicit or explicit prediction that the interacting other will reciprocally enact an anticipated role in relation to himself. Both poles of the RRP are noted in CAT and the joint enactment of the procedure analysed.

Psychological distress, symptoms and harmful forms of relating to others (such as a perpetrator who exhibits an *exploiting-to-abused* RRP toward a child during sexual abuse) and toward oneself (such as enactment of an RRP of *abusing-to-abused* in a self-to-self manner) are maintained by a failure to *recognise* and *revise* the harmful outcomes of enacting these types of RRPs. These patterns often defy revision and are maintained despite their repetitive, unhelpful complications. The process of changing procedurally derived RRP repertoires and their harmful implications requires the assistance of the therapeutic relationship and tools of therapy because of their resistance to spontaneous change.

When we consider the actions shown in criminal activities, the nature of the offender's RRP repertoire can be analysed. For example, a crime of homicide in which a victim is selected, pursued, captured and ritually killed may express the offender's RRP of *dominating/crushing* (the offender) in relation to *impotent/crushed* (the victim). In an offence of theft, the offender may be exhibiting an RRP of *manipulating/duping* (the offender) in relation to *exploited/fooled* (the victim). This simple level of analysis implies a relational component within the *offender-to-victim* unit and provides a means of formulating the offender's motivations, intentions and probable reasons for the act. The unique repertoire of RRPs identified for each individual facilitates an understanding of how the self, others, relationships and the world are perceived and approached. The nature and range of the repertoire of RRPs dictate the manner and options for relating to oneself and others, and which behaviours are chosen or automatically demonstrated. Psychological health can be conceived, therefore, as possession and demonstration of a wide range of positive, self-nurturing and adaptive RRPs that are expressed in a self-preserving and socially acceptable way, and that enhance personal growth and promote mutually beneficial relationships with others (*caring-to-cared for*, *nurturing-to-nurtured* RRPs, etc.). As illustrated in Fig. 1.1, an RRP can be enacted in several ways within the relationships with oneself and others.

In Fig. 1.1, a variety of permutations using the dominant RRP of *exploiting/manipulating-to-exploited/duped* can be seen. Enactment of the RRP may

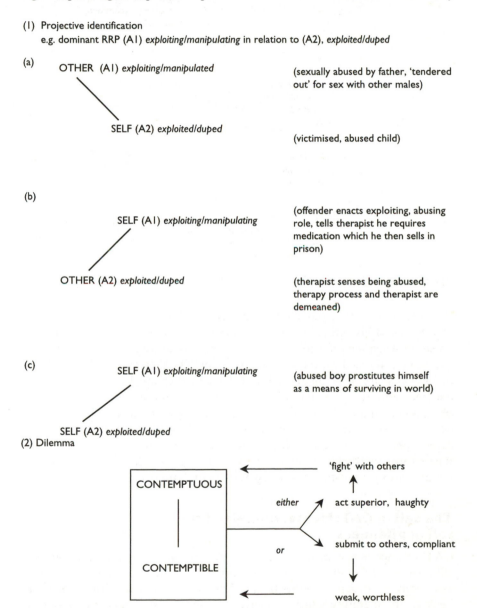

(1) Projective identification
      e.g. dominant RRP (A1) *exploiting/manipulating* in relation to (A2), *exploited/duped*

(a)   OTHER (A1) *exploiting/manipulated*   (sexually abused by father, 'tendered
                                                                     out' for sex with other males)

          SELF (A2) *exploited/duped*
                                                                     (victimised, abused child)

(b)
                                                                     (offender enacts exploiting, abusing
          SELF (A1) *exploiting/manipulating*   role, tells therapist he requires
                                                                     medication which he then sells in
                                                                     prison)

      OTHER (A2) *exploited/duped*   (therapist senses being abused,
                                                                     therapy process and therapist are
                                                                     demeaned)

(c)   SELF (A1) *exploiting/manipulating*   (abused boy prostitutes himself
                                                                     as a means of surviving in world)

      SELF (A2) *exploited/duped*
(2) Dilemma

                                                    'fight' with others

      CONTEMPTUOUS
                                             either   act superior, haughty

                                                    submit to others, compliant
                                             or
      CONTEMPTIBLE
                                                    weak, worthless

Figure 1.1 Reciprocal role procedures, dilemmas, traps and snags (*continued . . .*).

(3) Trap

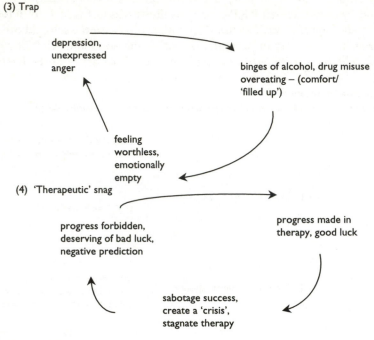

Figure 1.1 (cont.) Reciprocal role procedures, dilemmas, traps and snags.

have occurred during the child's experiences of sexual abuse by his father, who tendered his son for sex with others (point a). The same RRP may be apparent when the offender enacts the same procedure toward a therapist in lying to obtain medications and selling them. The therapist is likely to feel a reciprocal sense of being abused and demeaned (point b). As a self-to-self management procedure, the child may prostitute himself, allowing himself to be exploited and exploiting others at the same time (point c). These patterns can be noted to display a rudimentary RRP derived from this person's early experiences and internalised within his repertoire of procedures. These RRPs form the building blocks of the self in CAT, which focuses on their manifestation in self-to-self and self-to-other relationships.

The self in CAT: Mental models of the self in offenders

CAT advances a way of thinking about the self that is distinct from but also complementary to other theoretical and philosophical epistemologies. It is essentially constructivist rather than individualistic or rationalistic, and harks back to the literature which conceives the self to be a dynamic, dialogical network of interacting selves with no centralised, controlling entity. There are many 'I' positions which represent differing anchor points in a network of 'many-ness' conceived in space and time. Many tools such as diagrams invite the therapist and client to think about the personality as a spatialised ana-logue of the world (self, relationships, objects) and in the form of an 'imagi-nal landspace' or 'mind-scape' (Jaynes, 1986). The self is viewed as 'moving in time rather than existing in space' with no central, organising core, and mul-tiple versions of 'I' (self as subject) and 'me' (self as object) are possible, constituting a multifaceted, dynamic and narrative identity (Hermans & Kempen, 1993). Consciousness is defined as a product of the self-organising system of multiple selves and the function of a coalition of different self-states developed through two processes of *experiencing* and *narrating* (Kerby, 1991; p. 93). *Self-states* are defined as internalised RRPs that become, as identity coalesces, habitual *attractor states* (Whelton & Greenberg, 2002) and repeatedly experienced and observable structures influencing the stream of consciousness. Within each self-state is a distinctive RRP that affects the sense of self (how and who I think I am) and guides relating (how and who I think other people are in response to me).

Applying the metaphor of authored voices in novels, Bakhtin (1984) pro-posed that the self is composed of a 'polyphonic novel' of multiple 'voices', whereby, 'as in the polyphonic composition, the several voices or instruments have different spatial positions and accompany and oppose each other in a dialogical relationship' (p. 27). CAT depicts the self as a composition of often contrasting and even contradictory self-states (the habitual attractor states) that influence the conscious awareness and experience of oneself in such a multifaceted, dynamic and narrative way. As Herman (1993) suggested, the self is a multivoiced self-narrative with numerous, spatially separate 'positions' (forming the imaginal landscape or mind-space) with associated 'voices' that are in dynamic dialogue. Bakhtin (1984; p. 27) stated, 'it permits one individual to live in a multiplicity of worlds, with each world having its own author, telling a story relatively independent of the authors of the other worlds.'

The self can form narratives to structure its own experience in an idio-syncratic task of *emplotment*. This process is used to tell the story of the self through personal history and make sense of experiences and events. In CAT, the self is formed of relatively independent, identifiable self-states that are considered to be positions with associated voices and narrative histories. For example, the abused child is likely to be able to articulate a self-state and RRP which conveys and tells the story of his/her experience of being sexually victimised (self-state of the 'victim' labelled a 'rubbish bin' in relation to the 'perpetrator'). The person may be able to talk of particular memories (sens-ory, cognitive, affective responses such as flashbacks, auditory hallucinations, fear and self-loathing) associated with the role induced (e.g. an RRP of *crushed-to-abusing*) within a self-state of being a 'rubbish bin' with a self-evaluating voice commenting, 'I'm worthless and disgusting'. A specific narrative story is told from a given position with a relevant voice in the context of a reciprocal role (e.g. *abuser-to-victim*, the perpetrator perhaps described as 'the monster' in relation to 'the rubbish bin' self-state). It is important to state that 'the monster' as perpetrator also has a position, voice and state of mind. The nature and qualities of these self-states are explored and identified with the client to define the personality and its repertoire of relating to self and others.

If the self is conceived as multifaceted and formed structurally of a series of positions and voices (RRPs which form states of mind within self-states) embodying the personality, then *healthy functioning* can be construed as the individual's having access to and deployment of a range of self-in-the-world representations that can guide and predict action (Dimaggio & Semerari, unpublished; 2003). These selves are felt as dominant at different times. Often, access to and thinking about other positions are corrupted, and they cannot be accessed or thought about when in a given state of mind or RRP position. CAT aims to devise a *mental model* of the self through diagrams and the reformulation process, aiding identification of self-states, RRPs and associated states of mind. These portable tools encourage thinking and reflection about positions and their qualities as a form of metacognitive skill. If many theorists consider that we rely on these three-dimensional mental models (or portraits of scenes involving self and others as a narrative transaction unfolds) as tools to make rapid decisions, then indicators of personality dysfunction include the failure to identify one's own mental states and those of others, and an inadequate 'mapping function' to understand the complexity of social relationships and one's place within this world (Hermans & Dimaggio, 2004).

The most significant RRP and self-state to distinguish in CAT with offenders is that between offender and victim. This represents a fundamental *self-to-other* RRP characterising the 'position' and 'voice' that the offender has manufactured through his criminal actions. Even when the crime is spontaneous and reactive (e.g. a rage-type homicide), an underlying RRP (or RRPs within a number of self-states) can be determined that primed the offender to act. RRPs imply a motivational component of the criminal act and intention toward the victim, such as *destroying* (offender) to *destroyed* (victim), and *exploiting* (offender) to *used* (victim). The victim is induced or forced into a reciprocal counter-position as the RRP is enacted. The 'voice' associated with the role of the offender articulates the intent and motivation. For example, a rage-type killer who perceives his business partner as a threatening bully may state that, during an explosive act of fatal violence against the victim, he uttered or thought, 'Leave me alone! I can't take this anymore, I must get free of you!'

In summary, the basic units of inference in CAT are RRPs that are internalised through early care experiences with significant others. These RRPs form the templates for self-to-self and self-to-other relating. As these RRPs become cemented within the personality, a range of self-states emerge that can be labelled and that repeatedly guide perceptions of the self and others. These self-states can be thought of as 'positions' relative to others, with typical attitudes, affective states, 'utterances and voices' (Leiman, 2004), and ways of acting toward self and others. CAT focuses on the identification of this repertoire of RRPs and self-states and the nature of the patterns of relating shown. Of course, a person may exhibit positive and healthy RRPs and self-states (a 'good father' with an RRP of *nurturing/caring-to-cared for*) and display quite contradictory, unhealthy RRPs and self-states, such as the 'hard man' (*cruel/dominating-to-powerless*), during his criminal activities. The unique range of RRPs and self-states are defined during the reformulation phase of CAT.

Dilemmas, traps and snags

In CAT, neurotic or self-damaging ways of relating to oneself and others can be classified within three common patterns which cause harmful RRPs to fail to be revised (Ryle, 1979). *Dilemmas* are evident when the options for roles, choices or acts are restricted to falsely dichotomised alternatives where both alternatives are unsatisfactory and self-confirming. *Traps* represent negative beliefs that generate actions resulting in consequences that confirm the original beliefs, as in the notion of vicious circles. *Snags* occur when appropriate aims (e.g. to be in a rewarding relationship) are abandoned on the prediction (either rightly or wrongly) that their achievement will evoke negative consequences. Dilemmas, traps and snags, which are described in the Psychotherapy File (Appendix 1), represent the types of patterns that result in damaging, maintained, unrevised relating to oneself and others. Examples of typical dilemmas, traps and snags are shown in Fig. 1.1 (points 2, 3 and 4).

An overview of the CAT process: The three Rs of therapy

CAT as a therapy has three specific aims. These are termed the three Rs of therapy, namely, *reformulation* of the client's difficulties; his/her *recognition* of the harmful patterns of thinking, feeling and relating which cause and maintain these problems; and their *revision* through joint, collaborative work-ing between client and therapist. The goal is to assist the client to learn new ways of thinking, feeling and behaving. Fig. 1.2 lists the techniques and methods for reformulation, recognition and revision throughout CAT.

The process of reformulation

Reformulation stems from several varied sources, including a comprehensive history of the client; psychological testing; the therapist's 'naturalistic obser-vation' of how the client presents him/herself, communicates and interacts;

REFORMULATION

- presenting complaints, personal history, semi-structured interviews
- Psychotherapy File, self-monitoring diaries, psychometric testing, repertory grids, PSQ, SDP
- naturalistic observation of therapist–patient interactions, extraction of narrative themes from previous relationships, sequences and patterns of thinking, feeling and behaving
- presentation of Reformulation Letter, agreement about target problems (TPs) and underlying target problem procedures (TPPs)
- joint construction, discussion and refinement of sequential diagram, including identification and naming of prominent self-states and their RRPs

RECOGNITION

- recurrent use of diagram outside and within sessions to improve accuracy of reformulation
- review of themes within self-monitoring diaries
- ratings of recognition (and revision) for TPPs using TP Rating Sheet
- agreement about between-session tasks ('homework')
- reference to transference and counter-transference RRPs
- monitoring dilemmas, traps and snags

REVISION

- encouraging and practising new ways of thinking, feeling and behaving
- identifying 'exits' from TPs
- use of cognitive, experiential, behavioural and interpersonal techniques to achieve change
- use of transference–counter-transference understanding actively to avoid collusion
- breaking patterns within dilemmas, traps and snags
- discussion of termination of therapy and Goodbye Letter

Figure 1.2 The elements of reformulation, recognition and revision in CAT (the three Rs); adapted from Pollock (2001b).

and how the client describes the narrative episodes of his/her life experiences. Recurring patterns of relating, their sources and their maintenance are the essential materials of reformulation. Recognition of these patterns and the harmful procedures which cause them is not always achieved quickly. On occasion, the client may have difficulty in grasping the sequential pattern and its context. Clients often feel that they have 'gone around the same old circuit again' without being able to intervene successfully. As self-observation crystallises, the client can be encouraged to break these patterns with the help and guidance of the therapist. In a joint venture, the client and therapist share the duties and quest of a shared vision and outcome (the target problems to be worked on).

By the third or fourth session, the therapist comes to a provisional view of the origins and central features of the client's core problems. This is committed to paper in the form of a letter. The 'writing cure' (Bolton, Howlett & Lago, 2004) has become a feature of several therapies and is a central facet of CAT. The production of letters as forms of narrative description, catharsis and expression of emotion is a means to externalise internal states of mind in a similar way to our cultural creation of works of art, music, dance, etc. Transforming internal states of mind into a lexicon of some sort (words, musical composition, drawings, sculpture) can be thought of as a method of reformulation of 'states of being' in itself. The assessment sessions adhere to a usual psychotherapeutic protocol in the sense that they are relatively unstructured, allowing space for the offender to speak, be heard and understood, and for the therapist to attempt to make sense of patterns of transference and counter-transference. A number of techniques are used in CAT, including written letters, diaries, diagrams and sheets for target problems whereby ratings of the extent of recognition and revision can be monitored, and homework tasks outside sessions are employed.

The Psychotherapy File

Ryle (1990; 1995) created the Psychotherapy File (Appendix 1) as a means of introducing the offender to the recurring self-defeating and circular patterns of thinking, feeling and acting which produce distress and symptoms. The offender is encouraged to keep a self-monitoring diary of mood changes, occurrence of symptoms, interpersonal conflict and self-management problems. These areas are agreed between therapist and offender and reviewed regularly to extract new and repeated themes or issues in the offender's daily life. Thorough explanation and discussion, explaining the benefits of the data for the offender, should precede requesting the offender to keep a diary of any kind.

The offender is provided with a description of dilemmas, traps and snags in the file and a number of common patterns are included, the offender being asked to endorse the extent to which each pattern is relevant to him/her. Unique patterns of dilemmas, traps and snags can be interwoven into the file by the offender or therapist as they become apparent. A latter section of the file introduces unstable states of mind, mood variability and contrasting, conflicting and contradictory self-experiences. The Psychotherapy File is not a psychometric instrument, but does focus the therapy process in CAT, advancing and explaining where problems may emerge from for the offender.

The Reformulation Letter

Written 'letters' are used in CAT as a distinctive means of communicating the therapist's thoughts about the offender's internal and external processes, their source and how they are maintained, and to explicitly agree the work to be undertaken. A Reformulation Letter is produced and presented to the survivor in the early stages of treatment (typically during sessions 4 or 5), and a Goodbye Letter is compiled toward the end of the therapy, referring to the work completed to date, and acknowledging termination issues and problems which still require attention and monitoring.

The Reformulation Letter helps to cement the therapeutic relationship and check the accuracy of the client and therapist's perceptions of problems to be worked upon, and the derived problems to be targeted are written in the letter, which is shared with the client. The contents of the letter are drawn from several sources, including the client's narrative history of relationship episodes and events and how s/he coped, the observations of the therapist, and any problems emerging from the Psychotherapy File (Appendix 1) or psychological testing (e.g. repertory grids; see below). A number of features should be evident in the letter, although each therapist will express the issues to be included in his or her own personal style, taking into consideration the client's personality and likely response to the letter. Points to include are as follows:

(a) A succinct description of the relationship between the client's personal history and adversity, the emotional pain caused and the client's own subjective account of these experiences.

(b) Following on from (a), a description of the means used by the client to survive, cope or manage the pain experienced. Helping clients to recognise the link between the psychological pain and feelings endured as a result of events and how they coped as best as possible at that time promotes consideration as to how and why these patterns have become unhelpful and hard to break.

(c) Focusing on specific target problems (TPs) which emerge from the reformulation and defining the target problem procedures (TPPs) underlying them encourages the client and therapist to concentrate on specific areas to be addressed. These are listed in the letter, prioritised by both therapist and client, and named on a rating sheet to aid monitoring of the client's recognition and subsequent revision (see Fig. 1.3 for a version of the Target Problem Rating Sheet).

Typically, the Reformulation Letter comprises the following: a recapitulation of the presenting problem, an attempt to link the presenting problem to underlying procedural sequences, an attempt to name the underlying procedural sequences and an attempt to name or predict how those sequences may be acted out with the therapist. When appropriate, the meaning and significance or the ending of therapy may be anticipated as early as the Reformulation Letter. The introductory sessions are primarily concerned with understanding the offender's problems and concerns, setting them in a wider psychological context and agreeing the aim(s) of therapy. The assessment phase is brought to its conclusion usually at around the fourth session,

TP
Target Problem :
TPP
Target Problem
Procedure :

Patient's name :
Therapist's name :
Date :

		S4	S5	S6	S7	S8	S9	S10	S11	S12	S13	S14	S15	S16	f-up
A RECOGNITION Rate how skilled and quick you are at seeing the pattern	— more — same — less														
B STOPPING AND REVISING Rate how far you are able to stop the pattern and/or replace it with a better way	— more — same — less														

AIM
Alternatives or
exits.

Figure 1.3 The Target Problem Rating Sheet.

at which point the therapist presents his/her thoughts about the above in the form of a Reformulation Letter.

After the reformulation is read out by the therapist, the client's response is actively sought. Perceived inaccuracies are discussed and may be corrected, and agreement is sought about the focus of therapy and the TPPs. The Reformulation Letter is then given to the offender, and a copy is kept by the therapist. A common-sense approach is necessary when exchanging written materials within high-security settings, given anxieties about other parties obtaining access to or seizing sensitive information.

Explicit reference is made to how the procedures identified may affect the therapeutic relationship, particularly highlighting the expectations the client may have of the therapist (e.g. the *saving-to-saved* RRP) and placing these perceptions in a realistic light. Stating the 'holes in the road' where therapist and client may experience tension or stagnation can be useful. For example, it may be articulated that the client may perceive the therapist as demanding or tyrannical, leading to rebelliousness by the client.

Reformulation and narratives in forensic work

In conceptualisation of the offence and the underlying RRPs, the offender is assigned the role of protagonist/actor in the drama which has unfolded during the crime and of which s/he was the instigating author. The stories told (if at all) by offenders when asked to reflect on and explain their state of mind during offences tend to show many of the characteristics identified by Dimaggio, Salvatore, Azzara, Catania, Semerari & Hermans (2004) within the 'impoverished narratives' of many psychotherapy offenders. Of course, there can be many reasons and factors affecting the quality of offenders' descriptions (e.g. denial, feelings of shame, poor recall, a desire to sanitise the seriousness of the offence and its motivations, the effects of substance misuse at the time). Like the psychotherapy offenders reported by Dimaggio *et al.*, offenders show deficits in terms of a lack of access to internal states; an inability to describe others involved; a lack of thematic richness; no dialogue either internally or between victim, offender and extraneous others (e.g. the wife who ridiculed a rapist's sexual prowess, prompting him to assault a stranger sexually in a displaced offence); and poor pictorial quality. Promoting the enhancement of these aspects of the offender's inner narrative and constructing a mental model of the self in relation to others and oneself are critical components of CAT for offenders. The offender is guided through CAT reformulation to recognise prevalent RRPs, self-states and the range of positions under the format of 'I as . . .' (e.g. 'I as stalker') (see Hermans & Hermans-Jansen, 2004, for an illustration of the therapy for such an offender); motivations, intentions, 'voice' and attitudes ('utterances') associated with each state of mind and position are explored.

The use of all forms of assessment in CAT (i.e. the Psychotherapy File, clinical history taking, psychometric testing, analysis of crime scene and additional forensic data, and the naturalistic observation of the offender) permits the experiential material or 'life story' to be reformulated in a narrative style (e.g. incorporated into, for example, the Reformulation Letter) to identify the actors, authors and protagonist in the drama of the offence. Positions and voices are named through derived RRPs, and self-state grids with damaging, self-perpetuating patterns, such as dilemmas, traps and snags, are included in the diagrams. Through their joint construction, these psychological structures and processes are traced to their origins, understood, recognised and revised. Of course, the offender's *narrative* of events may indicate a deceptive 'cover story' or a defensively constructed account.

Analysis of the criminal acts

It is essential that the RRPs which define the *offender-to-victim* relationship are formulated. This is a difficult aspect of the therapy process for many offenders. Some are unable to contemplate the damaging way they acted toward the victim. Others, unable to exhibit sufficient theory of mind to project into the victim's experience, are unwilling or unable to consider the relevance of this procedure. Often the victim will be characterised as an object, vehicle or person (Canter, 1994), and the interactive qualities between offender and victim can be translated into these categories. The inference that interpreting the *inner narrative* of the offender can be done through his/her actions at the crime scene and tracing the decision, choices and behaviours demonstrated is relevant here. For example, the homicide offence and its elements can be viewed as a 'death tableau' that is a unique product of this narrative (Biven, 1997). The index offence and its scenario hold idiosyncratic information that can be considered a climactic end-state of the offender's personality functioning, and this can be examined as a 'snapshot' in suspended animation. An extensive analysis of all materials available, including crime scene evidence, autopsy findings, statements of witnesses and all relevant evidence should be undertaken to construct the offence scenario before asking the offender to provide his/her narrative account of the actions exhibited during the crime itself.

Identifying self-states and producing the diagram: Diagrammatic reformulation

In CAT, diagrams as devices and tools of reformulation are central to the joint scaffolding of the client and therapist's agreed understanding of the work to be addressed. CAT places an emphasis on identifying, recognising and addressing these recurring models or 'states of being', including them within a diagram called a *Sequential Diagrammatic Reformulation* (SDR) or a *Self-States Sequential Diagram* (SSSD). This diagram consists of the major distinct states of mind, the underlying RRPs, affective states and ways of thinking about oneself and others. It is generated with the client's collaboration and refined as therapy progresses.

The identification of distinct self-states that anchor the offender's perceptions of self and others is a pivotal exercise in CAT. A *self-state* appears as a recurring, dominant RRP that permeates the offender's experiences. These are named explicitly, and the offender monitors the content and triggers of their recurrence, the symptoms associated with them and the control of emotional regulation experienced (overcontrolled, undercontrolled). Similarly, Rowan (1990) proposed that we can identify 'subpersonalities' which function as semi-autonomous personalities. CAT differs from these conceptions of multiplicity of the self by explicitly cementing qualitatively contrasting and often contradictory states of mind within a relational framework.

Defining the RRP and naming the self-state provide a structural anchor point to trace patterns which tend to emerge from and circle back to each self-state in sequences of thinking, feeling and acting. Movement within and between states can be tracked through *role reversal, response shifts* and *state switches*, and symptomatic or avoidant procedures and dilemmas, traps and snags traced from one self-state to another.

Each state of mind is the named reciprocal pole of an RRP. For example, an RRP of *punishing-to-crushed* represents the underlying reciprocal ends of the same self-state, defining two states of mind. This RRP may be extracted from the interactions between rapist and victim in a sexual assault offence. A *response shift* is observed when a different, reciprocating reaction is made to the same RRP; for example, a compliant wife who begins to assert herself (from *complying* to *rebelling* in response to a controlling, bullying husband). A *role reversal* occurs when the person enacts the other end of the reciprocal role, perhaps acting aggressively through identifying with an abusing role to deal with his or her own victimisation (the abusing-to-victimised RRP). A *state switch* occurs when the person enters an entirely different self-state, as, for example, moving from idealising to rejecting another person.

The offender is encouraged to label or name the states of mind and self-state, using terminology and language which has personal meaning, and the therapist should not impose a lexicon of descriptors onto these states. Once named, the *procedural loops* (cyclical patterns from one self-state to another; see Fig. 1.4) of perceiving, feeling and behaving can be explored, and shifts and switches within and between states monitored. It is often advisable to start generating the diagram by focusing upon the offender's persisting and unresolved unmanageable feelings (referred to as *core pain*: hurt, pain, anger, unmet needs, etc.), the more or less adaptive methods that have been constructed to avoid or deal with these feelings (the *survival strategies* or *coping modes*) and the symptoms accompanying these coping strategies.

The tools which are generated through the reformulation assessment are used to structure and scaffold therapy in CAT and explicitly shared with the

SELF-STATE & STATES OF MIND

PUNISHING

|

CRUSHED

RRP = *punishing-to-crushed* form the distinct self-state: '*punishing*' and '*crushed*' represent separate states of mind with associated thoughts, feelings, perceptions and actions (e.g. a rapist assaults a female who rejected his amorous advances)

RESPONSE SHIFT

CONTROLLING

COMPLYING   REBELLING
(1) ⎯⎯⎯⎯→ (2)

(1) → (2) A compliant wife begins to assert herself toward a controlling, abusive partner, escalating violence between the couple

ROLE REVERSAL

ABUSING
(2)

|

VICTIMISED
(1)

(1) →(2) Victim rage expressed by attacking an abusing partner, the victim assuming the aggressive role through reactive, explosive violence

STATE SWITCH

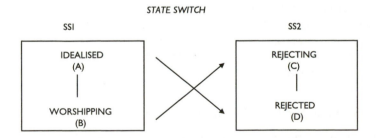

(A) ⎯⎯→ (D) An idealised partner is worshipped (SS1), then rejected (SS2) after disappointment in switching from one self-state to a different self-state.

Figure 1.4 Self-states, states of mind, response shifts, role reversals and state switches in CAT diagrams.

offender. Secretive insights are not held by the therapist and withheld from the offender. This stance is discussed to promote a forum of joint collaboration, and the offender's perceptions, views and opinions are requested, clarified and expanded throughout the process of CAT. The aim is to equip the offender with the 'tools' to think about and change his psychological processes and, importantly, to reduce risk, his potential to harm others through behaviours.

The relevance of 'doing things differently in the future' and 'not repeating certain acts' is emphasised, and the offender is encouraged to think about the crime(s) as the product of patterns of thinking, perceiving, feeling, relating and acting which are not automatic responses but can be understood and changed. Few offenders present with adequate, formulated insight into their own actions and the underlying psychological processes involved. Therefore, CAT encourages the acquisition of these tools to derive and improve the offender's insight, comprehension and modification of his/her psychological processes.

The objective of CAT is to promote improved self-reflection; identification of underlying processes; and tracing of the origins, naming, and resolution or control of self-states and damaging patterns of RRPs through acquisition of self-knowledge. Integration of the personality is achieved through helping the offender to generate the 'aerial map' (diagrams) of self-states and assume control over the healthy and pathological facets of the self. The formulation of self-states as 'positions' with 'voices' helps the offender to construct the dialogical basis of his/her personality and consider the nature and function of fantasies, and their source and origins.

Specific CAT assessment tools

A number of CAT-specific assessment procedures and measures are available in constructing a reformulation and directing the focus of the therapy itself. These include the Psychotherapy File, various types of repertory grids, the states description procedure (SDP) and the Personality Structure Questionnaire (PSQ). In combination with other assessment tools, these CAT methods can be used to generate an accurate reformulation and scaffold the therapeutic process. Here, each CAT tool is described, and an example is provided of its application to an offender.

Repertory grids in CAT for offenders

Repertory grids and construct theory (Kelly, 1955) have formed part of the foundation of CAT theory since its inception. The constructivist philosophy underlying CAT has persisted and developed. Two types of repertory grids are most often employed to establish the language used by the client to construct his perceptions of self, relationships and the world. A comprehensive description of the application and value of repertory grid analysis and personal construct theory and therapy in forensic settings is provided by Houston (1998) and Horley (2003), who report grid usage with violent, sexually and mentally disordered offenders and in institutions. The integration of personal construct perspectives with treatment programmes is detailed in

Horley's work, which claims that the constructivist approach permits an idiosyncratic and valuable insight into the offender's perceptions of himself, his crimes, others and the institutions in which they become embedded.

Examples of using this type of repertory grid with two female offenders who stabbed their respective partners are provided in Pollock & Kear-Colwell (1994), and outcome data from such grids were reported in Pollock (1996a) for a larger group of violent female offenders. A typical repertory grid of a sexual offender is shown in Fig. 1.5 and a self-states grid for the same offender in Fig. 1.6. Figure 1.5 is a spatial depiction of the 'mind-scape' and relations between significant people and selves in the offender's life. Certain elements such as the victim (a male child in this case) can be included, and the relationship between the offender and victim ('me as offender') examined, using the idiosyncratic constructs defined by the offender (e.g. self-hating, subnormal, disgusting). In Fig. 1.6, the self-states identified during CAT reformulation are entered into the self-states grid (Appendix 1) and rated with certain self and other orientated parameters ('Others attack me', 'I control others'), helping to provide a spatial analysis of affective states, such as 'rage', as well as self-states themselves ('sex beast' rated as out of control, wanting to hurt others, etc.).

Grids are excellent methods of eliciting both the idiosyncratic and pathological ways of construing self, relationships and the world, as well as more adaptive and healthier facets of the offender's personality and relationships. Often, the grid will show that certain elements such as *self-as-offender*, *victim* and *past self* are spatially close in distance and, perhaps, defined by constructs such as *aggressive-innocent*, *stupid-clever*, *in my control-out of my control*, *manipulative-gullible*, etc. These parts of the grid articulate the offender–victim construal of this core relationship. In addition, other parts of the grid often highlight that the offender has the capacity to attach, nurture and protect others, most typically their own children and family. The relationships as construed between the offender and other significant people (as well as facets of his own identity, such as *ideal-self*, *present-self* and *old-self*) are patterned in the grid and facilitate discussion between therapist and offender about the pathological and healthier parts of the self and how they relate to others. It is not uncommon to find that a sexual murderer, for example, who brutally killed an elderly woman in her home, would construe his relationship with his own grandmother as loving, emotionally close and special on a repertory grid. Similar findings have been noted for paedophilic offenders who are known to pride themselves in their role as a devoted father, yet abuse or kill other children.

Repertory grids permit a spatial analysis of the distance–closeness construed between offender and victim by a computer program (Tschudi, 1989). The RRPs which define the *offender-to-victim* dynamic are a core focus in CAT reformulation and therapy. For example, an offender's grid showed that self-as-offender and victim were spatially inseparable along a dimension

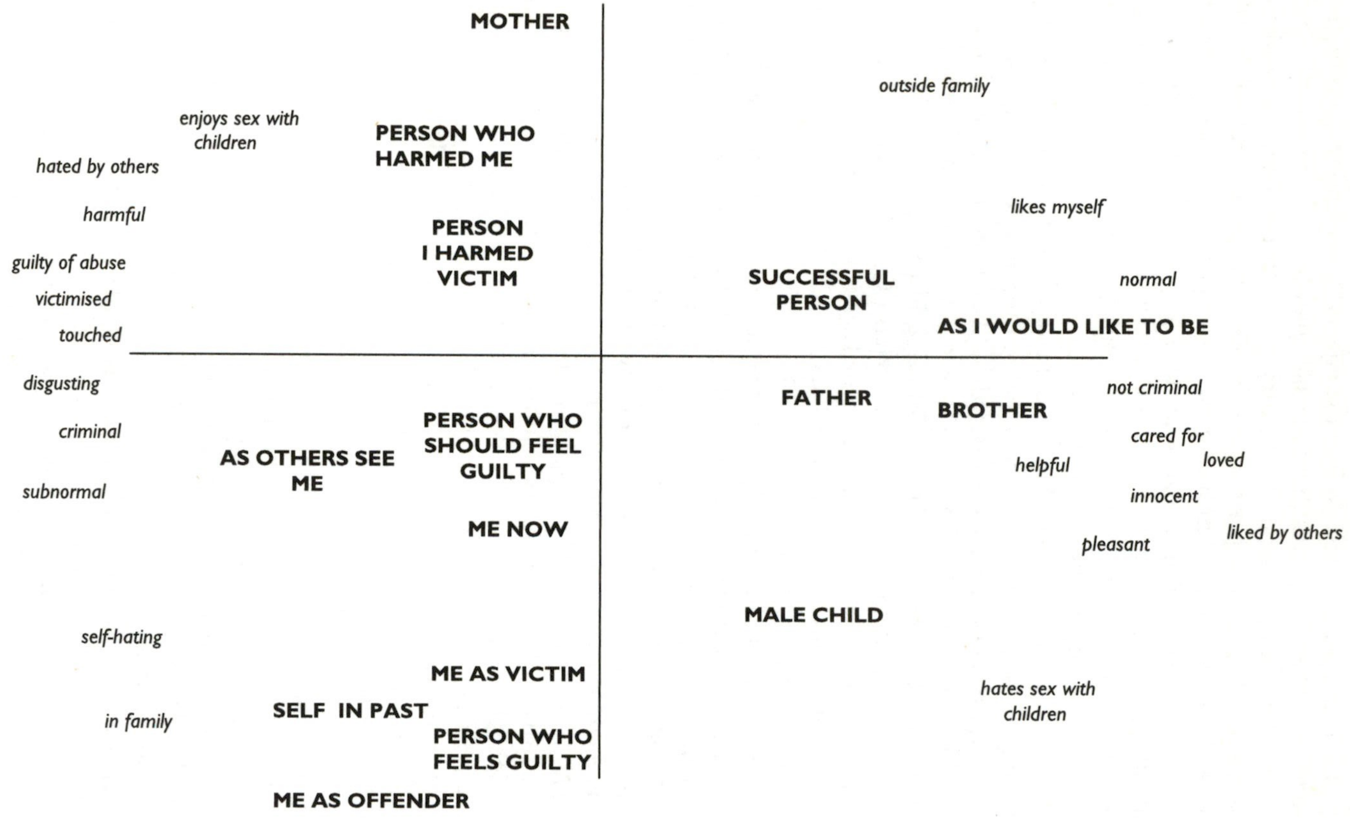

Figure 1.5 A sexual offender's repertory grid.

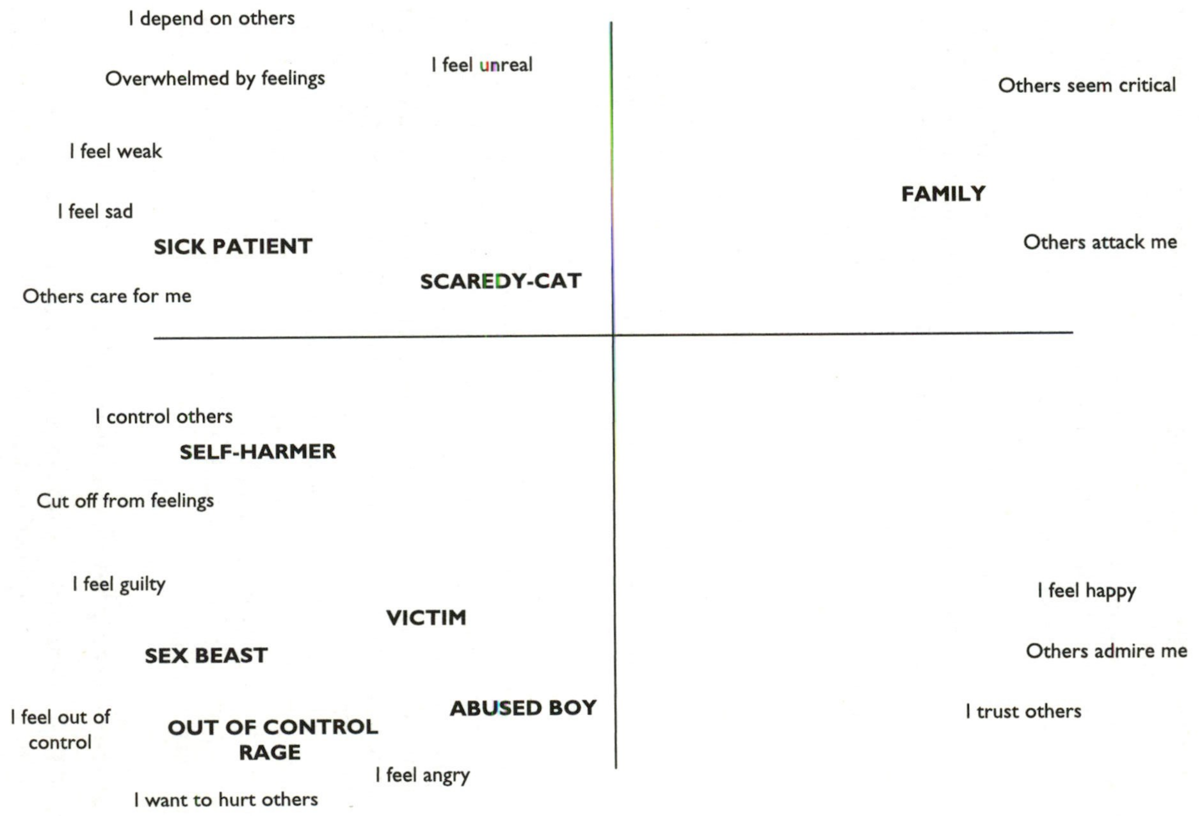
I depend on others
I feel unreal
Overwhelmed by feelings
Others seem critical
I feel weak
FAMILY
I feel sad
SICK PATIENT
Others attack me
SCAREDY-CAT
Others care for me
I control others
SELF-HARMER
Cut off from feelings
I feel guilty
I feel happy
VICTIM
SEX BEAST
Others admire me
ABUSED BOY
I feel out of control
OUT OF CONTROL RAGE
I trust others
I feel angry
I want to hurt others

Figure 1.6 A sexual offender's self-states grid.

consisting of the constructs of *control, stolen, invaded* and *surrender*. The victim had been selected, kidnapped, raped, facially mutilated, killed and dismembered, the offender disclosing that he had attempted to eat parts of the victim prior to disposal of the body at a local park where he played as a child. During discussion about the grid and its meaning, the offender declared that 'she's mine to own'. The construal on the grid and its significance when combined with the offender's explanation of his perceptions suggest a dimension of possession, ownership and use of the victim as an object for internal fantasy-driven sexual murder.

The grids elicit the offender's unique construction of the world and facilitate the naming of RRPs and self-states to structure diagrammatic reformulation and identification of target problems (TPs) and direct therapy. The RRPs (constructs) and self-states are combined with information from other sources to establish a working formulation of the anticipated transference and counter-transferences which are likely to emerge during therapy.

The Personality Structure Questionnaire (PSQ)

The PSQ (Pollock, Broadbent, Clarke, Dorrian & Ryle, 2001c) (Appendix 2) is a short, screening questionnaire designed to measure identity disturbances. It consists of 8-item pairs of contrasting descriptions of the self as stable or changeable, each item scored from 1 to 5 (stable to unstable in direction). The scores from normal samples range from 19.7 to 23.3, and cases of borderline personality disorder from 30.4 to 31.3. Correlations with other measures of psychopathology and identity disorder were observed, validating the PSQ. Research has shown that a PSQ score of 28+ warrants further exploration of the presence of facets of identity disturbance such as dissociation, amnesia, fragmentation and loss of behavioural control. Overall, the PSQ can be used to investigate the integrity of the client's identity. Positive changes in PSQ scores have been achieved through CAT for a group of sexually abused women survivors, with PSQ scores inflating when clients are presented with the complete CAT reformulation (i.e. Reformulation Letter, SDR or SSSD, and feedback about TPPs, dilemmas, traps, snags, etc.), most probably as an effect of explicit definition and stark analysis of the client's difficulties and psychological functioning.

The states description procedure (SDP)

The SDP (Ryle, Bennett & Pollock, in press) (Appendix 3) was developed to establish the degree of 'borderline-ness' of clients and to define the nature, frequency, transitions and quality of self-states. It aims to promote guided self-reflection in case reformulation. Like repertory grids, the SDP feeds into the construction of the SSSD and helps both therapist and client think about the transitions between self-states. The typical switches between contrasting and contradictory states experienced by those who show identity disturbances, as defined by the multiple self-states model (MSSM) (Ryle, 1997; see Chapter 2 for an illustration of this model). The SDP helps the therapist and offender to identify, recognise and monitor the 'movement' between states, their characteristics and their triggers. For example, states often noted with identity-disturbed offenders include a 'rage state', which may be characterised by feelings about oneself as 'out of control' and 'wanting to destroy others', and other people being perceived as 'do not care about me' and 'seem like threatening abusers'. Once a state is labelled, the frequency, duration and triggers which cause transitions (what starts the state, how it appears, how it ends, how the person gets out of the state) can be described, and the emotional and physical feelings associated with it considered.

A range of additional assessment techniques and tools are companionable with CAT and expand on the therapy-specific measures and methods described here. Actuarial assessment is entirely compatible with CAT case reformulation.

The process of CAT: Selection of cases

The issues of motivation to change and its enhancement are fundamental to the selection of clients for CAT, as they are to any other therapeutic endeavour (Kear-Colwell & Pollock, 1996). A variety of techniques and interventions can be employed to facilitate engagement with CAT, such as motivational interviewing approaches. The offender exhibiting indications of pre-contemplation should be afforded preliminary work prior to entrance into CAT.

Otherwise, CAT requires a degree of intellectual ability, yet it can be modified for those with cognitive and intellectual difficulties (see Chapter 8 as illustration). An offender experiencing florid psychotic symptoms or intoxication should be helped with other forms of treatment than, or before, CAT.

The time frame of therapy

As with other forms of brief psychotherapy, the meaning of time is important in CAT. The time frame is determined at the outset of therapy so that the ending of therapy can be confronted from the start. This structure, therefore, creates an environment in which issues of attachment and detachment can be adequately explored. Typically, CAT is offered once a week, for 16–24 sessions. Sixteen sessions might be allocated to more benign, neurotic problems, whereas 24 sessions might be offered to people presenting with, for example, significant levels of personality disturbance. Typically, a follow-up session will be offered subsequent to the completion of therapy. In the treatment of offenders with severe personality disturbance, the convention is to offer a series of staged follow-up sessions (Ryle, 1997; p. 121).

The time frame of therapy also influences the aims of CAT. Ryle states that major psychic restructuring is not the goal of CAT; rather, the aim is to facilitate the unblocking of stuck patterns of intrapersonal and interpersonal behaviour (Ryle, 1995). If this can be achieved, then deeper, underlying change might spontaneously occur. Unblocking is achieved through the delivery of the the 'three Rs' of CAT: reformulation, recognition and revision. This condenses the view that the various forms of reformulation deployed in CAT will facilitate a greater awareness of defective, problem procedures. In turn, this process of recognition will create a foundation that will allow for the revision of an array of unhelpful intra- and interpersonal patterns.

Recognition

Self-states and RRPs can be thought of as the 'positions' and 'voices' in CAT terminology. Of course, other theories have conceived of these facets of the self in a variety of ways, such as relational schemas (Baldwin, 1992), prototype narratives (Gonçalves, 1995) and voices in assimilation (Stiles, 1999). The diagrams (repertory grids, self-state grids, the SDR and SSSD) in CAT provide visual aids to help trace the origins, characteristics and functioning of different states of being, which can often alternate and vacillate in distinct state shifts. As Honos-Webb & Stiles remarked (1998; p. 448), 'it is not through eliminating conflicting perspectives or establishing intra-psychic unity but rather through promoting multifaceted complexity' that psychological health is achieved. Pizer (2002) considers the tolerance of the paradoxical nature of experience as a sign of health. When different states of mind and being are identified, Pizer refers to the need to develop an aerial map of the self-states as 'islands' with and, often without, 'bridges' between them, the goal of therapy being the acceptance of multiplicity rather than striving for an executive oneness. Bromberg (1998) suggests that 'health is the ability to stand in the spaces between realities without losing any of them, the capacity to feel like one self while being many' (p. 186). Therefore, health is judged to be the perpetual cycling between self-states in a seamless motion with the necessary illusion of being within one psychological skin. The metaphor of the individual narratives of each position is captured by thinking of the self as possessing the internal sophistication of counterpoint in complex musical arrangements.

Awareness of different self-states differs from individual to individual. Self-states which are named and personified within CAT terminology can be witnessed to have their own typical rhythms and transitions, depending upon how integrated the personality and identity are. The SDP is designed to track these changes and make them more predictable. Psychotherapy is the task of figuring out 'who' (self-state, position and voice) is speaking to whom at the given moment in time, and helping the offender to achieve insight into the narrating, dialogical, multiple nature of the self and its patterns. Bringing self-states into awareness and encouraging dialogue between them represent an important aim of psychotherapy.

Transference and counter-transference

In CAT language, both transference and counter-transference are understood in terms of RRP *enactments*, transference being an awareness of the offender inducting the therapist into a particular role (e.g. abusing therapist in relation to abused, victimised offender), and counter-transference being the therapist's awareness of the pressure to enact the role into which he has been inducted. In the course of assessment, the therapist may make immediate, yet not assumptive note of the RRPs which appear to materialise. The metaphor of the 'mosaic of hidden selves' woven in a tapestry of self-states illustrates the conceptualisation of the self and the emergence and manifestation of these self-states (Khan, 1989). Patterns of interaction are also detectable from clinical history of the offender and with reference to the past documented style of engagement with services (if recorded). The avoidance of collusive and damaging transference patterns is paramount for the safety and integrity of the therapist, offender, containing institution and the therapy itself, given the prevalence of 'manipulative cycling' (Bursten, 1972) and the possibility of the therapist's being deceived, compromised or induced into destructive or seductive relations.

Kiesler (1988) stated that a therapist 'cannot not be pulled in by the offender' (p. 38), referring to the manifestations of transference and counter-transference within the 'transitional game' that forms as the therapeutic dyad interact. Any ruptures to the alliance must be conceptualised, and impasses or stagnation in progress addressed. The therapist is required to undertake a task of internal observation regarding his/her own thinking, emotional reactions and perceptions of the client. Collusion with a client's self-perpetuating patterns of RRPs, dilemmas, traps and snags leads to stagnation and 'dropout' from therapy and reinforces the client's unhelpful ways of thinking, acting, feeling and relating.

Projective identification is another important process (Ogden, 1983) which underpins transference and counter-transference responses during therapy, and its conceptualisation within the CAT model is an important facet of clinical practice. Processes of enactments and inducements are observed within the projective identification system within the dyad of therapist and offender. Essentially, within this relationship, the dyad is a compound of a *projector* and a *recipient*. The projector enacts a certain role of an RRP, and the recipient is anticipated or induced (often in an implicit, controlling manner) to enact the reciprocal role affecting interpersonal activities and communication about internal affects and expectations in relationships. The naturalistic observation of the therapeutic alliance allows the therapist to gain a sense of the client's history, its impact and how the affect associated with these adversities is active and influential.

Ryle (1997) has specified a number of forms of transference and counter-transference that occur between therapist and offender and how these responses can be used to improve the planning of treatment. Analysis of the inducement of the therapist to assume a given role, the affect associated with it and the origin of the underlying RRP is a vital task of therapy. Offenders with greater fragmentation and identity disturbances often exert strong pressure upon others in general life and upon the therapist to collude by assuming the reciprocal role. If the offender's repertoire of RRPs is narrow, inflexible and restricted, the pressure to collude can be intense and controlling for the therapist (projection of a reciprocal role and a 'pull' to identify and reciprocate by the therapist as recipient). Collusion evidently reinforces the harmful, maladaptive RRP and maintains the fragmented structure of the offender's personality. Because the vast majority of RRPs are enacted automatically and implicitly learnt, repetitive patterns of damaging interpersonal procedures continue if they are not recognised and addressed. Ryle described a number of different forms of transference and counter-transference within the CAT model, including the following:

(1) An *identifying transference* occurs when an offender seeks to imitate, or become similar in role or manner, or physically to the therapist, akin to a mirroring transference. This may be observed by a change in the offender's physical appearance, use of language, attitudes and opinions, and mannerisms. To some extent, a loss of normal separateness and differentiation is likely to occur with this form of relating.

(2) A *reciprocating transference* represents a offender's attempts to induce the therapist to assume the reciprocal role of a given RRP. The offender's switching between these transference patterns and their underlying RRPs must be recognised, tracked and included within the SSSD.

The transference and counter-transference responses of the therapist are diagnostic in CAT to a degree when certain personalities (e.g. psychopathic) cause distinct reactions and effects, such as dermatological and pulmonary responses indicative of autonomic arousal provoked by evolutionary 'intra-species predation' (Meloy & Meloy, 2000). The therapist is advised to make immediate, yet not assumptive note of the RRPs that appear to materialise and the additional evidence supporting the hypothetical state's presence and relevance.

Regarding counter-transference (CT) patterns, Ryle (1997) proposed differing forms, including *personal*, and two types of elicited (*identifying* and *reciprocating*) CT. *Personal CT* is a feature of the therapist's own history, repertoire of experiences and RRPs, conflicts and early, unresolved issues. Knowledge of the nature and meaning of these CT reactions is vital to avoid becoming crippled or overwhelmed by the offender's current influence. As with all forensic psychotherapy, it is worth wondering why we choose to work with, not only damaged and disordered individuals, but those who are potentially harmful, destructive and dangerous to others and themselves. Psychotherapists who choose to work in forensic settings learn quickly how challenging and demanding therapy can be, professionally and personally. It is essential that each therapist undertakes a journey of self-exploration about the reasons for pursuing entrance into such settings and engaging with people who are defined as deviant, dangerous or 'evil'.

Motivations can include an infantile fantasy to understand the 'bogeyman', the 'monster', and to develop a sense of control over this adversary (Simon, 1997). A morbid fascination with evil is evident for some of us in the types of characters and archetypes; for example, those characters which are culturally communicated through fairy tales (Von Franz, 1995). The 'shadow' or 'demonic energies' of the disowned aspect of human existence captivates our attention, and many of us seek to understand these forces through self-exploration and interest in their depiction and personification in the media (Abrams & Zweig, 1991). In other instances, an attraction to working with dangerous and depraved offenders is a reflection of a sadistic identification with the offender, a factor which may enhance the therapist's empathic abilities, yet must also be thoroughly understood to avoid collusion and even danger. For others, an altruistic, self-righteous attitude can drive the therapist to believe that s/he is providing a service which guards society from the damaging and destructive actions of these people. As stated by Frey-Rohn, 'responsibility towards oneself always includes responsibility towards the whole' (1991; p. 267). Many therapists harbour a belief that working with the destructive potential of human nature permits a balanced appreciation of the different sides of our capacities and that changes are possible, a reflection of an enduring optimism, faith and hope regarding what is achievable by even the most wicked and 'evil' criminals. Guggenbühl-Craig declared that 'psychopaths provide fertile ground for the cultivation of our own shadow projections; when we do not pity them, we hate them, seeing in them our own destructive potential' (1991; p. 225). It is vital for our own personal heath that we reflect on our reasons for entering into a psychotherapeutic relationship with such individuals.

Elicited CTs are of diagnostic value for the therapist also. An *identifying CT* is indicative of empathic understanding, the therapist experiencing the role, state of mind and emotional responses of the offender, similar to the affective attunement of parent and child. The role and state of mind evoked in the therapist may represent a defensive or avoidant manoeuvre, which requires examination to discern the underlying state or role defended against. A *reciprocating* CT occurs when a therapist experiences him/herself drawn into or induced to assume the reciprocal role of a given RRP, the other pole being enacted by the offender. This is, essentially, a signal to the therapist that s/he has become part of a projective identification relation with a dominant RRP functioning.

These CTs are diagnostic to the extent that they permit the therapist to witness and experience directly RRPs of the offender. A particular skill in CAT is the ability to track the offender's switches, reversals and transitions within dominant RRPs and between different self-states. If this is not achieved, the interaction between therapist and offender can be experienced as confusion and unpredictability, and cause anxiety for the therapist and a lack of containment for the offender.

Projective identification and the offender-to-victim relationship

The projective identification which can occur between offender and victim requires consideration. In Fig. 1.7, part of an SDR is presented of a serial sexual murderer; this case is used to highlight self-states, RRPs and positions, projective identification within the offender-to-victim relationship, dialogical sequence analysis, the location of risk potential, and the types of dilemmas and traps that operate in offenders. The 21-year-old male offender was party to a relationship with a young woman who humiliated, controlled and derided him, using emotional blackmail and the threat of ending the relationship to obtain her wishes. For several months, the offender idealised his partner, whom he felt was socially and physically his superior. He cut his hair, dressed and avoided his friends to acquiesce in her requests, feeling 'like her poodle, not a man'. The offender felt de-masculinised, his partner belittling his sexual performance and comparing him negatively to previous boyfriends. The offender felt trapped in the relationship, and post-offence analysis during CAT showed that he felt weak and impotent as a male, humiliated, and harbouring unexpressed anger and a desire to retaliate against his partner. These feelings can be located in the lower part of self-state 1 (SS1) at the position *controlled/de-masculinised*, 'compliant poodle' (the short-hand name he gave to the self-state). His partner's role is assigned as 'Lady Muck' (his words), indicating his perceptions of her superiority and tendency to humiliate and control, the reciprocal role for the self-state. A dilemma (D1) is apparent in that, to deal with these negative feelings, the offender *either* remained in the relationship but chronically angry and weak, *or* he terminated the relationship and felt inadequate and lonely, giving up a much-wanted, esteem-elevating relationship. In many respects, the offender feels himself 'between a rock and a hard place' and caught in an ambivalent dilemma, experiencing unresolved conflict because of these positions. A trap (T1) is identified whereby the depressed, worthless feelings of the 'poodle' RRP are managed through alcohol misuse, only to engender exacerbated low mood and lack of resolution of the problems. The solution which emerged was one of expressing his anger through fantasies of revenge and retaliation

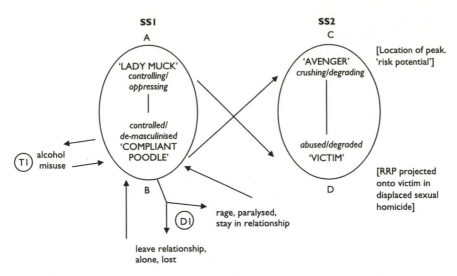

Figure 1.7 Projective identification in the offender-to-victim unit, dialogical sequence analysis and located peak, risk potential.

against his girlfriend through a displaced sexual killing of a local woman of the same age as his partner. The offender fantasised about the acts (a fantasy version of self-state 2; SS2) and, eventually, enacted the *crushing/degrading* (offender RRP) to the *devalued/punished* RRP (the victim's position) through the displaced sexual killing.

Dialogical sequence analysis (DSA)

Dialogical sequence analysis (DSA) of the offender's subjective states and RRPs is undertaken to track the transitions, shifts and switches that often occur as the risk potential reaches its climax or peak. Perceptions of the victim often change as the offender's state of mind and position change. Leiman (2004) described these procedures as *dialogical sequences* illustrating the ways in which RRPs, positions and states of mind with 'voices' can be articulated through analysis of the subjective experiences of individuals and identification of salient RRPs. The notion of the personal position repertoire and counter-position (Hermans & Hermans-Jansen, 2004) is reminiscent of the nature of RRPs. Dialogical sequence analysis is used to locate the *offence-dominant position* (self-state, RRPs), and the offender is made explicitly aware of its typical characteristics, the conditions for its emergence and the implied motivations. Its position within the SDR or SSSD is identified. Strategies to prevent its occurrence are discussed, and relapse prevention strategies are incorporated to promote better self-management of this state.

In Fig. 1.7, the example of the serial sexual killer, the dialogical sequence that could be extracted from his pre-crime thinking and subsequent offences indicated a pattern whereby his girlfriend is perceived as *controlling-oppressing* (position A; 'Lady Muck') in relation to *controlled/de-masculinised* (position B; 'compliant poodle') with associated thoughts, feelings and ways of coping (dilemma, D1; trap, T1). The displaced offence occurred after the offender could not resolve the dilemma, remaining within the relationship and experiencing mounting frustration, tension and unexpressed rage. The idea that killing was a solution emerged through the offender's transition to position C ('avenger', *crushing/degrading* of SS2), forcing another into position D ('victim', *abused/degraded*, SS2). Through projective identification, an RRP is induced or imposed onto the offender-to-victim relationship in the displaced homicide. The offender's entry to the SS2 position C of the 'avenger' represents his most heightened point of risk potential.

The dialogical sequence analysis that traced the offender's changing perceptions of his girlfriend, himself and the victim showed that utterances and voices associated with the RRPs, such as 'I must keep her happy or she'll leave me' (the 'poodle' position's voice), shifted to 'who do you think you are, treating me this way? You phoney slut, I'm going to knock you off your throne' (from the position of 'avenger'). The displacement of his aggression and assertion of his masculinity occurred through attacking a different woman, the offender placing a cushion cover over the victim's head during the offence, 'because she had a different colour of hair to my girlfriend'. The offender claimed that the victim 'spoke to me saying she loved me' after her death. The cycle of killing continued because of his inability to revise and resolve these patterns in that, while he remained within the relationship, tension built repeatedly and the same sequence of tension and relief recurred in a catathymic manner (Wertham, 1937). A process of projective identification is apparent in such an offence whereby the victim is forced into a role, as the offender's repertoire of RRPs is imposed onto the offender-to-victim relationship.

The dialogical facets of CAT have emerged as its theory has expanded (Leiman, 2004). The dialogical processes both within the offender's personality and those which can be distinguished through the offender's relationships require identification. The distinction between the 'healthy' and 'pathological' parts of the self (whether referred to as 'positions' with 'voices', self-states or 'parts of the personality') can be offered to help offenders think about the internal workings of their personality and the patterns of perceiving, feeling and acting that cause destructive behaviours to the self and to others. It is typical to encounter offenders who, at best, can reflect only vaguely on their own mental states (Bateman & Fonagy, 2004), and few have well-developed, formulated or coherent insights about how and why they think, feel and act as they do. Imagery work is often the best method to draw out and activate these self-states, generate the 'voices' which are associated and the feelings experienced, and facilitate various types of dialogical sequences both between and within self-states and across time lines (e.g. the newly formed, 'wiser' self-state now conversing with the destructive self-state which operated at the time of the offence, the 'healthy', post-offence self-states conversing with offender and victim during the crime).

For many offenders, the dialogical facets of personality have become disrupted or switched off, or are simply non-existent. Self-reflexivity (an observing 'I') (Cooper, 2003) is abandoned, and functioning occurs on the basis of a very much self-serving, narcissistic, need-driven self-state with minimal extension to thinking about one's actions and their effects. The narratives told and the characters which are acted out during the crime exhibit a *dominant* position, the position, voice, self-state and state of mind (RRP) accessible and focal at the time of the offence. This dominant self-state, when active, suppresses the dialogical voice of any other, more adaptive and conflicting states (e.g. a 'voiced' position which argues that harming a victim is not a solution). In many cases, a conflict- and conscience-free, dominant position or self-state controls the 'mind-scape' of the offender as his drive to commit the crime mounts. The climax of this position's influence is observed during the offence when it is permitted full expression, representing the height or climax of the offender's risk potential. Most often, it is apparent that, when asked to discuss the offence and tell the narrative story, the offender cannot articulate this dominant state of mind, and all manner of deficits are observed within the offender's narration of his thinking, feeling, intentions, inferred motivations and reasons for acting as he did.

Identifying risk potential

In many respects, when conducting CAT for offenders, we can define the targets for change (the 'symptoms') as behavioural patterns. It is surprising to find that many offenders cannot articulate what the concept of risk is and are unable to verbalise what might be conceived as 'very high risk' or 'low risk'. These offenders are unable or unwilling to contemplate their capacity to cause harm to others, and the targets of therapeutic work must be discussed to help the offenders understand what is being sought from them in terms of positive changes. The need to focus the offender on an agreed and proper conceptualisation of therapeutic targets and what risk actually represents for the offender represents a vital first step within therapy.

One tactic which is also important to incorporate into therapy at an early stage is the notion that terms such as 'risk' and 'dangerousness' are words used to define the *risk potential* that offenders harbour within their own personality, and that can be identified, understood, changed and controlled. This stance disqualifies the tendency of many offenders to claim that their crime was a product of external, situational factors entirely outside their locus of control, a facet of externalisation of blame and responsibility. The contributions of external factors are not denied, but the emphasis in therapeutic work is to target and address the relationship between the offender's personality and his actions. Therefore, terms such as 'risk' and 'dangerousness' are defined as explicit behaviours indicative of this potential and located within the personality of the offender. The interaction of static and dynamic factors which can be analysed from the crime is examined with this caveat in mind for both therapist and offender.

An important point emphasised in CAT for offenders is that what would typically be conceived of in therapy as change toward health and diminishing the influence of pathology is redefined as focusing on achieving changes which make the offender more responsible and in control of this *risk potential*. As offenders move from imprisonment to lesser security and into the community, where they are offered the opportunity to demonstrate changes or to reoffend, the value of this emphasis on their responsibility and control over this potential becomes of much greater importance. It could be argued that if a certain level of external supervision is necessary and professionals' anxieties are not assuaged sufficiently, the stated potential has not been modified enough to engender confidence that another offence is unlikely to occur.

The middle phase of CAT: From recognition to revision

Central to the middle phase of therapy is the reformulation which provides an agenda or 'scaffold' around which therapy takes shape. What is established at this earlier stage is knowledge of recurrent patterns of problematic RRPs. A focus is maintained on these procedures during this middle phase. A central task for the therapist is to encourage the recognition of these procedures through describing evidence of their enactments in the material which the offender brings to therapy. Evidence of enactments in both the offender's day-to-day life and in the relationship with the therapist is considered. Self-monitoring might be encouraged to facilitate the recognition of these patterns. An example of this in CAT might involve asking an offender to detail instances of relationship difficulties linked to a procedural pattern in which 'with others I remain safe by being wholly in control or, if my control slips, I feel weak, compliant and submissive'.

Often, awareness of these patterns forms the precondition for allowing the offender to explore alternative ways of relating to self and others. Recognition of the above pattern, for example, might allow offenders the opportunity to reality-test their belief that anything less than 100% control of others will have severely adverse psychological consequences. Bennett (1998) has developed an empirically refined model of how therapeutic activity in CAT might proceed. The model moves through various stages, beginning with the acknowledgement of a specific procedure, the linking of the procedure to a specific event or material, consensually linking procedural enactment to the offender's diagram, and concluding with a consideration of 'exits' from the procedural pattern.

Revision

The aim of CAT is to achieve insight and self-knowledge; to develop tools to help the offender understand, monitor, control and modify (revise) damaging patterns of relating; and to facilitate change in those facets of the self which generate harm to others and oneself. The three Ss of CAT with offenders, for want of an easier description, consist of enhancing *self-knowledge* and insight; developing a capacity to *self-monitor* and self-reflect; and, when opportunity to offend is available, developing *self-regulation/self-control*. As well as fostering the resolution of disorder associated with the offending, CAT actively addresses the task of diminishing the influence and expression of the offender's risk potential through analysis and modification of those structures and processes which have already caused and are likely in the future to cause harm to others and the offender him/herself. The contribution of CAT to relapse prevention (Laws, 1989; Pollock, 1996b) is evident, because CAT aims to equip the offender with the psychological tools to prevent a further offence.

The change processes in CAT can be noted to occur in the context of a non-collusive, collaborative, therapeutic alliance, whereby recognition and revision are scaffolded in what can be referred to as the 'zone of proximal development' (Ryle & Kerr, 2002). The new learning (self-knowledge; insight; recognition of procedures; new, revised ways of thinking and feeling; and alternative ways of relating and acting) achieved through CAT is encouraged by the extension of the client's psychological capacities, as the therapist scaffolds acquisition of portable tools which facilitate change. Attention is paid to the transference developments, and focus is placed on agreed target problems and the resolution and revision of their underlying procedures.

Ending therapy

While the end of CAT therapy is faced from the very first session, it is likely that termination will bring up unresolved issues for the offender. These issues might be associated with unresolved loss or with anger that, as therapy is ending, it has not proven to be the hoped-for experience of compensatory, perfect care. The *Goodbye Letter* written by the therapist and read out in the final session of therapy is an opportunity to address these concerns. Offenders are invited to do likewise and bring to the final session a letter which they, too, can read out. In addition to reviewing matters associated with the termination, the therapist's Goodbye Letter also offers a realistic review of how therapy has progressed, what has (and has not) been achieved during the course of therapy and some reflections on how therapeutic progress might be sustained.

The scope and evidence base for CAT

The accuracy of CAT reformulation methods (e.g. the SSSD) was explored by Bennett & Parry (1998), who compared the flow diagram created by therapist and offender from the same single case with data derived from two alternative formulation methods, namely, the case conflictual relationship theme (Luborsky & Crits-Christoph, 1990) and structural analysis of social behaviour–cyclic maladaptive pattern models (Benjamin, 1974). The findings of Bennett & Parry support the contention that accurate reformulation of a client's difficulties can be achieved by CAT without reliance upon complex, laborious methods. As a clinically sound process of reformulation, CAT can provide a comprehensive means of conceptualising the recurring damaging patterns of procedures and relating associated with an offender's difficulties.

Roth & Fonagy (1996) comment on CAT that the 'prime value of this technique is that it offers a structure for intervention by requiring the therapist to offer a parsimonious formulation of the offender's difficulties within an interpersonally focused schema-oriented framework' (p. 11). The diagrams generated during the reformulation process act as important tools for the work to be done in therapy and exemplify this technique. It is important that the diagrams are not overcomplicated and do not confuse the client. Creating the diagram in CAT requires a flexible and offender-unique approach from the therapist, and each diagram is typically as fundamentally unique as the offenders and their experiences and ways of coping with life's difficulties and relationships.

The development of research into CAT is described by Ryle (1995), Margison (2000) and Ryle & Kerr (2002). Ryle's 1995 text describes the processes of integration and evolution of CAT theory throughout the 1980s that in turn gave birth to a series of small-scale, uncontrolled, naturalistic studies throughout the 1990s. Examples from this phase include an account of a study by Garyfallos, Adampoulou, Saitis, Sotiriou, Zlatanos & Alektoridis (1993). This study involved the utilisation of a range of pre- and post-therapy measures allied to a series of qualitative measures applied to an outpatient population of a community mental health centre in Greece receiving CAT. Of those who completed therapy, significant Minnesota Multi-phasic Personality Inventory (MMPI) changes were recorded at both the post-therapy stage and after a 12-month follow-up period. Clarke & Llewelyn (1994) described the treatment of seven female survivors of childhood sexual abuse with CAT. This study used multiple outcome measures, including dyad repertory grid data. On the basis of repeated grid analyses, Clarke & Llewelyn concluded that two of the women changed the way in which they construed the relationship of men to themselves.

Duignan & Mitzman (1994) reported the use of CAT techniques applied in a group format to the treatment of a heterogeneous patient group drawn from a psychiatric outpatient population. Psychological difficulties identified by a range of psychometric measures included significant levels of personality disorder. Repeat testing of these measures at the conclusion of the group and at a 6-month follow-up indicated a statistically significant reduction in symptoms. Cowmeadow (1994) also reported the successful treatment of two deliberately self-harming patients. Success of therapy was measured both by the reduction in self-harming behaviour and by a reduction in general symptomatology as indexed by standardised psychometric measures. Golynkina & Ryle (2000) have reported the results of an uncontrolled study using CAT with a population of offenders with borderline personality disorder. Of the 27 patients who completed therapy, 14 were no longer found to meet the criteria for borderline personality disorder according to the Personality Assessment Schedule. The authors note the way in which these findings compare favourably with other longer-term treatments of borderline personality disorder. In a further study, Pollock (2001a) described an uncontrolled study of 37 offenders with histories of abusive experiences in childhood treated with CAT. A battery of psychological tests was administered before, after and at various follow-up intervals after the completion of therapy. Of the 36 offenders who completed therapy, statistically significant changes were identified by psychometric testing in a variety of domains, including areas of personality functioning, dissociative-type experiences, neurotic problems and other post-traumatic stress disorder-type phenomena.

While these previously reported studies comprise the general bulk of outcome work carried out within the field of CAT, there have been some attempts at carrying out controlled studies. Brockman, Poynton, Ryle & Watson (1987) describe the outcome of treatment in 48 patients randomly assigned to either 12 sessions of CAT or 12 sessions of treatment following the module of Mann & Goldman (1982). The CAT therapists involved in this trial were all trainees from a variety of professional backgrounds. Changes within the patients were indexed by a range of psychometric measures. Additionally, idiographic data such as repertory grid prediction scores and target problem (TP) and target problem procedure (TPP) ratings were also employed. Brockman *et al.* reported that differences in the rating of TPP between the two treatment conditions disappeared when initial score levels were taken into account. However, CAT produced significantly larger changes in the grid measures. Through the use of a series of case vignettes, Milton (1989) described the way in which emotional and psychological factors can impinge upon diabetic self-care. Building upon this, Fosbury (1994) compared the treatment of a non-compliant, poorly self-caring diabetic group by CAT and nurse education. The results of this controlled study show that the mean level of blood sugar improved under both treatment conditions. However, for patients receiving CAT, these changes were more significantly sustained at a 9-month follow-up appointment. A subsequent randomised, controlled trial of CAT with a similar group of poorly controlled diabetics (Fosbury, Bosley, Ryle, Sonsken & Judd, 1997), however, showed no significant difference between CAT and the comparison treatments. Ryle (1995) also describes a study in which CAT is applied to further medical problems. This study reports a randomised, control trial of CAT in relation to the treatment of a non-compliant group of asthma sufferers. Counselling provided the control group in this study. Whereas both interventions focused upon issues of general self-care, including asthma management, at a 12-week follow-up, there was a significant improvement registered in the group of patients receiving CAT.

Comparing CAT with other forensic psychotherapies

While CAT might claim a relatively established niche for itself within the wider infrastructure of general psychotherapy it can make no such claims in relation to the field of forensic psychotherapy. Currently, this field is dominated mainly by the psychodynamic and cognitive-behavioural paradigms, the former having a long tradition in the psychological understanding and treatment of the offender, and the latter an established evidence base. CAT's excursion into the world of forensic psychotherapy is at a very early stage, and it would seem unwise to make claims of its supposed advantages over either of these models. However, CAT does have a tradition and methodology for working with and conceptualising the hard-to-help, poorly integrated client. Add to this the fact that CAT offers not only a means of directly working with the offender but also, through the use of diagrammatic reformulation, a portable and communicable means for addressing relational issues that connect the offender to the wider forensic network, and there does appear to be potential for further development.

Chapter 2 provides an illustrative case study which describes the three Rs of CAT (reformulation, recognition and revision) and the assessment and therapeutic tools used throughout the three phases to promote the three Ss of such work with offenders (self-knowledge, self-monitoring and self-control/regulation).

References

Abrams, J. & Zweig, C. (1991). *Meeting the shadow: The hidden power of the dark side of human nature*. New York: Penguin.

Bakhtin, M. M. (1984). *Problems of Dostoevsky's poetics*. Edited and translated by C. Emerson. Manchester: Manchester University Press.

Baldwin, M. W. (1992). Relational schemas in the processing of social information. *Psychological Bulletin, 112*, 461–484.

Bateman, A. & Fonagy, P. (2004). *Psychotherapy for borderline personality disorder*. Oxford: Oxford University Press.

Benjamin, L. S. (1974). Structural analysis of social behaviour. *Psychological Review*, *81*, 392–425.

Bennett, D. (1998). Deriving a model of therapist competence for good and poor outcomes in the psychotherapy of borderline personality disorder. Unpublished PhD thesis, University of Sheffield.

Bennett, D. & Parry, G. (1998). The accuracy of reformulation in cognitive analytic therapy: A validation study. *Psychotherapy Research*, *8*, 84–103.

Biven, B. (1997). Dehumanisation as an enactment of serial killers: A sadomasochistic case study. *Journal of Analytic Social Work*, *4*, 23–49.

Bolton, G., Howlett, S. & Lago, C. (2004). *Writing cures: An introductory handbook of writing in counselling and psychotherapy*. London: Taylor & Francis.

Brockman, B. & Smith, J. (1990). CAT in forensic services. Chapter 9. In A. Ryle (Ed.), *Cognitive analytic therapy: Active participation in change: A new integration in brief psychotherapy*. Chichester: Wiley.

Brockman, B., Poynton, A., Ryle, A. & Watson, J. P. (1987). Effectiveness of time-limited psychotherapy carried out by trainees: Comparison of two studies. *British Journal of Psychiatry*, *152*, 602–610.

Bromberg, P. M. (1998). *Standing in spaces*. Hillside, NJ: Analytic Press.

Bursten, B. (1972). The manipulative personality. *Archives of General Psychiatry*, *26*, 318–321.

Canter, D. (1994). *Criminal shadows: Inside the mind of the serial killer*. London: HarperCollins.

Clarke, S. & Llewelyn, S. (1994). Personal constructs of survivors of childhood sexual abuse receiving cognitive analytic therapy. *British Journal of Medical Psychology*, *67*, 273–289.

Cooper, M. (2003). 'I–I' and 'I–Me': Transposing Buber's inter-personal attitudes to the intra-personal plane. *Journal of Constructivist Psychology*, *16*, 131–153.

Cordess, C. & Cox, M. (Eds) (1996). *Forensic Psychiatry: Crime, psychodynamics and the offender patient*. London: Jessica Kingsley.

Cordess, C., Riley, W. & Welldon, E. (1994). Psychodynamic forensic psychotherapy: An account of a day-release course. *Psychiatric Bulletin*, *18*, 88–90.

Cowmeadow, P. (1994). Deliberate self-harm and Cognitive Analytic Therapy. *International Journal of Short-Term Psychotherapy*, *9*, 135–150.

Crittenden, P. M. (1985). Maltreated infants: Vulnerability and resilience. *Journal of Child Psychology and Psychiatry*, *26*, 85–96.

Dimaggio, G., Salvatore, G., Azzara, C., Catania, D, Semerari, A. & Hermans, H. J. M. (2004). Dialogical relationships in impoverished narratives: From theory to clinical practice. *Psychology and Psychotherapy*, *76*, 385–410.

Dimaggio, G. & Semerari, A. (2003). Disorganised narratives: The psychological condition and its treatment: How to achieve a metacognitive point of view restoring order to chaos. (unpublished).

Duigan, I. & Mitzman, S. F. (1994). Measuring individual change in offenders receiving time-limited cognitive analytic therapy. *International Journal of Short-Term Psychotherapy*, *9*, 151–160.

Fosbury, J. A. (1994). Cognitive Analytic Therapy with poorly controlled insulin dependent diabetic offenders. In C. Coles (Ed.), *Psychology and diabetes care*. Chichester: PMH Production.

Fosbury, J. A., Bosley, C., Ryle, A., Sonken, P. H. & Judd, S. L. (1997). A trial of cognitive analytic therapy in poorly controlled type I offenders. *Diabetes Care, 20*, 959–964.

Freud, S. (1957). Some character types met in psychoanalytical work. *Standard Edition* (vol. 14). London: Hogarth Press.

Frey-Rohn, L. (1991). How to deal with evil. Chapter 57. In J. Abrams & C. Zweig (Eds), *Meeting the shadow: The hidden power of the dark side of human nature*. New York: Penguin.

Garyfallos, G., Adampoulou, M., Saitis, M., Sotiriou, M., Zlatanos, D. & Alektoridis, P. (1993). Evaluation of cognitive analytic therapy (CAT) outcome. *Neurologia et Psychiatria, 12*, 121–125.

Golynkina, K. & Ryle, A. (2000). Effectiveness of time-limited cognitive analytic therapy for borderline personality disorder: Factors associated with outcome. *British Journal of Medical Psychology, 73*, 197–210.

Gonçalves, O. F. (1995). Cognitive narrative psychotherapy. In M. J. Mahoney (Ed.), *Cognitive and constructive psychotherapies*. New York: Springer.

Guggenbühl-Craig, A. (1991). Why psychopaths do not rule the world. Chapter 47. In J. Abrams & C. Zweig (Eds), *Meeting the shadow: The hidden power of the dark side of human nature*. New York: Penguin.

Hermans, H. J. M. & Dimaggio, G. (Eds) (2004). *The dialogical self in psychotherapy*. London: Brunner-Routledge.

Hermans, H. J. M. & Hermans-Jansen, E. (2004). The dialogical construction of coalitions in the personal position repertoire. In H. J. M. Hermans & G. Dimaggio (Eds), *The dialogical self in psychotherapy*. London: Brunner-Routledge.

Hermans, H. J. M. & Kempen, H. J. K. (1993). *The dialogical self: Meaning as movement*. San Diego, CA: Academic Press.

Honos-Webb, L. & Stiles, W. B. (1998). Reformulation of assimilation analysis in terms of voices. *Psychotherapy, 35*, 23–33.

Horley, J. (2003). *Personal construct perspectives on forensic psychology*. Hove: Brunner-Routledge.

Houston, J. (1998). *Making sense with offenders: Personal constructs, therapy and change*. Chichester: Wiley.

Jaynes, J. (1986). Hearing voices and the bicameral mind. *Brain and Behavioural Sciences, 9*, 526–537.

Kear-Colwell, J. & Pollock, P. H. (1996). Confrontation or motivation? Which approach to the sex offender? *Criminal Justice and Behaviour, 24*, 20–30.

Kelly, G. (1955). *The psychology of personal constructs*. New York: Norton.

Kerby, A. P. (1991). *Narrative and the self*. Bloomington, IN: Indiana University Press.

Khan, M. M. R. (1989). *Hidden selves: Between theory and practice in psychoanalysis*. London: Karnac.

Kiesler, D. J. (1988). *Therapeutic metacommunication. Therapist impact disclosure as feedback in psychotherapy*. Palo Alto, CA: Consulting Psychologists Press.

Laws, R. D. (1989). *Relapse prevention for sexual offenders*. New York: Guilford.

Leiman, M. (2004). Dialogical sequence analysis. In H. J. M. Hermans & G. Dimaggio (Eds), *The dialogical self in psychotherapy*. London: Brunner-Routledge.

Leiman, M. & Ryle, A. (1995). How analytic is CAT? In A. Ryle (Ed.), *Cognitive analytic therapy: Developments in theory and practice*. Chichester: Wiley.

Luborsky, L. & Crits-Christoph, P. (1990). *Understanding transference: The CCRT method*. New York: Basic Books.

Maden, A., Williams, J., Wong, S. C. P. & Leis, T. A. (2004). Treating dangerous and severe personality disorder in high security: Lessons from the Regional Secure Centre, Saskatoon, Canada. *Journal of Forensic Psychiatry and Psychology*, *15*, 375–390.

Mann, J. & Goldman, R. (1982). *A case book of time limited psychotherapy*. New York: McGraw-Hill.

Margison, F. (2000) Editorial: Cognitive Analytic Therapy: A case study in treatment development. *British Journal of Medical Psychology*, *73*, 145–150.

McGauley, G. & Humphreys, M. (2003). Contribution of forensic psychotherapy to the care of forensic offenders. *Advances in Psychiatric Treatment*, 117–124.

McGuire, J. (1995). *What works: Reducing reoffending*. Chichester: Wiley.

Meloy, J. R. & Meloy, M. J. (2000). Autonomic arousal in the presence of psychopathy: A survey study of mental health and criminal justice professionals. *Journal of Threat Assessment*, *2*, 21–33.

Milton, J. (1989). Brief psychotherapy with poorly controlled diabetics. *British Journal of Psychotherapy*, *5*, 532–543.

Ogden, J. H. (1983). The concept of internal object relations. *International Journal of Psychoanalysis*, *64*, 227–241.

Pizer, S. A. (2002). The capacity to tolerate paradox: Bridging multiplicity within the self. Chapter 5. In J. C. Muran (Ed.), *Self-relations in the psychotherapy process* (pp. 111–130). Washington, DC: American Psychological Association.

Pollock, P. H. (1996a). Clinical issues in the cognitive analytic therapy of sexually abused women who commit violence offences against their partners. *British Journal of Medical Psychology*, *69*, 117–127.

Pollock, P. H. (1996b). Self-efficacy and sexual offending against children: Construction of measure and changes following relapse prevention treatment. *Legal and Criminological Psychology*, *1*, 215–228.

Pollock, P. H. (1997). Cognitive Analytic Therapy with an offender with borderline personality disorder. In A. Ryle (Ed.), *Cognitive analytic therapy and borderline personality disorder: The model and the method*. Chichester: Wiley.

Pollock, P. H. (2001a). Cognitive analytic therapy for borderline erotomania: Forensic romances and violence in the therapy room. *Clinical Psychology and Psychotherapy*, *8*, 214–229.

Pollock, P. H. (2001b). *Cognitive analytic therapy for adult survivors of childhood abuse: Approaches to treatment and case management*. Chichester: Wiley.

Pollock, P. H. (2003). Cognitive analytic therapy for adult survivors of childhood abuse: Changes to identity disturbance during and after therapy. (unpublished).

Pollock, P. H. & Belshaw, T. D. (1998). Cognitive analytic therapy for offenders. *Journal of Forensic Psychiatry*, *9*, 629–642.

Pollock, P. H., Broadbent, M., Clarke, S., Dorrian, A. & Ryle, A. (2001c). The Personality Structure Questionnaire (PSQ): A measure of the multiple self-states model of identity disturbance in cognitive analytic therapy. *Clinical Psychology and Psychotherapy*, *8*, 59–72.

Pollock, P. H. & Kear-Colwell, J. (1994). Women who stab: A personal construct analysis of sexual victimization and offending behaviour. *British Journal of Medical Psychology*, *67*, 13–22.

Roth, A. D. & Fonagy, P. (1996). *What works for whom? A critical review of psychotherapy research*. New York: Guilford.

Rowan, J. (1990). *Subpersonalities: The people inside us*. London: Routledge.

Ryle, A. (1978). A common language for the psychotherapies. *British Journal of Psychiatry*, *132*, 585–594.

Ryle, A. (1979). The focus in brief interpretive psychotherapy: Dilemmas, traps and snags as target problems. *British Journal of Psychiatry*, *135*, 46–64.

Ryle, A. (1982). *Psychotherapy: A cognitive integration of theory and practice*. London: Academic Press.

Ryle, A. (1990). *Cognitive analytic therapy. Active participation in change: A new integration in brief psychotherapy*. Chichester: Wiley.

Ryle, A. (Ed.) (1995). *Cognitive Analytic Therapy: Developments in Theory and Practice*. Chichester: Wiley.

Ryle, A. (1997). The structure and development of borderline personality disorder: A proposed model. *British Journal of Psychiatry*, *170*, 82–87.

Ryle, A. & Kerr, I. B. (2002). *Introducing cognitive analytic therapy: Principles and practice*. Chichester: Wiley.

Simon, R. I. (1997). *Bad men do what good men dream: A forensic psychiatrist illuminates the darker side of human behaviour*. Washington, DC: American Psychiatric Press.

Stiles, W. B. (1999). Signs and voices in psychotherapy. *Psychotherapy Research*, *9*, 1–21.

Tschudi, F. (1989). *Flexigrid*. Oslo: University of Oslo.

Van Schoor, E. (1996). The 'technique-technology' of brief psychotherapy. *Free Associations*, *6*, 258–275.

Von Franz, M.-L. (1995). *Shadow and evil in fairy tales* (2nd edn). London: Shambhala.

Vygotsky, L. S. (1978). *Mind in society: The development of higher psychological processes*. Cambridge, MA: Harvard University Press.

Welldon, E. V. & Van Velsen, C. (1998). *A practical guide to forensic psychotherapy*. London: Jessica Kingsley.

Wertham, F. (1937). The catathymic crisis: A clinical entity. *Archives of General Neurology and Psychiatry*, *37*, 974–977.

Whelton, W. J. & Greenberg, L. S. (2002). The self as a singular multiplicity: A process-experiential perspective. In J. C. Muran (Ed.), *Self-relations in the psychotherapy process* (pp. 87–106). Washington, DC: American Psychological Association.

From theory to practice

Cognitive Analytic Therapy for an arsonist with borderline personality disorder

Philip H. Pollock

The language and concepts of Cognitive Analytic Therapy (CAT) theory can be cumbersome at first, and its translation into practice requires illustration. Chapter 1 aimed to provide the reader with a synopsis of CAT theory and practice in forensic work. A case study is presented here of an offender with borderline personality disorder (BPD) to animate the main concepts, reformulation processes, and tools and therapy techniques of CAT. The therapy described comprises all of the methods and techniques that would, typically, be part of individual CAT with an offender. Firstly, the CAT model of BPD is briefly described.

Borderline personality disorder (BPD): The diagnosis

BPD is included in the *Diagnostic and statistical manual of mental disorders* (fourth edition (DSM-IV)) (American Psychiatric Association, 1994) within Cluster B of 'dramatic and erratic' personality disorders. Nine criteria are used to describe the disorder, with five criteria required for the formal, categorical diagnosis. It is a heterogeneous concept in that there are 256 possible combinations for the disorder. Sensitivity and reliability problems have been described when diagnosing the disorder, whether using categorical or dimensional approaches.

CAT for borderline conditions

Ryle (1997a and b) introduced the multiple self-states model (MSSM) for BPD to describe the different levels of personality damage observed in this disorder. According to this model, the key features of BPD are that the person (1) exhibits a limited, narrow repertoire of harsh reciprocal role procedures (RRPs) at level 1 of the MSSM, (2) tends to experience partial dissociation into a number of limited and separate self-states (level 2), and (3) shows impaired and disrupted capacity for self-reflection (level 3). These levels describe the linked damage underlying the personality disorder and, in particular, the discontinuities, changeability, unpredictability and inconsistency subjectively felt and noted in responses and behaviours. The nine diagnostic indicators of DSM-IV which define the psychological and behavioural disturbances of BPD can be accounted for by the MSSM model. In particular, the central features of the disorder include a degree of instability in self-construing and experience, identity disturbance, and associated affective states and symptoms (e.g. chronic emptiness, inappropriate and intense anger, dissociative symptoms, emotional lability) with interpersonal markers such as intense, unstable relationships (shifts from idealizing to devalued), frantic efforts to avoid abandonment, paranoid decompensation when stressed and dysfunctional behaviours (impulsivity, self-harming and suicidal tendencies). The MSSM explains these BPD signs within a CAT framework in the following manner:

(1) Patterns of relationships (enactment of reciprocal role procedures (RRPs) in self-to-other exchanges) and of self-management (self-to-self) are frequently extreme and rigid, and are prone to elicit similarly extreme responses from others. These patterns usually stem from early neglect and abuse, either repeating what was experienced through enacting reciprocal role procedures such as *abusing-to-victim* (in which either pole may be played by the individual) or representing partially or wholly dissociated symptomatic, restricted, but less extreme alternatives.

(2) The partial dissociation (or complete dissociation; dissociative identity disorder (DID)) (Pollock, 2001a) between different RRPs, which originates as an escape from noxious and toxic experiences, produces a fragmented self in which a small number of patterns or multiple *self-states* become established and alternate in organising experience and action. A lack of integration in experience, self-construal, perceptions of others and behaviour is observed. *Switches* between such states occur in an abrupt and confusing manner, and their provocation is not always evident or appropriate. Switches between self-states occur, as for example, between an idealised state with RRPs of *ideally caring-to-fused* and another contrasting self-state such as *abusing-to-victimised*. A *response shift* is observed when a person perceives him/herself to be, for example, *punished* and shifts response to the same reciprocal role from *punished* to *resisting/avenging* in relation to a *punishing* other. A *role reversal* occurs when the patient oscillates to abusing from victimised (see Chapter 1 for explanations of these patterns). The inconsistency and discontinuities of the disorder can be explained through these patterns and their changes.

(3) As a result of these switches, and also as a consequence of a lack of concern from others during childhood, self-reflection is poorly developed and is disrupted at the very times when most needed, namely, when switches into destructive or otherwise dysfunctional procedures occur.

Implicitly, the background context of the development of BPD is dysfunctional parenting and care-giving, which, with later additional environmental failures, leads to the development of a fractured, disturbed and fragmented identity with partially dissociated, multiple self-states. Limited integration in identity is achieved. The person with BPD displays a narrow range of RRPs, which are often of an *abusing-to-victimised* quality (Pollock, 2001a). The lack of integration between states is evident in abrupt switches between contrasting states, changing responses to others and reversals. Dissociative symptoms are observed in association with these unpredictable shifts, the person's experiences being confusing, hard to self-monitor and lacking the smoothness of transition in mood, perceptions of self and others, and behavioural reactions. In many ways, the 'glue' or 'oil' of the personality is absent and the changes between states and responses are similar to a needle on a record being repeatedly scratched between songs (self-states, positions, etc.). Both the patient and therapist's experiences of dialogue and interactions can be confusing and difficult to track unless a proper reformulation is made of these psychological states and the procedures affecting them.

Recognising dissociated states: CAT methods

Pollock, Broadbent, Clarke, Dorrian & Ryle (2001) and Pollock (2001a) reported an investigation into the conceptualisation of identity disturbance as proposed by the MSSM, using several measures including a self-report measure. The Personality Structure Questionnaire (PSQ) was designed as a screening measure to assess identity-like disturbances. This scale is reproduced in Appendix 2 and consists of eight pairs of contrasting descriptions of the self as stable or changeable, each item being scored between 1 (stable) and 5 (changeable). Scores range from 8 to 40, higher scores indicating greater reported disturbance. The mean scores of samples of normal subjects are in the range 19.7–23.3, whereas for cases of BPD they were shown to be 30.4–31.3. The BPD patients in this study showed similar levels of multiplicity of self (number of identifiable self-states) to patients with DID, yet less dissociative symptoms and experiences, supporting the thesis that BPD as a disorder represents a personality exhibiting multiple, fragmented self-states which are partially dissociated, without amnesia and severe dissociation evident (as seen in those with DID). The extent of multiplicity of self-states was not dissimilar for BPD or DID patients, yet the degree of dissociation was significantly different. Pollock (2003), in a study investigating the relative change in PSQ scores for women who had histories of childhood abuse and were receiving individual CAT compared with a no-treatment group, reported that PSQ scores showed an increase after the first stages of the CAT reformulation process. A subsequent decrease in PSQ scores and identity disturbance was noted throughout additional sessions of CAT.

A second method to identify the types of self-states in BPD was proposed by Golynkina & Ryle (1999), using repertory self-states grid material from 20 BPD patients (see Appendix 1 for this grid). The authors found that certain typical self-states, among others, could be ascertained for this group of patients including *ideal, abuser rage, victim, coping states, zombie* and *victim rage* states. The link between the development of BPD and a history of childhood adversity has been proposed, and it is likely that, among other causal and contributory factors, this type of childhood experience can compromise the optimal achievement of a consistent, stable and integrated identity (Johnson, Cohen, Brown, Smailes & Bernstein, 1999). Not all victims of childhood abuse and adversity are traumatically compromised (Pollock, 2001b), yet there is evidence of the influence of developmental roots in the emergence of BPD (see Bateman & Fonagy, 2004, for a succinct review). Abused and victimised self-states are often observed using self-states grid data for BPD, and the grid permits identification and analysis of the nature of these states.

The states description procedure (SDP) (Bennett, Pollock & Ryle, 2004) was devised as a measure of 'borderline-ness' and a method of defining and tracking the partially dissociated self-states observed in BPD, and as a therapy tool to promote improved self-reflection (MSSM, level 3). The SDP is reproduced in Appendix 3. The SDP consists of two parts. The first part describes a number of typical states such as an 'OK state', 'victim/abused' state, etc. The patient recognises or identifies the experienced states with the therapist's help and lists the characteristics under two headings of 'I feel' and 'people in my life'. Once identified, the features and subjective experiences of the state are noted in terms of frequency, duration, emotional and physical attributes, etc. The SDP helps conceptualise and identify the switches, shifts and reversals often observed as part of the identity disturbances and the relational 'pull' of BPD whereby the therapist and others are drawn into collusive reinforcement and enactment of the reciprocal role of dysfunctional RRPs.

The Reformulation Letter and diagrammatic tools in CAT help the therapist and patient to construct a retrospective, autobiographical narrative of the offender's history and identify critical RRPs and the 'core pain' within the patient's experiences. It has been stated that the person with BPD is overwhelmed by intolerable affects and psychological pain that cannot be regulated and repeatedly fractures the sense of identity and colours relating. Holmes (1998) remarked that producing a coherent self-narrative helps to organise the patient's experiences and self-story, and is a target for therapy.

Research evidence for CAT with BPD

Several case studies describe the use of CAT for patients with BPD with moderate success (Dunn, 1994; Ryle & Beard, 1993; Marlowe & Ryle, 1995; Ryle, 1997a). Within forensic settings, Pollock (1997) described CAT for a sexual offender who was diagnosed with BPD, and who had a significant history of offending and self-harm; the outcome was positive in terms of diminishing many dysfunctional indicators of BPD. Pollock & Belshaw (1998) reported two forensic case studies of offenders with BPD which identified the types of RRPs (e.g. particularly offender-to-victim RRPs), procedural loops, dilemmas, traps and snags that explained these offenders' criminal actions. Pollock (2001a) described the CAT reformulation and treatment of a female patient who stalked and attempted to kill her therapist and showed evidence of a condition termed 'borderline erotomania' (Meloy, 1989), the therapy achieving reduction in psychological symptoms and improved integration in identity and dissociation symptoms, more stable interpersonal relationships, and an absence of offending subsequently. These case studies highlight the utility of CAT for treatment of BPD.

In terms of case series studies, Ryle & Golynkina (2000) reported the application of a 24-session CAT programme for patients with BPD, the results demonstrating that half of the patients in the series did not show diagnostic criteria for the disorder 6 months after termination of therapy, and average scores on questionnaires revealed continuing improvement at 18 months after therapy. Severity of disorder at intake was associated with poorer outcome and progress. Wildgoose, Clarke & Waller (2001) proposed that personality fragmentation and dissociative processes are core features of BPD. These authors reported evidence that CAT promoted personality 'integration' and reduced dissociative symptoms in a series of BPD patients through strengthening awareness and control over these fragmenting processes.

The CAT model for BPD has been compared to other theoretical stances. For example, Bateman & Fonagy (2004) reviewed the similarities between their mentalisation-based treatment (MBT) of BPD and CAT, commenting that 'CAT shares a number of features with MBT' (p. 132), yet numerous differences in the emphasis of developmental reasons for the deficits in the personalities of those with the disorder are noted. Judd & McGlashan's (2003) developmental model of BPD and the treatment course and outcomes achieved during the Chestnut Lodge study identify causal and contributing factors, such as genetics, environment, disorganised attachment systems, temperamental traits, history of maltreatment and chronic stress, leading to integrative processing problems such as dissociation, and three modes of dysfunction (cognitive, emotional and behavioural). In addition, intense, unstable relationships and identity diffusion are explained. As in CAT, Judd & McGlashan (2003) identify the significance of multiple models of predominantly insecure, disorganised and poorly integrated attachments as central features of the disorder. It is proposed that, under conditions such as stress, the predominant relationship 'model' collapses with subsequent cognitive, emotional and behavioural disorganisation and dysregulation. The authors suggest that the insecure attachment and degree of disorganisation under stress predict the variations in BPD course and severity of impairment. They also report an impaired capacity in reflective functioning and metacognitive monitoring and knowledge, which is similar to Bateman and Fonagy's developmental failures in mentalisation as explanatory mechanisms for the indicators of BPD. Both theories and therapies are psychoanalytically informed and differ from Linehan's biosocial dialectical behaviour therapy (DBT) (Linehan, 1993), which places emotional dysregulation as the core, causal problem of the disorder. Other established forms of psychotherapy for BPD, such as transference-focused psychotherapy based on Otto Kernberg's (1967; Kernberg, Clarkin & Yeomans, 2002) theory of borderline personality organisation, are difficult to compare with CAT, given their differences in conceptualisation and treatment emphasis. Young, Klosko & Weishaar's (2003) schema therapy model of BPD implies that BPD can be notated to show early maladaptive schemas (EMS), such as defectiveness, abandonment and abuse/mistrust, which are often expressed through characteristic 'schema modes' such as the *angry child*, *vulnerable child* and *detached protector* modes. Jeffrey Young's original model of schema therapy is a therapist-attractive and patient-friendly approach which explicitly incorporates ways of conceptualising the therapeutic relationship and the reasons for its rupture. The unpredictable and bewildering confusion experienced by the person with BPD is understood to be caused by switching between schema modes.

The CAT model for BPD aims to improve self-knowledge, self-monitoring and self-regulation through the integration of the identity of the offender's personality. This is accomplished through use of several tools and methods, with attention paid to constructing a narrative reformulation, identifying and improving control over affective instability and impulsive acting out, and the attenuation of damaging and destructive procedures that lead to harm for self and others. The illustrative case described here applies the MSSM and links the model to the therapeutic work within this individual CAT intervention.

An arsonist with BPD: Saul

Saul, a 34-year-old Caucasian, was placed in a medium-secure psychiatric hospital unit for arson of a local Social Services building. His criminal and psychiatric histories were extensive. His past convictions included criminal damage, arson (11 offences), driving while intoxicated, shoplifting and assault. He had been hospitalised on 13 separate occasions since the age of 17, mostly because of serious incidents of parasuicide, self-harm and depression. His psychiatric notes queried bipolar disorder with personality disorder. At the time of the index offence, Saul's lifestyle was reported to have been aimless, chaotic and vagrant; he lived in squats and derelict housing in the inner city, misusing alcohol and drugs on a daily basis. At no time in his life had Saul gained employment, and he had numerous unsuccessful episodes of inpatient drug and alcohol rehabilitation. His lifestyle was generally antisocial and driven by his substance dependency. Saul stole from other vagrants or shops and had robbed persons at knifepoint on several occasions to obtain money to satisfy these needs. His episodes in prison were characterised by attendance at mental health services for medication, and transfer to prison hospital for cutting his wrists and attempted hanging. Prison records documented that Saul was viewed as a vulnerable, inadequate personality who tended to ingratiate himself with imprisoned paramilitaries for self-protection (e.g. delivering warning messages from paramilitaries to other prisoners. In one instance of extreme violence, he slit the throat of a child sex offender to pay off a tobacco debt).

Saul was referred for psychological assessment by the multidisciplinary team of the unit. At first interview, Saul presented as a thin, somewhat socially inadequate and inarticulate individual who was fidgety and distracted. He expressed his suspicion about attending and repeatedly asked why he was in the hospital, claiming that he was not mentally ill. He voiced his intention to abscond at the first opportunity. He did not like the hospital environment, commenting, 'They're all loons in there – are you trying to drive me mad as well?' Nursing staff reported that Saul was troublesome, complaining and disruptive. They queried his motivation to engage with any treatment and his continuing usage of prescribed and illicit substances. He was non-compliant with prescribed medication and tended to try to misuse drugs at every opportunity.

Saul proved to be a poor historian. It was apparent that his account of his personal history was an example of an impoverished narrative with limited reflection on past events and autobiographical memories (Dimaggio, Salvatore, Azzara, Catania, Semerari & Hermans, 2004). Information was obtained from case materials and documentation in the first instance. Saul's early life history was fraught with trauma and adversity. He was brought up by his grandmother and a woman he believed to be his sister, the latter actually his mother, Saul being informed about this when aged 10. His reaction to this disclosure consisted of acting out, conduct problems and aggression toward himself and others. His father was absent throughout his upbringing, and Saul had been told that his father was a paedophile who had died of a heart attack many years previously. His grandmother was alcoholic and the care afforded him was neglectful and lacking in affection or concern, Saul learning to fend for himself for survival. Saul's relationship with his 'sister' was limited (she had been 14 years old when he was born). Saul's description of his upbringing did not leave the assessor with any sense that he had forged significant nurturing relationships.

Saul was placed in statutory care when aged 11 after his grandmother's death, losing all contact with his mother, whom he had never seen since this time. He recalls that he reacted indifferently to the death of his grandmother and did not feel any grief or sadness. Within school, Saul was considered to be an unruly, ill-disciplined child who acted out in temper through destroying furniture, hitting other pupils whom he bullied and flaunting school rules with disregard for the consequences. He engaged in several instances of self-injury, cutting his wrists, attempting to hang himself and overdosing on Prozac, records suggesting that these incidents were appraised as manipulative gestures. Saul did not achieve academically and truanted frequently from school, preferring to steal cars, abuse solvents and drink alcohol, mostly with other youths, but often alone. He was described in Social Services records as a conduct-disordered 'hustler', well known for his criminal guile and manipulation of others. He was detained in Borstal and youth prisons for a variety of offences, usually being transferred to the hospital wing for medical treatment after acts of self-harm. Diagnoses of conduct disorder and antisocial personality disorder had been previously made in court reports.

Saul began setting fires when 15, mostly as a means of soothing his distress. Saul commented, 'I remember the first time I lit a fire, I was on my own, there'd been arguments in the house, I lit the fire and stared at it, it fascinated me, it made me feel warm inside my stomach, like it took away all the pain, fire became important to me, attracted me.' At these times, he did not light fires to destroy. The event which triggered his fire-setting against others occurred when he was sitting in a local public house drinking and the perpetrator of sexual abuse against him in childhood (a friend of his uncle) approached him, stating, 'I'm back to see all my boys, I'll pay this time.' Saul experienced an anxiety state and fled the public bar, recalling, 'I was dizzy, couldn't settle myself, sick in the stomach.' Two hours later, in a fit of ruminative rage, Saul set fire to refuse bins behind a hostel, standing watching for some time. He was later informed that a number of people from the hostel were ill because of smoke inhalation. A second encounter with his abuser occurred some months later. On this occasion, Saul was leaving the toilet of a public bar and the perpetrator blocked his exit from the doorway. Saul reported, 'I just flipped, lost it. I started to strangle him, got him on the floor, bit him on the face, then some people dragged me off. I would've killed him.' Saul admitted that, in the following weeks, he began to fantasise about killing the perpetrator and did seek him, before being told that he had left the local area because of threats from within the community. Saul claimed, 'I felt good. It was as if the community had stood up for me and protected me.'

The diagnosis of BPD in Saul's case was made with the Structured Interview for DSM-IV Personality, a semi-structured interview schedule (Pfohl, Blum & Zimmerman, 1997). Saul completed the PSQ and obtained a score of 33 (above the cut-off score of 28), suggesting that additional exploration of identity problems and dissociative symptoms was required. His Millon Clinical Multiaxial Inventory–III (MCMI–3) (Millon, Millon & Davis, 1994) showed elevations on the borderline, sadistic, antisocial, paranoid and dependent scales with symptoms of mood disturbance, anxiety, depression, substance misuse and post-traumatic stress. His intelligence was assessed as within the low average range with no neuropsychological impairment or dysfunction detected. Saul refused to complete projective testing. His profile on the Dissociation Questionnaire (DIS–Q) (Vanderlinden, Van Dyck, Vandereycken, Vertommen & van Verkes, 1999) showed elevations on scales measuring identity fragmentation and loss of behavioural control.

Interviews with Saul detected that he would frequently vacillate in attitudes, mood and emotional reactions. For the most part, his presenting states of mind were either angry and paranoid, despondent and self-hating, or agitated and expressing a desire to harm others through reckless, impulsive acting out. On many occasions, Saul would accuse the therapist of failing to help him, disparaging the use of therapy and blaming him for his distress and for being detained. He voiced his perceptions of others as unfairly and maliciously victimising him. His anger would typically shift to a state of desperation, despondency, and child-like vulnerability, pitying himself for the suffering existence he had endured. At these times, he would beg for help and assistance to rid him of the psychological pain he felt. Over the period of the first four sessions of assessment, Saul had engaged in many instances of self-injury on the ward, including swallowing batteries, cutting his wrists and going on 'hunger and thirst strike' to protest at his perceived mistreatment. Nursing staff reported that they considered Saul's self-harm to be manipulative and attention-seeking rather than genuine attempts to kill himself. The therapist's counter-transference responses varied from anxiety about the strength of Saul's threats to harm himself or others when angry to an urge to comfort, soothe and absorb his emotional pain and helplessness when begging for help. It was felt that these counter-transference responses were likely to be enactments of two RRPs within Saul's repertoire of relating. The therapist was also wary of Saul's tendency to manipulate care and felt that ruptures could occur in therapy.

Saul completed the Psychotherapy File and the self-states grid (Fig. 2.1). The self-states grid showed a number of definable RRPs, positions and self-states. Professionals were labelled as 'do-gooders' (RRP of *helping/giving-to-cared for/needy*) and characterised as helping, but devalued and duped. Other elements (self-states) of the grid were labelled, such as 'fire/unleashed hell' (RRPs of *destroying-to-destroyed* and *soothing-to-calmed*) and the 'victim' state, which was described as hated, worthless, weak, hurt, guilty and associated with rage. The 'lost soul' state was perceived as abandoned, anxious and agitated. 'Fire' (RRP of *destroying/calming*) represented being in control, powerful, soothing, punishing and harmful, close spatially to 'monster'. It was decided that these states should be amalgamated and the link between Saul's 'unleashed hell' and 'fire' states examined. Being in the 'zombie' state and 'drunk' were indicative of cut-off, unfeeling, unlovable states. The 'hustler' was included as a survival strategy, which Saul had developed as a means of coping with being alone, neglected and abandoned.

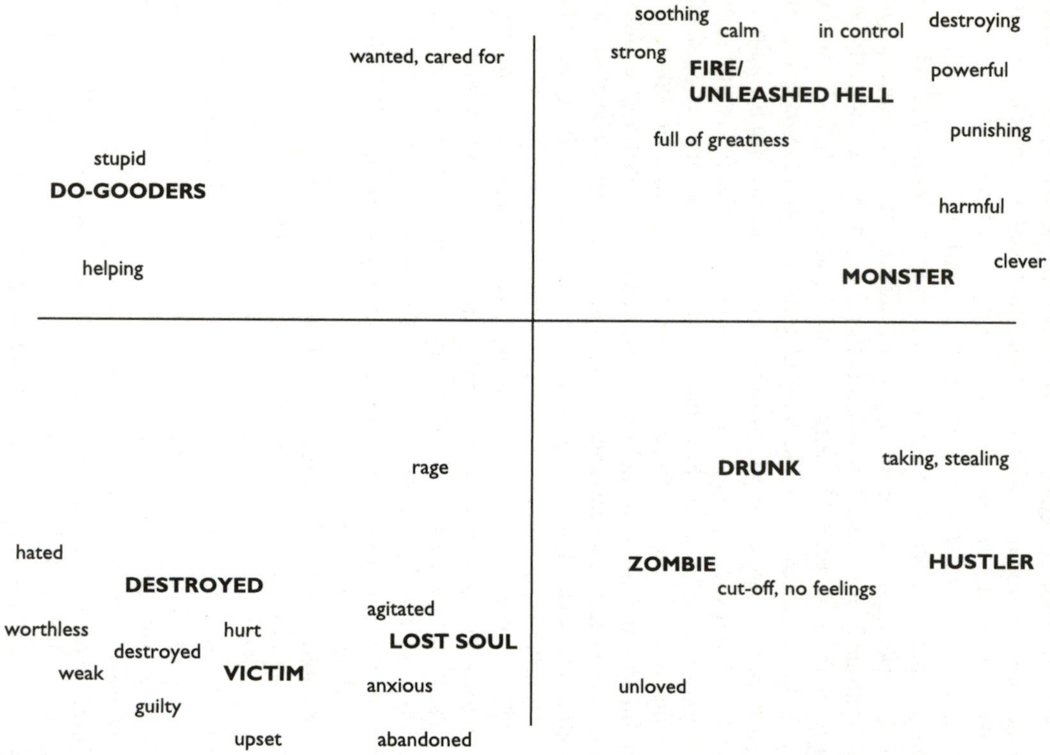

Figure 2.1 Saul's self-states grid.

The Reformulation Letter attempted to provide a narrative account of Saul's past history as follows:

Dear Saul,

As promised, I am writing this letter to put together what we have discussed so far and to help you make sense of the difficult life that has led you to this point. I also hope we can use this letter as an initial means of thinking about the reasons for the crimes and how you have come to act in such a harmful way toward yourself and others.

Growing up was a difficult time for you. You lived with your grandmother and 'sister', your sister really being your mother. You were not given this information until you were 10. It appears that you were not emotionally close to your mother or grandmother, and your grandmother's death did not cause you any particular distress. You drifted in the care system and lost touch with your mother. School was a time of getting into trouble, and you started criminal activities and drug and alcohol misuse, ending up in prison. You are aware that you were known as a 'hustler', capable of surviving on your own without anyone's help, and managing to survive through stealing and robbing from others. You consider yourself to have been a talented criminal and stated, 'If there was one life jacket on a boat of people, I'd get it.' Your life has generally been aimless and without direction, living by your wits and crimes. From an early age, setting fires became a means of soothing yourself and making you feel different inside, calming your anger and distress.

A significant incident seems to have occurred when the man who abused you (you have never told anyone about these events until recently) returned to the local community and threatened you. You attacked him in a fit of rage and recall that you became emotionally upset and irritable, with mood swings and depression. At this time, you began to set fires to destroy rather than to soothe yourself, feeling that setting fires gave you a sense of power and allowed you to express destructive feelings as well as calming you inside. Setting fires has become habitual in your life. I think it would be helpful to explore what fire means to you and the connection between your views of yourself, others, the world and setting fires.

It seems as if your feelings about yourself are difficult to understand and make sense of, causing you confusion and stress. You state that your feelings change quickly and without any pattern, resulting sometimes in harming yourself severely because of your dislike for yourself. At times you have harmed yourself, and at other times felt like harming other people. Who you feel you are is not consistent or stable for you. At other times, you have felt depressed without understanding the reasons for these changes within yourself. When very distressed, you will seek refuge in alcohol or drugs, or 'shut down' when you don't feel anything.

I have observed that you seem to believe that no one will give you care (as if you are not worthy of it); sometimes, you beg for help, because of the emotional pain you feel. On other occasions, you have accused staff and me of mistreating you and victimising you for no reason. We must be aware of these patterns within the therapy relationship.

I suggest that we discuss working together to address the following areas:

- *the thoughts, feelings and decisions which lead to setting fire behaviours; the 'fire/unleashed hell' you have labelled, its destruction and effects on victims*
- *helping you understand and stabilise how you feel within and about yourself; making sense of your own experiences and permitting you to feel more predictable inside*
- *helping you understand the reasons for the self-hatred you feel and find ways of dealing with your self-injury (being a 'monster' to yourself and victimising yourself)*
- *helping you obtain care from others and feel that you are worthy of care and do not need manipulation to get it (without using self-harm to get care, then rejecting it as 'not good enough'; coping with being independent and meeting your own needs without crimes)*
- *helping you resolve your anger, depression and the ways you deal with it through alcohol, drugs and 'shutting down'*
- *helping you learn to consider living a different, purposeful and more productive life rather than pursuing criminal activities and being a 'hustler'.*

We can discuss and alter any of these suggested problems, and I hope we can work jointly to understand these confusing experiences, ways of relating to others and acting in the world.

Best wishes

Saul's SSSD is shown in Fig. 2.2. Saul's self-harm was construed as an expression of the internalisation of this *self–other* RRP of SS2 enacted against himself (*neglecting/cruel* RRP position C to *harmed/neglected* of D). Saul was able to discuss the psychological pain he associated with the 'victim' state and how certain patterns emerged from this state. Firstly, Saul reported an angry, destructive, raging state of mind that prompted him to want to act out impulsively and recklessly against others ('victim' rage of SS2). It was clear that the majority of Saul's destructive crimes were linked to this state and its attitudes, feelings and behaviours. The placement of 'fire' as an element within the self-states grid close to 'unleashed hell' indicated that setting fires was a potent, symbolically important method of expressing destructive feelings for Saul, and was related to his emotional control and regulation of his internal states. 'Fire' was depicted as a multifunctional and powerful ally for Saul that he used to enact a 'destroying' procedure toward others (SS1),

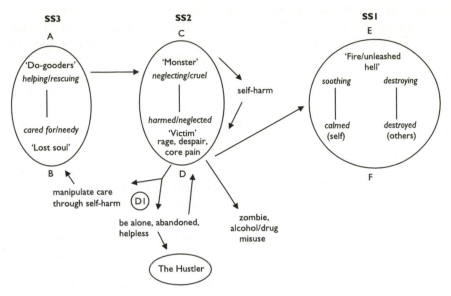

Figure 2.2 Saul's self-states sequential diagram (SSSD).

expressing his rage, but also inducing feelings of being soothed emotionally and enveloped.

The *offender–victim* state (the 'fire/unleashed hell' state of SS1) was conceptualised as a means of transforming his psychological pain, expressing his destructive impulses and altering his painful feelings. Saul could not articulate in any way the impact of arson upon others, as victims, concentrating solely upon the internal regulation this act provided for him. Early on in his development, arson had provided Saul with a powerful means of self-management of internal states. This 'fire/unleashed hell' state represented the *dominant offence position* implicated in Saul's destructive crimes, and he could voice his intentions and motivations as 'I'm going to hurt you like I hurt'. The dialogical sequence analysis of Saul's case could be traced from the 'victim' position (D, SS2) to the 'fire/unleashed hell' self-state as his destructive rage incubated. The 'fire/unleashed hell' position (E, SS1) represented the height of his risk potential and the location of peak dangerousness for Saul.

At other times, Saul reported feelings of despondency, depression and hopelessness, which he could manage only through self-injury. It was apparent that Saul had often used self-injury to express his self-hatred (a *self–self* enactment of RRPs within SS2) but also as a vehicle to elicit sympathy, care, and coerced affection and attention. He labelled this position and self-state the 'wee lost soul' (B, SS3), associated with displaying vulnerable, childish and pitiable distress. When in this state, he mentioned thinking 'please help me' followed by 'you fools', referring to professionals. This is indicative of a shift from 'victim' of SS2 to 'lost soul' of SS3, as he used self-harm to manipulate care. Professionals were portrayed as 'do-gooders' (A, SS3) who, stupidly from Saul's perspective, tried to rescue him, but were denied by either his withdrawal from help or his sabotage of their efforts (a snag). This vacillation between SS3 and SS2 occurred rapidly and confused both Saul and the therapist initially until reformulation was completed. The potential influence of these patterns on the therapeutic relationship was noted. Stagnation or rupture of the therapeutic alliance was anticipated, and the therapist observed his presentation to avoid being drawn into patterns of collusion with Saul's style of relating.

Saul completed the SDP, which verified that he experienced abrupt and marked shifts in terms of his self-experience, mostly from victim rage (harmed/neglected of 'victim', causing a risk of impulsive acting out against others to abusing/neglectful of the 'monster' and self-harm) through to dependent/manipulating care to a dissociated, zombie state, in which he reported a withdrawal from human contact and 'not thinking or feeling' (this represents a *procedural loop*; see Chapter 1). Alcohol and drug misuse occurred frequently as coping reactions. Through the SDP, he explained that the victim/abused state was experienced frequently, was of long duration, caused him to feel angry and despairing, emerged abruptly in response to someone's statements and ended gradually. A role reversal was apparent in that he would perceive himself as victimised, and this then led to enactment of the 'fire/unleashed hell' RRP of *destroying* toward others. A significant *state switch* occurred from SS2 'victim' state to SS1 'fire/unleashed hell' state, representative of his position of peak *risk potential*. For Saul, to be alone elicited feelings of dread and desperation, yet he found relationships with others to be either clinging and insecure in relation to a strong provider and protector or risking harm through abuse or neglect (the dilemma of relating, D1).

From the PSQ, self-states grid, SDP and the Reformulation Letter and Self-States Sequential Diagram (SSSD), it is apparent that Saul's personality suggests identity disturbance, borderline personality features and deficits at all three levels of the MSSM in terms of the restricted, narrow repertoire of RRPs, dissociation and fragmentation, with many shifts and switches and a lack of self-reflective capacity.

Saul's response to the reformulation was, initially, ambivalent and indifferent. Efforts were made to facilitate Saul's consideration of the various states identified and the location of his risk potential. With perseverance, Saul's engagement improved and a target problem (TP) list and target problem procedures (TPPs) were constructed jointly with him. These TPs included the following:

(1) Developing awareness of the link between his arson behaviours, his internal states and the nature of the RRPs and positions underlying these actions. Saul was helped to contemplate the significance of his victim

rage, the *destroyer-to-destroyed* RRP and the perceptions he held about fire *(identifying RRPs, positions, self-states and the dialogical sequences).* The aim was to resolve Saul's victim rage and to promote adaptive methods of self-soothing and emotional control.

(2) To help Saul understand the enactment of the cruel, harming RRPs of SS2 expressed through self-harm and self-neglect, and to improve his sense of self as worthy.

(3) To analyse Saul's patterns of relating (the dilemma, D1) through either manipulating care and requesting rescue, and then rejection of help and sabotage or clinging dependency/anxious to a strong protector who abuses.

(4) To examine the association between Saul's feelings of depression and anger and his coping strategies of bingeing on substances or transition into a dissociated, zombie state.

(5) To help Saul construct an appreciation of the destroyed reciprocal role of the victim and its destructive potential when recklessly and impulsively acting out. Saul's empathic concern for his victims was absent and clouded by his egocentric viewpoint.

(6) Improvement in his sense of self to combat the likelihood of a return to a chaotic, aimless, disorganised and neglectful lifestyle (e.g. the 'hustler' survival strategy).

CAT for Saul proved to be a testing endeavour. He was offered 24 sessions of individual CAT, but his attendance was sporadic and time was spent trying to focus Saul's attention on target problems. During this initial phase of therapy, he demonstrated turbulent, acting-out behaviour on the ward such as drug-taking, conflicted relationships with staff and patients alike, and withdrawal from all programmes for periods of time because of 'stress' and becoming paranoid and angry.

The SSSD, list of target problems and underlying TPPs were presented to the multidisciplinary team that nursed Saul, who consented to this information being openly exchanged, and he expressed his hope that the nursing staff would better understand his behaviours and motivations (a reflection of his 'lost soul' state). The sharing of diagrammatic reformulations has been discussed by others and the advantages for devising care plans considered (Kerr, 2001), permitting a contextualised reformulation for all staff. It was clear from the discussion with nurses on the unit's ward that Saul had become a frustrating and challenging patient for them, many expressing their annoyance about his manipulation and the provocative escalations in his self-injuring. The RRPs which underpinned these counter-transference reactions were identified, and the shifts and vacillations in Saul's own subjective experiences were traced with the SSSD. It was decided by professionals that the SSSD would be used to construct a plan of action for responding to Saul's self-injury. It was accepted that this behaviour served differing functions at different times; for example, it was an expression of self-hatred (self-to-self enactment of the *neglecting/cruel-to-harmed/neglected* RRP) and a method of manipulation of care, which he later complained bitterly about (Saul's inducement of staff into a *helping/rescuing* RRP). It was apparent that the staff had very contradictory impressions of Saul, some labelling him a 'manipulative psychopath' prone to reckless, angry and malicious acting out, and others perceiving him as a person who deserved all of their effort and sympathy. These perceptions were located on the SSSD as indicative of Saul's vacillation and shifts between self-states. The deliberations between professionals applying the SSSD as a graphic depiction of Saul's personality allowed attuned and responsive nursing and more sensitive management of his conduct on the ward. This contextual use of the diagram was to promote consistent, helpful and non-collusive patterns of relationship between staff groups and Saul.

Within individual therapy, similar patterns of transference and counter-transference were observed, particularly Saul's rageful accusations against the therapist of mistreatment, Saul alleging, 'Why do I have to do this? All you are interested in is making me worse.' The therapist was perceived as abusing and insensitive to Saul's psychological pain, victimising him (an enactment of the RRPs of SS2). On other occasions, Saul would present as inconsolable, crying and pleading for help and 'somebody or something to take this hurt away'. The therapist's counter-transference responses ranged from frustration at Saul's lack of focus and inability to sustain his attention to therapy tasks without shifting states, to a desire to reach and absorb his piteous and wretched psychological state and distress. The therapist felt the 'pull' to help Saul, yet remained cautious of his rejection of this care and devaluing of help as 'not good enough'. Saul demonstrated significant problems in identifying his own and others' state of mind and ascribing motivations and feelings to other people. His narratives of past events were disjointed and splintered, becoming confused and entangled as Saul's distress overwhelmed him. Supervision was vital for the therapist throughout contact with Saul, considering the demanding presentation and complexity of his fragmented identity. The potential ruptures and stagnations within the alliance, which were predicted by the SSSD, became evident at differing junctures.

A decision was made at the earliest stages of CAT actively to name and acknowledge Saul's tendency to act destructively toward himself and others and to identify the 'therapeutic snag' (Pollock, 2001b) whereby the patient feels that s/he does not deserve to rid him/herself of the psychological pain and distress, and sabotages any progress made. The therapeutic snag can be an obstruction to progress which frustrates the clinician's efforts and hinders the patient from sustaining any gains in therapy which are seen as beneficial, the patient destroying and undermining positive achievements. Saul was helped to identify this snag and agreed to monitor its emergence. Saul felt that he did not deserve 'good things' such as progress and improvement, a reflection of his neglecting RRP toward himself (SS2).

The focus on this self-defeating pattern led to further exploration of the position and 'voice' which caused Saul to feel depression and rage. He acknowledged that his depression and self-hatred were associated with the 'victim' state and its RRP, and he was encouraged to think about the perceptions, feelings and view of others which were related to this state. Saul declared that he viewed himself as 'cornered, like a cat that's been chased and is now in a corner. I'm beaten but gonna scratch, fight back, but I feel helpless to do anything, so I just let it simmer. I think, "My time will come, you're gonna get your come-uppance, I want to kill." I hate everybody when I'm like that.' Bingeing on substances was an emotional survival strategy to avoid thinking and feeling. The zombie state tended to occur as a secondary reaction when alcohol and drugs had failed to function for Saul, and it indicated a dissociative, switched off, emotionally shut-down withdrawal from reality.

Saul's self-hatred was a prominent feature of his presentation and, when this was discussed with him, he could reflect that he would manipulate care from others through self-injury because he felt that this represented the only means of guaranteeing attention and care, of which he had been deprived in the past by abusive and neglectful carers (the TP regarding care-seeking). This care-seeking dilemma was observed as a self-perpetuating procedure which did not achieve its goal (D1) because it alienated others, who felt manipulated, and prevented them from providing proper care. These actions gave Saul a momentary sense of glee rather than forging caring relationships. With nursing staff, Saul jointly constructed a plan of action to encourage him to request care and attention appropriately from staff (an hourly session with his key worker) when he felt it necessary, which would be given only on the condition that he did not engage in any form of drug misuse or self-injury. Despite Saul's minimal expectations of the nursing staff's ability to provide attention and care, this strategy was successful and reduced the frequency of self-injury (TP regarding self-injuring).

The *offence-to-victim* RRPs and Saul's arson were given significant focus within CAT sessions. It became apparent that Saul's unresolved rage and the destructive potential he felt were critical targets for therapy. The link between the powerless, 'cornered' and abused RRP, the position of weakness and defilement ('victim' state), and his anger were connected to his fascination with and relationship to fire and arson. Developmentally, fire had become multifunctional for Saul as a powerful means of expressing his rage and destroying others (or objects symbolic of hate and targets for his anger such as the Social Services buildings, etc.), and as a comforting, soothing transitional function which shored up his identity and absolved his feelings. Saul had labelled this self-state as 'fire/unleashed hell', and the elements of this state of mind were explored at length. He was enrolled in art therapy classes, which he felt provided a different mode of expression, Saul concentrating on defining what fire meant to him and its significance for him. It became obvious that Saul's rage and anger were of an extreme intensity and that he often ruminated about past events and fantasised about 'causing the biggest fire ever seen – it would be swirling, like a blazing angel, eating up everything, purifying all the Earth, like something out of the Bible'. These fantasies were recognised as the springboards for offence planning. Saul was encouraged to think about the positive functions and attributes of fire and how he wished in fantasy to attain a sense of self which was comparable to fire, yet less destructive. He was helped to learn new methods of alleviating his angry arousal, comforting himself without resorting to binges on alcohol or drug misuse, and to develop a new, adaptive RRP which he could employ in self-to-self nurturing, with an acceptance that such actions were tolerable. The *destroying-to-destroyed* RRP of SS1 was explicitly identified as his 'most risky' state of mind, and Saul learned to manage the perceptions, feelings and responses to the raging, painful 'victim' state to prevent shifting to SS1 and committing an offence.

Initially, Saul's victim empathy was very poor; he could not articulate any thoughts about the victim's position or plight, and empathic concern was absent. His thinking was egocentric and self-absorbed. When the SSSD was jointly constructed, a question mark was placed for the victim RRP (SS1, *destroyed*), and, despite lengthy exploration, Saul could not offer any coherent thoughts about the victims' likely experiences. The reciprocal nature of abusing experiences was used as a way of helping Saul contemplate how his actions had affected others. Pollock (2001b) highlights how the victim internalises the perpetrator-to-victim RRPs and can configure his way of dealing with abuse through identification with the perpetrator RRP because it is a potent, powerful and forceful position compared with the weak, disabled and helpless victim RRP. Saul was invited to undertake an internal dialogue between his 'victim' state and that of the perpetrator (the 'monster'), and to compare this experience with his fire-setting 'fire/unleashed hell' state and the probable experiences of the victims he created. This exercise allowed Saul to distinguish the similarities and differences between these states and increase his awareness of the attributes of the victim roles. Saul found this task difficult, yet did show evidence of an improved appreciation that his victim rage led to victimisation of others through his reckless and destructive identification with an avenging, perpetrator role. It was considered that Saul did develop a degree of victim empathy and concern for those he had harmed, borne out by his comment that 'hurting other people doesn't work, it just keeps it all going, the suffering'.

The function of the SSSD was vital as a containing and holding tool for Saul. The shifts and vacillations which suggested that Saul's identity disturbance was problematic could be attributed to deficits at all levels but particularly level 3 of the MSSM, in that he had, through his adverse childhood experiences and parenting from others, failed to develop metacognitive abilities to self-reflect and think about his own subjective experiences and states of mind. Saul's disparate and contradictory states of mind, his switching of positions within self-states RRPs, caused confusion and distress for him. The SSSD was repeatedly referenced as a tool for making sense of these experiences. The therapist asked Saul to think about how the therapist felt and thought about Saul's mental states, encouraging an empathic identification and internalisation of the therapist as a new, attuned, constant, consistent and mirroring RRP. Saul did state that he would engage in internal, imaginary dialogue with the therapist during times of stress, although this disclosure occurred after therapy. Furthermore, Saul was helped to recognise the cyclical, self-perpetuating patterns of procedures that failed to become revised and ensured his misery and distress. It is not uncommon that patients will 'go around the same cycles' until recognition and revision are achieved. After repeated reference to the SSSD, Saul was able to notice that patterns were recurring, that he was sequentially moving through harmful procedures, and that dilemmas and traps were occurring. Exits were established through a variety of methods for Saul only after he was able to note the presence of these procedures. His ratings on the Target Problem Rating Sheet indicated improved recognition of the majority of TPs after 16 sessions.

Saul's history suggested that he had failed to develop a coherent identity with defined aims and goals or a directed lifestyle. His chaotic, neglectful background and his lack of guidance and identification with any positive figures rendered him unable to structure his lifestyle, so that he had resorted to living as a vagrant and misusing substances, surviving through acts of theft and robbery. This was presented to Saul as a self-to-self management enactment of the *neglecting/cruel-to-neglected/harmed* RRP and its associated coping strategies. The 'hustler' survival strategy was established as the only feasible way of coping with the adversity he had endured. He had also learned to dislike himself and express his hatred through self-injury. Saul reported that he experienced a pessimistic, depressed and hopeless state of mind, believing that the only care available, if any at all, had to be coerced from others or met through his own resources. Saul felt that reliance upon others was a dangerous option that would only lead to abuse, and he remained vigilant and detached from relationships. A part of therapy focused upon helping Saul develop positive perceptions of himself and take time to devise an 'inner gyroscope' of actions for his self-development (TP regarding self-development and lifestyle). Gravitation to a criminal lifestyle had been this offender's only salvation of identity, offering a sense of direction (as 'the hustler'), acceptance of and affiliation with other criminals, and a sense of purpose. Saul completed careers counselling and entered educational work for employment as a chef within the prison, successfully pursuing this career after release. Saul did show a capacity to work in partnership with professionals within the prison, and his reluctance and anxieties about attachment to others were explored and acknowledged as an additional, understandable and rational coping strategy that he had used to manage his circumstances when younger.

In terms of risk prediction, Saul's *dominant offence position* and the location of his most potent state were identified in the SSSD as position E of SS1, termed 'fire/unleashed hell'. In *dialogical sequence analysis* terms, Saul's potential to harm and commit an offence could be traced through the identified self-states from position B ('lost soul') to feeling victimised (position D, 'victim'), and then to position E (SS1, 'fire/unleashed hell'). The sequential patterns of procedures and conditions which led to this position could be traced, and triggering situations and external circumstances noted. Saul was informed about the link between his ruminative anger when experiencing the victim state and his fantasies of destroying others through setting fires. His fantasising inflated his risk potential greatly, and he was taught techniques to prevent these fantasies from overriding his reasoning. A relapse prevention plan was devised, based on the SSSD and the cycles of states and procedures identified, to facilitate Saul's maintenance of changes made and prevent re-offending. The relevance of 'the hustler' survival strategy was apparent when forecasting any return to criminal activities.

Progress and outcome

At the completion of CAT, this offender had rated progress on all of the TPs considered. Post-therapy psychometric testing indicated a decline in PSQ scores to 21 (within normal range), a decrease in dissociation (less identity fragmentation, improved behavioural control scales and fewer recordings of the 'zombie' state) and no incidents of self-injury. A repeated SDP revealed that his subjective experiences were less unpredictable and intensely felt, with fewer rapid shifts between states. The aim of CAT with BPD is to enhance the development of certain capacities that did not develop, such as self-reflection; to improve the patient's sense of integration; and to decrease dissociation, impulsivity, anxiety and depressive symptoms. Targeting interpersonal relationships and achieving insight and control over self-damaging procedures can be witnessed through CAT as emotional stability is acquired. These types of changes were achieved with Saul, who presented unique challenges within a difficult therapy.

Termination of therapy was anticipated to be difficult for Saul, given the investment he had made in addressing these problems and the strength of the working alliance that had been forged. Saul did voice a sense of disappointment that therapy could not continue, even intermittently for support. The therapist's concern about the ending was that Saul might sabotage progress to avoid the loss of a positively internalised RRP with the therapist that had been developed throughout contact. The Goodbye Letter for Saul was as follows:

Dear Saul,

We are approaching the final three sessions of our agreed work in therapy. I am writing this letter to help both of us think about what the ending of therapy might mean for you and help us handle your feelings without you suffering a setback. It is important that we understand that therapy will end and that you have made positive progress in many ways and achieved a great deal.

Firstly, you have entered a relationship with a professional, a relationship which you have used properly and constructively. I have formed great respect for your attempts to overcome a challenging background, and you have worked hard to correct the difficulties and problems that had developed from this past. You are clearer in your own mind about the reasons for your setting fires and other destructive behaviours, better able to think about and understand that you have, in the past, caused harm to others, as others have hurt you. This cycle cannot continue, and I feel that you have taken ownership of this task, working to end your criminal career. I think you understand why you set fires, the meaning of fire for you, how it made you feel, and the impact it has had on your life and that of other people.

Secondly, I feel that you have developed a better idea about who you feel you are; your moods, feelings about yourself and control of your behaviours are more stable and generally positive, as you have learned to think for yourself and act in your best interests. You do not feel the need to injure yourself and have discarded the idea that because other people have made you feel bad about yourself, you need to follow those rules and hate yourself.

There is further work to be done. In particular, I must emphasise to you that the danger you have posed to others lies within you, and you are aware of the states of mind when this is likely to occur and appear. It is your job to watch and be aware of yourself, to notice when these states of mind are emerging and to act to control them before an offence does occur. I recommend that you refer to the diagram we made when you feel that your reactions and situations are becoming difficult for you.

Saul responded positively to the letter and discussed his goals for the future without sabotaging the gains made or trying to induce the therapist to extend the work. It was judged that CAT had achieved as much progress as could be made while Saul was imprisoned. Saul was released from prison and has gone 2 years without committing a crime. Supervising professionals in the community report that he is in full-time employment and has established a productive lifestyle without reversion to target problems as addressed in therapy. He consumes alcohol, but not at a problematic level.

Commentary

It is not easy to convey accurately the intricacies of therapy, and this case is simply illustrative of the CAT language, model, methods, tools and processes involved. CAT terminology is rarely used explicitly with the patient, but information and concepts are translated into accessible and appropriate language. A diagram, piece of art work or even songs and music can be substituted for the core language used in CAT if they provide a user-friendly lexicon to prompt change for the patient (Pollock, 2001b). The confusing subjective experiences and lack of self-reflection apparent with the BPD patient require the containing function of reformulation with enough structure and agreement about target problems and goals within a flexible therapeutic space to allow the exploration and the playing with thinking and feeling that are often so lacking in the early care of these people during their development.

References

American Psychiatric Association (APA) (1994). *Diagnostic and statistical manual of mental disorders* (4th edn) (DSM-IV). Washington, DC: APA.

Bateman, A. & Fonagy, P. (2004). *Psychotherapy for borderline personality disorder: Mentalization-based treatment*. Oxford: Oxford University Press.

Bennett, D., Pollock, P. H. & Ryle, A. (2004). The states description procedure: The use of guided self-reflection in the case formulation of patients with borderline personality disorder. *Clinical Psychology and Psychotherapy*, *12*, 50–57.

Dimaggio, G., Salvatore, G., Azzara, C., Catania, D., Semerari, A. & Hermans, H. J. M. (2004). Dialogical relationships in impoverished narratives: From theory to clinical practice. *Psychology and Psychotherapy*, *76*, 385–410.

Dunn, M. (1994). Variations in cognitive analytic therapy technique in the treatment of a severely disturbed patient. *International Journal of Short-Term Psychotherapy*, *9*, 1151–1160.

Golynkina, K. & Ryle, A. (1999). The identification and characteristics of the partially dissociated states of patients with borderline personality disorder. *British Journal of Medical Psychology*, *72*, 429–445.

Holmes, J. (1998). Defensive and creative uses of narrative in psychotherapy: An attachment perspective. In G. Roberts & J. Holmes (Eds), *Healing stories: Narrative in psychiatry and psychotherapy* (pp. 49–68). Oxford: Oxford University Press.

Johnson, J. G., Cohen, P., Brown, J., Smailes, E. B. & Bernstein, D. P. (1999). Childhood maltreatment increases risk for personality disorders during early adulthood. *Archives of General Psychiatry*, *56*, 600–605.

Judd, P. H. & McGlashan, T. H. (2003). *A developmental model of borderline personality disorder: Understanding variations in course and outcome*. Washington, DC: American Psychiatric Press.

Kernberg, O. F. (1967). Borderline personality organisation. *Journal of the American Psychoanalytic Association*, *15*, 641–685.

Kernberg, O. F., Clarkin, J. F. & Yeomans, F. E. (2002). *A primer of transference-focused psychotherapy for the borderline patient*. New York: Aronson.

Kerr, I. (1999). Cognitive analytic therapy for borderline personality disorder in the context of a community mental health team: Individual and organisational psychodynamic implications. *British Journal of Psychotherapy*, *15*, 425–438.

Linehan, M. M. (1993). *Cognitive behavioural treatment for borderline personality disorder*. New York: Guilford.

Marlowe, M. & Ryle, A. (1995). Cognitive analytic therapy of borderline personality disorder: Theory and practice and clinical and research uses of the self states sequential diagram. *International Journal of Short-Term Psychotherapy, 10*, 21–34.

Meloy, J. R. (1989). Unrequited love and the wish to kill. Diagnosis and treatment of borderline erotomania. *Bulletin of the Menninger Clinic, 53*, 477–492.

Millon, T., Millon, C. & Davis, R. D. (1994). *Millon Clinical Multiaxial Inventory–III*. Minneapolis, MN: National Computer Systems.

Pfohl, B., Blum, N. & Zimmerman, M. (1997). *Structured interview for DSM-IV personality*. Washington, DC: American Psychiatric Press.

Pollock, P. H. (1996). Clinical issues in the cognitive analytic therapy of sexually abused women who commit violence offences against their partners. *British Journal of Medical Psychology, 69*, 117–127.

Pollock, P. H. (1997). CAT for an offender with borderline personality disorder. In A. Ryle (Ed.), *Cognitive analytic therapy and borderline personality disorder: The model and the method*. Chichester: Wiley.

Pollock, P. H. & Belshaw, T. D. (1998). Cognitive analytic therapy for offenders. *Journal of Forensic Psychiatry, 9*, 629–642.

Pollock, P. H. (2001a). Cognitive analytic therapy for borderline erotomania: Forensic romances and violence in the therapy room. *Clinical Psychology and Psychotherapy, 8*, 214–229.

Pollock, P. H. (2001b). *Cognitive analytic therapy for adult survivors of childhood abuse: Treatment approaches and case management*. Chichester: Wiley.

Pollock, P. H., Broadbent, M., Clarke, S., Dorrian, A. & Ryle, A. (2001). The Personality Structure Questionnaire (PSQ): A measure of the multiple self states model of identity disturbance in cognitive analytic therapy. *Clinical Psychology and Psychotherapy, 8*, 59–72.

Pollock, P. H. (2003). Cognitive analytic therapy for adult survivors of childhood abuse: Changes to identity disturbance and outcome. (unpublished).

Ryle, A. & Beard, H. (1993). The integrative effect of reformulation: Cognitive analytic therapy with a patient with borderline personality disorder. *British Journal of Medical Psychology, 66*, 249–258.

Ryle, A. (1997a). *Cognitive analytic therapy and borderline personality disorder: The model and the method*. Chichester: Wiley.

Ryle, A. (1997b). The structure and development of borderline personality disorder: A proposed model. *British Journal of Psychiatry, 170*, 82–87.

Ryle, A. & Golynkina, K. (2000). Effectiveness of time-limited cognitive analytic therapy for borderline personality disorder: Factors associated with outcome. *British Journal of Medical Psychology, 73*, 197–210.

Vanderlinden, J., Van Dyck, R., Vandereycken, W., Vertommen, H. & van Verkes, R. (1993). The Dissociation Questionnaire (DIS-Q): Development and characteristics of a new self-report scale. *Clinical Psychology and Psychotherapy, 1*, 21–27.

Wildgoose, A., Clarke, S. & Waller, G. (2001). Treating personality fragmentation in borderline personality disorder: A pilot study of the impact of cognitive analytic therapy. *British Journal of Medical Psychology, 74*, 47–55.

Young, J. E., Klosko, J. S. & Weishaar, M. E. (2003). *Schema therapy: A practitioner's guide*. New York: Guilford.

Chapter 3

States and reciprocal roles in the wider understanding of forensic mental health

Mark Stowell-Smith

This chapter seeks to illustrate how some of the conceptual innovations from CAT can be linked to the wider context of forensic mental health care. Firstly, I describe how forms of reciprocal roles are embedded in our thinking about forensic mental health issues. I enlarge on the notion of the reciprocal role by taking it from the level of the micro (the internal world of the individual) to that of the macro (that of the individual in the context of wider social organisation). I argue that at this macro-level, implicit reciprocal roles, that is, versions of self and the other, can be conceptualised as a series of binary oppositions constituting a conceptual space that either opens up or delimits particular therapeutic actions or discourses, and that awareness of this conceptual space is important, as it has practical consequences for those populating such systems. Secondly, I adapt the self-states model of psychological organisation to an examination of a forensic institution, the high-secure hospital. The high-secure hospital can be likened to a type of container or repository into which society deposits the dangerously disturbed. At one level, this seems a legitimate function for the high-secure hospital; however, at another level, the pressure to contain and segregate this group splits the hospital off from a society that is increasingly risk-obsessed and that often has unrealistic expectations of the management or elimination of those risks. I consider this as the background to a contextual reformulation of the high-secure hospital that I depict as a system of interconnected states within which individuals can easily become mired.

Reciprocal roles in the theory of CAT

Reciprocal role procedures (RRPs) are described by Ryle (1990) as an internalised model of self-other organisation that evolves in relation to early caregivers. Out of early experience, the individual develops a capacity to predict and adapt to the acts of the other These experiences are acquired from early family interactions and from the wider culture in which the person grows up. The capacity to predict the other's behaviour in this way becomes integrated into what might be considered an enduring psychological structure, template or procedure. Hence, the child who grows up in an abusive family environment internalises a view of himself or herself as an abused victim and of the other as an attacking abuser.

Ryle suggests that RRPs provide one of the cornerstones of the self, organising an array of procedures for both intra- and interpersonal management. This brief account of RRPs suggests that they become integrated into the psyche through a process of internalisation. That is to say, while they are psychological structures that end up as part of the individual's 'inner world', they are incorporated into that 'inner world' from external reality. Having been incorporated in this way, they operate outside consciousness, pervading the sense that individuals make both of themselves and of their relationship to others.

Further understanding of how this process of internalisation operates is supported by the work of the theorist Mikhail Bakhtin (Holquist, 1995). Bakhtin's theory has become increasingly influential in CAT and illustrates how psychic structures are realised in the external reality of language and culture. His ideas also help us to understand the developmental process by which we become both the objects and subjects of language. Bakhtin argues that it is through the external relationship with language that the subject's internal world is created, a view expressed by Volishinov in the following terms:

> The subjective psyche is to be localized somewhere between the organism and the outside world, on the borderline . . . but the encounter is not a physical one; the organism and the outside world meet here in the sign. Psychic experience is the semiotic expression of the contact between the outside world and the organism.
>
> (Volishinov; quoted in Ryle, 1997)

Psychic experience takes shape at the interface between the sign and the organism: mental experience requires a living, sentient organism, but the nature and form of that experience is influenced by those signs which are culturally available to that organism. For example, how we think and reflect upon and experience ourselves is partly determined by what categories or narratives are available to us both in culture and within the more specific parameters of our lives. The necessary role of language and external narrative in this process gives rise to a process of 'decentring' in which the self becomes an object for reflection both for the self and for others only through being located in the language of the other (the term 'other' is used here to represent culture and society as well as an individual 'other'). Sampson (1993) describes this as a biphasic process in which the self first exists as a prereflective 'I' and then a 'me'. The prereflective phase of the 'I' is one in which we exist in a state of unmediated unity and are not self-consciously aware of our acts. However, in order to become consciously aware of our acts, we must find a way of reflecting upon ourselves as an object, as a type of second person – a 'me'. Language is the means by which we are able to achieve this, so that 'I' develop a descriptive vocabulary through which I can think and talk about 'me'. It is at this point, however, that we become fixed in the already existing categories of language. Holquist (1995; p. 28) restates this idea in the following terms:

> In order to see ourselves, we must appropriate the visions of others . . . the Bakhtinian just-so-story of subjectivity is the tale of how I get myself from others: it is only the others' categories that will let me be an object for my own perceptions . . . In order to forge a self, I must do so from *outside*. In other words, *I author myself*.

Bakhtinian theory, therefore, helps us to think about the way in which categories of self and the other take shape and are inseparable from the categories and narratives available within wider culture. These categories or 'visions of others' influence in a pervasive, but often unseen way how we understand both ourselves and others. An important premise in this account is that it is important to make these categories visible, as CAT is both a theory and therapy about the self, and obviating the roles within which the self has become ensnared is a precondition of attempting to effect change.

Visions of self and the other in the conceptual landscape of the criminolegal complex

What visions of self and the other might we find in the field of forensic mental health? Welldon (1993) states that the practice of forensic psychotherapy involves three interested parties: the therapist, the patient and the criminal justice system. A fourth, equally influential party is represented by societal attitudes and beliefs about, for example, both the victim and the offender. Young (1996) suggests that we can visualise this matrix of societal beliefs as a type of network constituting a 'criminolegal complex'. This complex compels us to see crime, the offender and the criminal act as a series of binary oppositions. Examples of these binary pairs include guilty/innocent, victim/perpetrator and rational/irrational. I will argue here that these forms of opposition are roughly analogous to the notion of the RRP inasmuch as they mark out a psychological space for both self and the other. I will also suggest that some of these oppositions combine with a range of social stereotypes to create influential, highly polarized, self–other locations.

Welldon (1993) provides a number of examples of how this process of binary categorisation occurs, noting how one category is always kept logically distinct from the other. For example, there are offenders and there are victims. Society views the former as being the product of 'evil forces', whereas the latter are treated sympathetically and their treatment is encouraged. Conceptual confusion arises, however, when the victim expresses negative, hostile attitudes toward the perpetrator, as this does not fit in with the sentimental manner in which victims are viewed. Hence, expression of such feelings is discouraged, often leading to a desire for revenge. Welldon makes further observations as to how these oppositions are intertwined with gender stereotypes. For example, men are cast as perpetrators and women as victims. Whereas there are ready-made categories for the victimising man, confusion arises when we are confronted with the female offender. According to Welldon, this confusion becomes particularly intense in the case of the female sexual offender ('Nobody wants to hear about her predicament, and nobody takes her too seriously' (1993; p. 488)), as the idealisation of motherhood in our culture means that there is no space to form an adequate understanding of deviant female sexual behaviour (Welldon, 1998).

Even harder to place within the victim–perpetrator opposition are the families of perpetrators. Do they, too, suffer adverse consequences as a result of the perpetrator's actions, and are they therefore also to be regarded as victims, or should they be considered as contributors to the offender's psychopathology, and therefore be considered an influence upon the perpetration of the criminal act? The conceptual unease that surrounds the categorisation of these conflicts means that such families, too, find it difficult to have a voice or to gain adequate understanding of their needs (Shannon, 1999).

Within the context of the legal system, the binary pair 'rational–irrational' and the associated couplet 'responsible–not-responsible' both have a long ancestry (Forshaw & Rollin, 1990). Within the context of contemporary forensic mental health, they have been given added impetus by the 'cognitive revolution' that has gained momentum within the forensic world throughout the 1990s. In practice, this revolution has led to the large-scale adoption of offender-focused treatments based upon cognitive-behavioural methods (e.g. Ross & Fabiano, 1981; Maguire & Priestley, 1985). Kendal (2004) suggests that such approaches be premised upon the idea that criminogenic cognitions are influenced by a variety of environmental factors (e.g. stress, abuse, peer influences) that, in turn, distort or impair thinking processes or skills. However, as cognitions are learnt, rather than innate, there is the possibility of repair through techniques such as cognitive restructuring and cognitive skills training. Such approaches equip offenders with the skills required to make responsible, evaluative choices about future actions. Kendal sees the adoption of cognitive-behavioural therapy in the treatment of the offender as a form of paradigm shift sustained not on the basis that it is an approach that has delivered demonstrably successful results, but on the grounds that it is compatible with a particular set of norms in neo-liberal culture. These norms are said to centre upon the idea that people can be equipped to make rational, responsible choices about actions and, furthermore, that such choices can be made from the position of a particular 'level playing field' within an ethical community (a position that denies the existence of structural inequalities and power relationships) (Kendal, 2004).

In what ways does the 'rational–irrational' opposition map on to social stereotypes? In *Justice unbalanced*, Allen (1987) sought to explain some of the discrepancies in sentencing practice for male and female defendants through an examination of the implicit psychological models deployed by medicolegal personnel. In her study, Allen found that female defendants were more likely than men to be the subject of psychiatric reports, to be perceived of as insane or of diminished responsibility, and, on conviction, to receive psychiatric treatment instead of a penal sentence. Analysis of the relevant case reports, judicial instruments and institutional practices suggested a considerable emphasis in court reports upon the mental life of women, something that was considerably less apparent in relation to the male reports. To repeat Allen's description, the focus of the reports of the male offenders is on 'what he does, where he participates, how he acts in the world' (Allen, p. 40). As such, Allen depicts a conceptual landscape in which female offenders are seen as irrational, and therefore potentially suitable for corrective psychological interventions, while male offenders are regarded as more calculating and rational, and therefore are more likely to be made the recipients of a punitive intervention that will control their behaviour.

Arguably, a similar polarisation takes shape around the idea of race. Sampson (1993), for one, has described how an ideal self often emerges through a dialectic with a version of the other, and Miles (1989) has argued that representation of the (black) other has become a necessary counterpoint to our experience of an ideal (white) self. A similar argument has been advanced within psychoanalytic theory, which contends that racial distinctions, based around a black–white dichotomy, are maintained as a means of projecting unwanted aspects of the ideal white self into the denigrated, black subject. The black self becomes a container into which are projected hated, disavowed parts of the white self, so that

> the person who wishes to feel masterful, civilised, and superior and in control of his object world, and despises feeling inferior, uncivilised and invaded, has a readily available projection route to get rid of such feelings, if he is able to identify with being white.
>
> (Timimi, 1996; p. 184)

This position was earlier developed by Fanon (1986), who has depicted the colonial situation as a context in which the black man was located as hypersexual and hyperphysical, but low in intelligence. There are also clear links here with contemporary representations of black men as high in physicality divorced from emotions and intelligence (Rutherford, 1988).

Overall, these ideas distil into a version of reality in which it is 'naturally' easier for us to focus upon the internal life of the white male offender and the physicality of the black offender. By contrast, what is less available to us is an understanding of the internal reality of the black offender. The following anonymised segments of psychiatric reports illustrate this point. The first segment is taken from a report on a black, male offender being considered for admission to a special hospital under the legal category of psychopathic disorder; the second is from a report on a white, male offender whose admission is being considered under the same category:

> He told me that at this time he was regularly carrying a knife, being a hunting knife with a nine- or ten-inch blade. He would put it into the pocket of his jacket or trousers. At around this time, apparently, Mr Johnson moved back to the probation unit in Jackson Street. [He] told me that he thought Mr Johnson was in prison. However, on Saturday he said that he was planning to go back up north to look for his girlfriend. He went for a last look around town and went to a supermarket, where he said he saw a friend, who told him that Mr Johnson was back at the hostel. He said, 'I want to see that bastard.' He said he said this in a friendly way. He apparently saw Mr Johnson and they spent some time together. They watched the parade on the High Street, and then bought some cans of beer and a bottle of cider. They were apparently seen in the town square, laughing and joking together. [He] says that he remembers suddenly that Mr Johnson was shouting at him right in his face. He said that things happened, but he could not further describe this. Apparently, Mr Johnson was stabbed and was pronounced dead on arrival at hospital. [He] stated that he could remember nothing for approximately the next five hours. He remembers coming to his senses realising that his knife was gone and that there was blood on his hands. He gave himself up to the police at this stage.

> I think it is likely that, at some level, he was aware that his relationship with Julie was deteriorating and unlikely to last and he also realised that he was dependent on her. I suspect that this was the main cause for his anxiety and depression, his increased drinking and his retreat into fantasy. I also believe, though he would strenuously deny it, that at some level he deeply resented Julie as the cause of his dependency and for being about to end their relationship. This I believe was the cause of the hostility to her, which must have been behind his violence.
> (quoted in Stowell-Smith & McKeown, 1999)

As will be seen, there are a number of points within the first account when the subject, as a dynamic centre of awareness, almost seems to disappear: there are few attributions of intention and little speculation regarding the patient's inferences around the time of his offence. By contrast, the white report is replete with psychological terminology, contains a commentary about his internal states and attaches a psychological meaning to the offence.

These segments of text are taken from a larger piece of qualitative research (Stowell-Smith & McKeown, 1999) which argues that this physical-mental dichotomy is broadly representative of the way in which mental health professionals organise their thoughts about prospective black and white male clients. Potentially, this has significant implications for forensic practice: it lays the conceptual foundation that legitimises the use of more physical, constraining interventions with the black male offender (Lawson *et al.*, 1984; Prins, 1993; Mason, 1994), makes it appear less appropriate for him to receive talking therapy and reduces the likelihood of categorising him under the legal-diagnostic category of psychopathy (Stowell-Smith & McKeown, 1999), a diagnosis which requires some level of psychological inference in order to establish 'a disability of mind ... which results in abnormally aggressive or seriously irresponsible conduct on the part of the person concerned' (HMSO, 1983; p. 2).

Contextual reformulation and the high-secure hospital

Recent work in CAT (Walsh, 1996; Dunn & Parry, 1997; Kerr, 1999; Ryle & Kerr, 2002) has also built upon the intrapsychic model of RRPs in other ways in order to open up an understanding of how RRPs might operate at a wider, organisational or institutional level. Walsh (1996), for example, illustrated how organisational functioning could be represented through the medium of the SDR. She conceptualised a district surgical theatre unit as a work environment structured around the reciprocal pairings of overcontrolling, rejecting managers in relation to crushed, rebellious and angry staff. Her account suggested that this environment was a harmful one on the grounds that procedures emanating from this core, although self-defeating and non-productive, were never adequately revised. Subsequently, both Dunn & Parry (1997) and Kerr (1999) have described the dysfunctional, 'as if' type relationship that might form between the hard-to-help, challenging client and elements of the mental health system. Processes such as splitting, idealisation and denigration (which can be conceptualised in CAT terms as dissociated reciprocal roles) that occur in individual therapy might be enacted more freely and destructively in a relationship with an often fragmented and poorly integrated professional network. The explicit detailing of how these processes are enacted by both the patients and the staff team can be represented in the form of a 'contextual reformulation' (Kerr, 1999; Ryle & Kerr, 2002).

Personal experience of the high-secure hospital suggests to me that both staff and patients are subject to a number of seemingly irreconcilable psychological experiences. The manner in which these experiences are configured can be both psychologically damaging and confusing to the point where it might justifiably be claimed that the high-secure hospital constitutes what Walsh (1996) has termed a 'psychologically harmful work environment'. However, rather than having a type of neurotic structure – a unitary core around which various defective procedures revolve – the high-secure hospital can better be represented as having what Ryle (1997) describes as a more borderline structure, that is, a series of defensively dissociated, psychological states that hang together in a fragmented way. The following sections offer a descriptive and then diagrammatic account of how these states fit together.

Separateness and exclusion

The UK high-secure hospitals, previously known as 'special hospitals', 'exist in order to provide treatment in conditions of security not available elsewhere' (Hamilton, 1990; p. 1363). They exist on the understanding that they provide an environment for 'persons subject to detention under the Mental Health Act 1983 who in his [the Secretary of State for Social Services] opinion require treatment under conditions of special security on account of their dangerous, violent or criminal propensities' (Gostin, 1986; p. 57). The security requirements of the hospitals, high perimeter fencing, locked wards and a regime of constant surveillance, provide the most conspicuous distinguishing features which mark them off from other National Health Service (NHS) psychiatric hospitals. The physical reality of these security features creates an environment which is compatible with Goffman's description of the 'total institution', whose 'encompassing or total character is symbolised by the barrier to social intercourse and to departure that is often built right into the physical plant, such as locked doors, high walls, barbed wire, cliffs, water, forests or moors' (Goffman, 1960; p. 15).

Despite recent changes which have seen the high-secure hospitals merge with NHS mental health trusts, their concentration into only three sites, allied to their physical characteristics, tends to maintain this sense of separateness. The themes of separateness and segregation are echoed in some of the characteristics of the patient population. An earlier study by Gostin (1986) stated that 50% of the total high-secure hospital population had been detained for 5 years or more and 5% for more than 20 years. Subsequently, Maden et al. (1993) suggested that the average length of stay was 8 years while a more recent review by Williams et al. (1999) on academic literature on the characteristics of the high-secure hospital population noted some variation in length of stay within particular demographic and diagnostic groups. For example, the length of stay for women was slightly longer than that for men, and the length of stay for those assigned to the legal category of mental impairment was significantly longer than for those assigned to the other categories.

Separateness is further enhanced by the fact that the patient's stay in a high-secure hospital is typically characterised by relatively infrequent contact with the outside world. There is restricted contact between high-secure hospitals and other health service resources. Bowden highlighted the difficulty in persuading Regional Health Authorities to accept labour-intensive and potentially 'risky' patients (1981; p. 344). Gostin (1986) described a large number of high-secure hospital patients whose officially authorised transfer or conditional discharge had been delayed due to a lack of agencies willing to provide supervision, rehabilitation or accommodation.

The state of separateness of the high-secure hospital is also enhanced through a variety of social processes. Deacon (2004) has argued that the containment of dangerous individuals in high-secure hospitals serves the purpose of establishing a physical and psychological separation from the public, something that, in turn, creates an illusion of safety. In this respect, the work of the high-secure hospital mirrors one of the psychological processes at work in horror films, wherein the audience achieves a safe distance from that which is fear provoking (but also exciting) through its projection onto the safety of the movie screen (McKeown & Stowell-Smith, in press). Deacon (2004; p. 88) suggests that, in a risk-obsessed culture, the high-secure hospital appears to provide a sense of 'safety in concreteness' by marking out a physical boundary between the 'dangerously mad' (i.e. those incarcerated in the high-secure hospital) and the wider society. She continues:

> Those contained within the walls of the high-secure hospitals are visibly captive and available to receive such unconscious social projections, with little opportunity to accept or return them. As such they become powerful symbols of the evil in society, demonized in the press and collective unconsciousness.
>
> (p. 93)

Young (1996) has something similar to say about this process. She discusses how popular discourse about offences that are hard to explain often seems to express the desire for a parental surrogate to appear in the form of a 'stern lawgiver'. The task of the lawgiver is to re-establish identity and order through, among other things, the outlawing and exclusion of the perpetrators of the aberrant act. According to Young, this process of exclusion serves a symbolic purpose, as it 'purifies and strengthens our attachment to a cleansed, imagined community in which we can re-experience the modernist desire for oneness and unity' (1996; p. 10).

Hence, one way of beginning the contextual reformulation of the high-secure hospital is to consider it as the place of exclusion to which certain types of dangerous offenders are consigned. The act of exclusion establishes a sense of safety in the now-purified wider community.

Claustrophobic dependency

The functional, legal requirements of the high-secure hospital, allied to its psychological and symbolic purpose, contribute to the establishment of a long-stay population. In turn, this gives rise to a claustrophobic atmosphere that can feel suffocating for both staff and patients. Tensions are heightened by the fact that within this context the isolation and segregation confound traditional notions of care and treatment. This is significant as, 'Traditional Western medical accounts of illness tend to presume a normal state of independence interrupted by a discrete, time-limited period of abnormality and dependence', and that 'Appropriate care seeking and caregiving aim to restore normality and independence' (Adshead, 2002; p. 40). It becomes difficult to apply this model in the high-secure hospital where, as previously noted, the average length of stay is approximately 8 years. In this context, notions of 'normal dependency' and treatment that aims to restore independence start to fall apart.

Adshead (2002) notes how a number of seemingly irreconcilable dilemmas emerge around the receipt and provision of professional care within the high-secure hospital. For example, in order to function within the framework of traditional medical care, professional staff require patients to assume a particular role in which they are dependent upon a more knowledgeable other to help treat psychopathology that, by its very nature, has proven resistant to self-cure or self-management. To this extent, dependence is tolerated; however, at some point, the requirement for reliance upon expert professional help comes into conflict with a less medicalised, more 'offence-focused' discourse which exhorts offenders to take responsibility for their offences. As earlier described, this set of ideas has taken shape around the cognitive-behavioural paradigm, something which Kendall (2004) associates with the neo-liberal doctrine of 'responsibilisation'. Issues of normal dependence and independence are further skewed by the fact that, as previously noted, a variety of influences may conspire to ensure that patient discharge or transfer is often contingent upon factors other than the apparently successful completion of a treatment programme. The political, legal and resource issues that can influence and delay the discharge or transfer of patients heighten feelings of stagnation and tension.

Control

I have described how societal demands for the control of dangerous offenders provide part of the impetus for the establishment and continuation of the high-secure hospital. The societal need for the literal and symbolic control of dangerous offenders also helps to shape a psychological context in which the traditional medical concepts of dependency and treatment start to unravel, and in which staff and patients can feel suffocated, impotent and helpless. In this context, the issue of control features at another level, namely, as an attempt to manage feelings generated within the institution that might otherwise seem unmanageable. This idea draws upon the notion of the 'social defence system', a concept originally propounded by Jaques (1955) and defined by Hinshelwood in the following way: 'If the nature of a certain kind of work is particularly effective at raising anxieties, the social structure may tend towards developing specific cultures – that is, modes of doing the work – which help the individual from those anxieties' (Hinshelwood, 1993).

In her classic study of a London teaching hospital in the late 1950s, Menzies Lyth (1998) illustrated how such structures evolved within nursing practice to reduce the levels of anxieties that nurses might otherwise experience in their contact with often severely ill or dying patients. Menzies Lyth noted that the core of nurses' anxiety lay in the direct relationship that they might have with their patients. Hence, a variety of institutional practices, such as a concentration on ritual task performance and the removal of individual nurse responsibility for patient care, emerged to split up or at least dilute the intensity of the nurse–patient relationship. According to Menzies Lyth (1998), these cultural practices functioned as a social defence system, as they had the cumulative effect of reducing the nurses' level of anxiety provoked by their relationship with the suffering patient.

Ethnographic studies of the high-secure hospitals have suggested how this defensive use of control might apply both to staff and patients groups. For example, in a study of a ward for personality-disordered patients in Ashworth Hospital, Richman (1998) noted how the maintenance of control was an important construct for the patient group, pervading their relationship with staff members, with peers and with other patient subpopulations. By its very nature, the bringing together of large numbers of dangerous people is a task that requires careful management and orchestration. However, experience of the high-secure hospital suggests that this level of organisation can shade into the form of regimented control described by Menzies Lyth. This is often deemed evident, for example, in the interface between the therapeutic needs of the patients and their participation in other scheduled activities, such as education classes and vocational workshops. A common grievance of staff within the high-secure hospital who were involved in psychological work concerned the perceived privileging of routine hospital activities over the apparent therapeutic needs of the patients. Attendance at such activities was facilitated by an escorted hospital 'movement'. Often, situations arose in which patients would not be available for individual psychotherapy, group sex offender treatment or anger-management training, as escort staff were committed to the routine movement of patients and were unavailable for other forms of escorting. This was both frustrating and seemingly paradoxical inasmuch as people with histories of antisocial, sexually aggressive behaviour, admitted to 'hospital' for the treatment of such behaviour, would become adept at, for example, art, tailoring and bricklaying, but would have diminished opportunities to address offence-related behaviour. One way of understanding this apparent paradox was that the hospital routine privileged these forms of activity over activity that might excite a greater level of excitement or psychological distress, thereby challenging stability and order.

Issues of control and order were also played out at the level of the hospital ward. Here, a perspective articulated by the more traditional, longer-serving nursing staff suggested that it was dangerous to stir up patients by encouraging the exploration and expression of underlying psychological issues. Even manualised psychological treatments, such as cognitive-behavioural anger-control training, were held to be potentially subversive, as they encouraged the expression rather than suppression of feelings. Such views were not universally held by all ward-based staff, but did appear to constitute a significant body of opinion within the staff group.

Emotional numbness

Hinshelwood (1987) has argued that staff and patients in mental hospitals have one thing in common, 'a fear of mad violence and of other states of personal fragmentation and obliteration', and Cox (1996) has suggested that fears such as this are particularly heightened in the high-secure hospital. In response to these fears, a defensive set of attitudes emerge in which 'any spark of initiative, any emotional responsiveness between people is dangerous and will lead to a serious disruption of one's own mind' (Hinshelwood, 1994; p. 286). Within the high-secure hospital, the deadening effects of regimentation and control appeared to provide one escape route from this fear; by contrast, the provision of a therapeutic environment that invited exploration and reflection appeared to offer the reverse.

A consequence of this process was that the hospital appeared to function as if crudely subdivided into two different psychological zones: in one zone, patients lived, received medical treatment, worked and were educated; in another zone, patients reflected upon their lives, thought about their offences, had their 'offending behaviour' confrontationally challenged and were encouraged to express difficult thoughts and feelings. The first zone could be seen as characterised by a form of psychological numbness: functional activity took place there, but it had some of the sterile, non-therapeutic qualities described in some user accounts (e.g. George, 1998). The second zone, while offering the possibility of opening up the type of exploration and spontaneity described by Hinshelwood, was small in comparison with the first, and a common frustration voiced among the patient population concerned, for example, the lack of psychologists, psychotherapists and therapeutic groups. This pessimism is picked up in a comparative study of the quality-of-life issues in English high-secure hospitals and Dutch TBS clinics treating personality-disordered patients (Swinton et al., 2001), where it is suggested that lack of therapeutic optimism in the high-secure hospital may partly be related to the lack of therapeutic resources. Furthermore, the scarcity of these resources in this zone, combined with the fact that it was envisioned as the place in which all psychological issues were resolved, contributed to a feeling of pessimism, stagnation and numbness.

The relationship between these different states or domains is illustrated in Fig. 3.1. This structural model offers separation and segregation as the

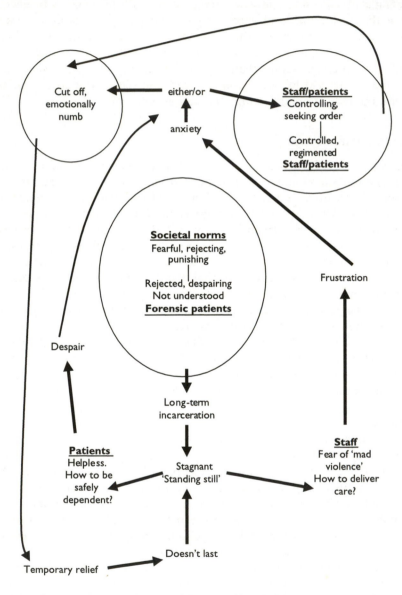

Figure 3.1 Contextual reformulation and the special hospital.

primary state. This creates a sense of stagnation, out of which emerge a number of related anxieties for both staff and patients. The anxieties engendered here a dissociative-like process that leads to the formation of two further states, one organised around the theme of control, and the other linked to the theme of emotional disconnectedness. The model illustrates how these defensively derived states provide some form of temporary respite from unwanted feelings but ultimately contribute to the sense of stagnation or hopelessness, which might be described as the chronically endured pain of the high-secure hospital.

Ryle & Kerr (2002) argue that a common aim of providing this form of contextual reformulation is to engender a greater understanding of the self-reinforcing role enactments of individuals and agencies that often centre upon or revolve around a particular, often hard-to-help, client or patient. If this can be achieved, a less judgemental view can be established of the individual within the system. This, in turn, opens up the possibility of working through negative, hostile feelings and unblocking entrenched, stuck, circular patterns of behaviour. While the reformulation offered here is deindividualised in the sense that it presents the institution as the 'patient', it does highlight areas in which the individual can become subject to unwanted anxieties and locked in collusive, self-perpetuating patterns of behaviour. Hence, in this way, it offers a type of aerial perspective that might facilitate thinking about and addressing these patterns in a more joined-up way.

References

Adshead, G. (2002). Three degrees of security: Attachment and forensic institutions. *Criminal Behaviour and Mental Health, 12*, 31–45.

Allen, H. (1987). *Justice unbalanced: Gender, psychiatry and judicial decisions*. Milton Keynes: Open University Press.

Bowden, P. (1981). What happens to patients released from special hospitals? *British Journal of Psychiatry, 138*, 340–345.

Cox, M. (1996). Psychodynamics and the special hospital: 'Road blocks and thought blocks'. In C. Cordess & M. Cox (Eds), *Forensic psychotherapy: Crime, psychodynamics and the offender patient*. London & Philadelphia: Jessica Kingsley Publishers.

Deacon, J. (2004). Testing boundaries: the social context of physical and relational containment in a maximum secure psychiatric setting. *Journal of Social Work Practice, 18*, 81–97.

Dunn, M. & Parry, G. D. (1997). A formulated care plan approach to caring for borderline personality disorder in a community mental health team. *Clinical Psychology Forum, 104*, 19–22.

Fanon, F. (1986). *Black skin, white masks*. London: Pluto Press.

Forshaw, D. & Rollin, H. (1990). The history of forensic psychiatry in England. In *Principles and practice of forensic psychiatry*. Edinburgh: Churchill Livingstone.

George, S. (1998). More than a pound of flesh: A patient's perspective. In T. Mason &

D. Mercer (Eds), *Critical perspectives in forensic care: Inside out*. London: Macmillan Press.

Goffman, I. (1960). *Asylums*. London: Penguin.

Gostin, L. (1986). *Institutions observed*. London: King's Fund Centre.

Hamilton, J. (1990). *Special hospitals and the state hospital. Principles and practice of forensic psychiatry*. Edinburgh: Churchill Livingstone.

Hinshelwood, R. D. (1987). The psychotherapist's role in large psychiatric institutions. *Psychoanalytic Psychotherapy*, *2*, 207–212.

Hinshelwood, R. D. (1993). Locked in role: a psychotherapist within the social defence system of a prison. *Journal of Forensic Psychiatry*, *4*, 427–440.

Hinshelwood, R. D. (1994). The relevance of psychotherapy. *Psychoanalytical Psychotherapy*, *8*, 283–294.

HMSO (1983). *The Mental Health Act, 1983*. London: HMSO.

Holquist, M. (1995). *Bakhtin and his world*. London: Routledge.

Jaques, E. (1955). *Social systems as a defence against persecutory and depressive anxiety*. In M. Klein, P. Heinman & R. E. Money-Kyrle (Eds), *New directions in psychoanalysis*. London: Tavistock.

Kendal, K. (2004). Dangerous thinking: A critical history of correctional, cognitive behaviouralism. In G. Mair (Ed.), *What matters in probation*. Cullompton, Devon: Willan Publishing.

Kerr, I. (1999). Cognitive analytic therapy for borderline personality disorder in the context of a community mental health team: Individual and organisational psychodynamic implications. *British Journal of Psychotherapy*, *15*, 425–438.

Lawson, W. B., Jerome, A. & Werner, P. D. (1984). Race, violence and psychopathology. *Journal of Clinical Psychiatry*, *45*, 294–297.

Maden, A., Curle, C., Meux, C., Burrow, S. & Gunn, J. (1993). The treatment and security needs of patients in special hospitals. *Criminal Behaviour and Mental Health*, *3*, 290–306.

Maguire, J. & Priestley, P. (1985). *Offending behaviour: Skills and strategies in going straight*. London: Bristol.

Mason, T. (1994). Seclusion in a special hospital: A developmental study. Unpublished PhD thesis, Anglia Polytechnic University.

Mason, T. & Alty, A. (1995). *Seclusion and mental health: A break with the past*. London: Macmillan.

McKeown, M. & Stowell-Smith, M. (in press). The comforts of evil: Dangerous personalities and high secure hospitals and the horror film. In T. Mason (Ed.), *Evil in forensic psychiatry*. London: Humana.

Menzies Lyth, I. (1998). *Containing anxiety in institutions: Selected essays* (vol. 1). London: Free Association Books.

Miles, R. (1989). *Racism*. London: Routledge.

Prins, H. (1993). *Report of the Committee of Inquiry into the death in Broadmoor Hospital of Orville Blackwood and a review of the death of two other Afro-Caribbean patients: 'Big, black and dangerous?'* London: Special Hospitals Service Authority.

Richman, J. (1998). The ceremonial and moral order of a ward of psychopaths. In T. Mason & D. Mercer (Eds), *Critical perspective in forensic care: Inside out*. London: Macmillan Press.

Ross, R. & Fabiano, E. (1981). *Time to think: Cognition and crime, limitation and remediation*. Ottawa: Department of Criminology, University of Ottawa.

Ryle, A. (1985). Cognitive theory, object relations and the self. *British Journal of Medical Psychology, 58*, 1–7

Ryle, A. (1990). *Cognitive Analytic Therapy: Active participation in change*. Chichester: Wiley.

Ryle, A. (1995). *Cognitive Analytic Therapy: Developments in theory and practice*. Chichester: Wiley.

Ryle, A. (1997). *Cognitive Analytic Therapy and Borderline Personality Disorder: The model and the method*. Chichester: Wiley.

Ryle, A. & Kerr, I. B. (2002). *Introducing Cognitive Analytic Therapy: Principles and practice*. Chichester: Wiley.

Sampson, E. (1993). *Celebrating the other: A dialogic account of human nature*. Hemel Hempstead: Harvester Wheatsheaf.

Shannon, C. (1999). Families talking about homicide: A discourse analytic approach. Unpublished MSc dissertation, University of Liverpool.

Stowell-Smith, M. & McKeown, M. (1999). Race, psychopathy and the self: A discourse analytic study. *British Journal of Medical Psychology, 72*, 459–470.

Swinton, M., Carlisle, J. & Oliver, J. (2001). Quality of life for patients with a personality disorder – comparison of patients in two settings: An English special hospital and a Dutch TBS clinic. *Criminal Behaviour and Mental Health, 11*, 131–144.

Timimi, S. (1996). Race and colour in internal and external reality. *British Journal of Psychotherapy, 13*, 183–192.

Walsh, S. (1996). Adapting cognitive analytic therapy to make sense of psychologically harmful work environments. *British Journal of Medical Psychology, 69*, 3–20.

Welldon, E. (1993). Forensic psychotherapy and group analysis. *Group Analysis, 26*, 487–502.

Welldon, E. (1998). *Mother, madonna, whore: The idealisation and denigration of motherhood*. London: Free Association Books.

Williams, P., Badger, D., Nursten, J. & Woodward, L. (1999). A review of recent academic literature on the characteristics of patients in British special hospitals. *Criminal Behaviour and Mental Health, 9*, 296–315.

Young, A. (1996). *Imagining crime: Textual outlaws and criminal conversations*. London: Sage.

Chapter 4

The adjunctive role of Cognitive Analytic Therapy in the treatment of child sexual offenders in secure forensic settings

Mark Stowell-Smith, Aisling O'Kane & Arthur Fairbanks

In this chapter, we explore the potential advantages of using Cognitive Analytic Therapy (CAT) as an adjunct in the treatment of the child sexual offender. We begin by examining some current theories and treatment approaches. We then examine the role that CAT might play in facilitating the treatment of the child sexual offender, arguing that a CAT-informed approach may have particular relevance to treatment within in-patient settings such as special hospitals and regional secure units. We develop this argument by looking at some of the links between CAT, attachment theory and attachment-based understandings of child sexual offending. We argue that combining these theoretical frameworks creates the potential for an approach that adequately conceptualises the dynamics of child sexual offending. We also argue that this approach offers the potential for clinicians to conceptualise how those dynamics might be enacted in a range of parallel, institutional behaviours.

Some current theories on the treatment and understanding of child sexual offending

Current theories of sexual offending broadly fall within the psychodynamic and cognitive-behavioural paradigms. The origins of the former can be located in Freud's (1957) notion of 'perversion' as a sexual instinct that is perverted from the normal aim of sexual intercourse with a heterosexual partner. Freud went on to note how deviation from this aim, in one form or another, was common and was not in itself damaging. However, in instances where such practices tended to predominate and override feelings such as shame and guilt, they were regarded as pathological. This account has been criticised for the way in which the definition of 'perverted' sexuality relies heavily upon contemporary notions of morality and normality.

Wood (2003) notes how other psychoanalytic theorists have attempted to move away from this trap by looking beyond purely behavioural descriptions of aberrant sexuality toward the underlying motives for that behaviour. An example of this approach is provided by Stoller (1986), who illustrates how sexuality can be used both to express hostility and attain a sense of mastery. Stoller's focus is mainly upon adults with gender dysphoria, where he describes a process of transformation through which the trauma in male children of unwanted feminisation is revisited, but triumphed over, through the act of adult, voluntary feminisation. As Wood notes, Stoller's model moves more into an interpsychic understanding of sexual offending. Glasser's (1979; 1988) notion of the 'core complex' extends this further and is particularly relevant to a dynamic understanding of child sexual offending. According to Glasser, the core complex is a psychological configuration comprising a group of interrelated characteristics which have their origin at an early stage of development. The starting point for the complex is the ordinary human need for emotional closeness with the other. However, in certain cases, rather than being enriching, this contact threatens to annihilate the self, as there is an expectation that contact will result in the self being taken over to the point where it ceases to exist as a separate entity. This distortion may occur, for example, in patients whose early histories have been characterised by abusive, intrusive caregiving. In such individuals, a conflict may be set up between wanting and fearing contact. One response to this conflict may be withdrawal, but this, in turn, may activate feelings of abandonment, depression and desolation.

According to Glasser, the 'perverse solution' to this dilemma entails sexualising the aggression elicited by the perceived threat of the other, so that the intention to destroy is converted into a desire to hurt and control. This allows the self to retain contact with the other, but at a safe distance – a distance which precludes trust and intimacy (Glasser, 1988). This form of relationship is apparent in 'perversions' such as paedophilia, where contact with the other is maintained at the expense of denying his/her individuality. This is chillingly expressed in Glasser's statement, 'One might say his [the pedophile's] "love" for the child is predominantly like that of the dog for the bone' (1990; p. 744). Glasser's concept of the core complex identifies conflicts between the desire for and fear of intimacy. Within a contemporary CAT framework, this dilemma could be expressed as the consequence of child-derived, restrictive reciprocal role procedures (RRPs) based on abandonment and engulfment. In this framework, the offence becomes the procedure that allows some resolution, albeit at the expense of the child victim, of the emotional pain associated with these internalised roles.

The application of some of these concepts under the heading 'forensic psychotherapy' has been detailed by Welldon & Van Velsen (1998) and Cordess & Cox (1996). The model is presented as the offspring of forensic psychiatry and psychoanalytic psychotherapy, and it aims to provide a psychodynamic perspective to the understanding, management and treatment of the offender. The overarching aim of forensic psychotherapy is to help offenders understand, and take responsibility for, their actions in order to reduce the likelihood of reoffending (Cordess et al., 1994). In this respect, a central focus is maintained on both the intra- and interpsychic meaning and consequences of the criminal act, which may be assumed to be something equivalent to a neurotic symptom, the expression of a severe, underlying psychopathology or a defence against an underlying depression (Welldon, 1998; p. 15). When it is conceptualised in this way, the therapist may address the offence with the patient as, for example, an attempt to gain 'symptom relief' or as an attempt to resolve a conflict arising from a basic primary event.

While there is an extensive case study literature describing the application of this model to the treatment of the child sexual offender, there is, at present, a dearth of either controlled or naturalistic outcome studies. This is a criticism that does not apply to the cognitive-behavioural treatment of the child sexual offender. Of the various models which have been used to explain sexual offending, Finkelhor's (1984) 'four-stage model' has provided the conceptual underpinning to cognitive-behavioural models of sex offender treatment. It conceptualises sexual thoughts and emotions, including sexual arousal, as the basis for motivation to offend. Within Finkelhor's model, inhibition of offending is reduced through the development of cognitive distortions by the individual. Thinking and behaviour are then directed toward a plan for the offence, which includes strategies for overcoming the victim.

While this theory has been useful in aiding the understanding of processes in the approach to offences, it does little to explain the wider function of sexual violence for the perpetrator. Hall & Hirschman's (1991) quadripartite model addresses this deficit by classifying offenders according to the hypothesised underlying reason for their sexual violence. The first group comprises 'true paedophiles', who seek sex with children because it is their primary sexual orientation. By contrast, the offences of the second group are seen as deriving from distorted beliefs and thinking. Of the remaining two groups, one is seen as acting out emotional antecedents, such as anger or anxiety, using sexual offending as comfort or as an expression of core emotions, while the final group is driven by underlying personality pathology manifest in the attitudes and interpersonal difficulties associated with their offending. Critiques of the model have commented on its failure to account for the variance among sex offenders, as each of the four stages is likely be seen in most child sexual offences. Nonetheless, it offers a unifying language and framework for the various elements of multimodal treatment approaches.

Another, more interpsychic model focused more closely on the role of 'hostile masculinity' in sexual offending is defined by Malamuth et al. (1991; 1993). Their description of this construct is typified in the controlling, adversarial male attitude toward women. Such men frequently aim to dominate sexual partners in an attempt to manage feelings of hurt and anger that they associate with rejection. While Malamuth et al.'s model was not designed to explain sexual offending against children, the theme of acting out sexually with a controlled other (a process that approximates to the objectification of the victim in Glasser's core complex) often seems to occur in many sexual offences against children. Moreover, the personality traits alluded to by Malamuth *et al.* are found among those who commit such acts. Malamuth *et al.*'s model also addresses the issue of sexual promiscuity, seen in parallel to a wider antisocial personality trait. This brings in issues such as entitlement, disregard for rules and use of sexual behaviour to enhance self-esteem, elements which may have some relevance to understanding the child sexual offender.

Marshall & Barbaree (1990) proposed a multifactorial model that integrated biochemical and genetic factors relating to the role of social learning. They hypothesise that sex offenders have early life experiences that confound the differentiation between sex and aggression. These experiences are the source of vulnerability or risk of committing acts of sexual violence, which can be further influenced by social factors such as cultural values and, more specifically, pornography. In explaining the final stages of individuals' thinking and behaviour in their approach to offending, the model then utilises constructs similar to those set out by Finkelhor.

The most integrative theory of child sexual abuse to date is that of Ward & Seigert (2002), commonly referred to as the 'five-pathways model'. This model builds upon Hall & Hirschman's model. However, rather than viewing factors as separate parts of diverse typologies, it favours the notion of a coming together of multiple factors. The four key constructs, which combine a range of inter- and intrapsychic components, include distorted sexual scripts (implicit, maladaptive learning about the nature of sex itself and the social rules which govern it); difficulties in managing emotions; cognitive distortions, particularly deeper-core belief and schema which affect the top-down processing of the offender's perception of the victim; and deficits in intimacy and social skills. According to Ward & Seigert (2002), the last are associated with histories of childhood abuse and neglect. This influences the development of an insecure adult attachment style that predisposes offenders to seek sex with a child not out of preference to an adult but because they see it as the only available means to meet intimacy needs.

As with psychoanalytic approaches to child sex offending, a cognitive-behavioural paradigm has emerged out of the above explanatory models. Laws and Marshall (2003) name Abel as the person who first included a cognitive component in behavioural treatments for sex offenders. Abel, together with his colleagues in the USA, developed a treatment programme which incorporated cognitive mediating processes into behavioural therapy (Abel, Blanchard & Becker, 1978; Abel, Becker & Skinner, 1983; Abel, Osborn, Anthony & Gardos, 1992). Abel and his colleagues have focused on the identification of offence precursors or sexual offence cycles. This is treated in offenders by examination of their distorted thinking patterns, control of their deviant fantasies, enhancement of their victim empathy and development of their social competence and skills. Marques (1982; 1984) further extended this model by annexing the concept of 'relapse prevention' specifically to develop strategies for addressing future risk situations. Implicit in much of this work is the assumption that targeting procriminal beliefs will reduce offending behaviours. This development has been particularly influential in relation to an understanding of procriminal thinking and the role played by cognitive distortions in the acquisition and maintenance of sexual offending.

Attachment issues and the relevance of the treatment environment

Overall, the outcome of sex offender treatment studies indicates that treatment can be effective, out-patient samples showing a greater effect size than those which are institutionally based (Hall, 1995). While some of this difference may be accounted for by the fact that incarceration may be dealing with more dangerous sex offenders, it also seems likely that the context of the treatment is significant. However, perhaps a limitation of both psychoanalytic and cognitive-behavioural models is that they make little, if any, reference to the context in which treatment is delivered. Arguably, contextual factors are important, for, as we will discuss later, a significant amount of child sexual offender treatment takes place in secure psychiatric settings with patients who have demonstrable difficulties in forming secure attachments (Bumby & Hansen, 1997; Marshall *et al.*, 1997). We might therefore expect this client group to have a diminished capacity for forming straightforward, collaborative relationships, not only with the therapist and other individuals in a treatment group, but also with the institution as a whole. We might also assume that issues concerning attachment and engagement might be either exacerbated or improved by the institution's capacity to act as a base that will contain some of these difficulties.

The significance of the treatment environment in sex offender work has been illustrated in a descriptive study by Ragsdale (2002). This qualitative study examined a number of treatment-related factors. Among other things, these included an account of factors which offenders identified as proving helpful in therapy, changes that offenders had seen in themselves since they began treatment, perceptions of themselves before and after treatment, information they thought therapists who work with sex offenders should know, perceptions of what they thought in their past contributed to their sex offending and information about their relationships with significant others. Thematic coding was used to analyse the data. An important theme to emerge from this research concerned the importance that offenders ascribed to having a safe, secure place to discuss their behaviours and to have others in similar situations to talk with. They detailed the importance of the group treatment process to their progress. Included in this process were trust of other group members, listening to others in the group, participation in and attendance at long-term group therapy, and the group members displaying honesty and monitoring their risk. They used the group therapy situation as a place to acquire feedback from peers and therapists regarding inappropriate beliefs and behaviours. Such studies suggest the importance of perceived safety for sex offenders in engaging in group treatments. They also serve to underline the importance of the therapeutic relationship for these individuals. Some of the more confrontational techniques which have been used in the past have led some researchers to conclude that such approaches used to confront and challenge perpetrators assume guilt and treat the individual as if he were the 'contemporary witch' (McConaghy, 1989).

Do treatment environments provide a sense of safety and security to the offender? If not, what impact might this have upon child sexual offender work and how can some of the issues which arise within treatment environments be addressed? Before tackling these questions, we will briefly review what we regard as some of the more salient ideas from the field of attachment theory.

Attachment theory is an idea originally developed by Bowlby (1969) and given expression in a variety of forms by a number of contemporary theorists. Drawing upon the work of ethnologists such as Harlow (1958), Bowlby's early expression of theory emphasises the way in which the human infant is born with an innate drive for attachment that has a survival function, securing proximity to the caregiver, and thereby lessening the chances of predation. The 'primary attachment relationship' that emerges at around 7 months in the human infant mediates physical proximity to the caregiver: when the infant is under threat, it moves nearer to the caregiver; when the attachment relationship is threatened by separation, the infant protests by crying. Gradually and under sufficiently benign conditions, the infant comes to experience the caregiver as providing a 'secure base' from which it can begin to explore the world. The security engendered in this relationship allows the child to leave the base in order to explore the world. If a level of secure attachment has been established with the caregiver, the infant will feel enabled to return to the caregiver without fear that the 'secure base' has been removed or destroyed. Holmes (1993) says that as this form of internal working model in the securely attached infant becomes internalised, it provides the bridge between the position of childhood, immature dependence and both mature, adult dependence and mature, adult 'emotional autonomy' (Holmes & Lindley, 1989).

Less benign environments, however, produce less secure patterns of attachment. Two notable, insecure attachment styles delineated by Ainsworth *et al.* (1978) are those of the 'insecure-avoidant' and 'insecure-ambivalent' attachment. Research derived from the Adult Attachment Inventory (Main & Goldwyn, 1994) has labelled the insecure-avoidant style as 'dismissing' on the grounds that avoidant adults respond defensively to failed or frustrated attachment with adult caregivers by devaluing and minimising the significance of interpersonal relationships to their lives. By contrast, ambivalent adults are described as 'preoccupied', as they display patterns of intense, emotional overinvolvement with others. This may reflect early histories in which they have been embroiled in enmeshed relationships with caregivers. Holmes (1993) cites research that estimates the prevalence of secure attachment in a north European sample to be about 65%, insecure-avoidant at 20% and insecure-ambivalent at 14%.

Attachment problems in forensic populations

Adshead (2004; p. 35) summarises a body of research that has illustrated how unresolved and dismissing attachment styles tend to be overrepresented in forensic populations. She notes: 'Since a dismissing style is associated with attempts to negate or ignore affective distress in self or others, it is not surprising to find that this pattern of attachment would be common in a group who have behaviorally demonstrated a capacity to ignore distress' (Adshead, 2002; p. 35).

In two related papers, Adshead (1998; 2004) describes how attachment concepts can be usefully applied in relation to treatment organisations, such as psychiatric hospitals and forensic institutions. Her analysis suggests that attachment ideas are relevant in several ways, not least as there is evidence that people with histories of failed, insecure attachment are more inclined to find their way into psychiatric hospitals, prisons and special hospitals (Coid, 1992; Van Ijzendoorn et al., 1997).

By its very nature, the process of admission to institutions such as a prison, a regional secure unit or a special hospital involves the necessity of detachment and attachment. The probability of the attachment system's being activated is high then, as admission to such environments usually occurs at a time of crisis (e.g. during a period of psychiatric disturbance, after a court appearance, after an offence has been perpetrated), a time when Bowlby (1969) envisaged the individual's attachment needs as heightened. The possibility of toxic forms of attachment pattern being enacted is enhanced by the fact that, as we noted earlier, the forensic population tends to have an overrepresentation of individuals with histories of insecure attachment. Two possibilities seem to present themselves here. Firstly, insecure-avoidant offenders may find it difficult to engage psychologically with professional carers and therefore fail to engage adequately in treatment. Secondly, insecure-ambivalent offenders may develop overly close, fused relationships with carers and find it difficult, among other things, to disengage from the therapeutic relationship.

To what extent might attachment-related issues be relevant to the child sexual offender? Important work by Marshall and his colleagues (1993) in Canada has focused upon what they refer to as the 'vulnerability' of the offender. They propose that this lies in a dimension with strong resilience at one end and extreme weakness at the other. These attributes develop over the lifespan and can be altered by experience. An individual who is high in vulnerability offends because he is more likely to create, recognise or give in to opportunities to offend. They propose that the beliefs, cognitive and behavioural skills, and emotional dispositions associated with vulnerability and resilience are acquired in childhood, particularly in the context of the relationship with parents. Such assertions are supported by Marshall *et al.*'s work (1993) on the role of attachment and the subsequent development of sexual offending. They describe how insecure parent–child attachments can result in the child's developing fearful or avoidant attitudes and behaviours toward closeness to others. These children develop features that persist into adulthood such as unfriendliness, low self-esteem, social uneasiness, and lack of warmth. Marshall (1993) concludes that these characteristics make the person vulnerable to becoming a sexual offender.

Furthermore, research on the backgrounds of sex offenders indicates that rates of sexual and physical abuse in this group are higher than for non-offenders. Laws and Marshall (2003) propose that, taken together, a modelling effect and a distortion of the internal working model of intimate relationships lead to feelings of loneliness and problems in establishing intimacy that contribute to the development of a template according to which the child will later seek intimacy through an abusive sexual relationship.

Attachment issues and the professional helper

The effects of working with clients who have been victimised have been investigated under several theoretical models such as burn-out (Freudenberger & Robbins, 1979), secondary traumatic stress (Figley, 1999), counter-transference reactions (Dalenberg, 2000) and vicarious traumatisation (McCann & Pearlman, 1990). Noffsinger & Resnick (2000) assert that while increasing numbers of treatment groups for sex offenders are now being run in different settings in the UK, the majority of these are cognitive-behavioural in orientation, and there has been little reported in the literature about the complex processes and dynamics that occur in these groups. Cognitive-behavioural therapy has been criticised for insufficient attention to the therapeutic process compared with therapy of other persuasions (Schaap, Bennun, Schindler & Hoodguin, 1993). This is potentially problematic, given the relevance of the therapeutic relationship and the fact that counter-transference issues are reportedly common with clinicians working with this population.

Given the nature of attachment difficulties within the forensic population, it could be expected that considerable emotional demands would be placed upon professional helpers. Under optimum conditions, a relationship between the patient and professional staff might provide an opportunity for the development of a more secure form of attachment. But what if professional staff also have their own unresolved attachment issues? There seem to be a number of ways in which unresolved attachment problems within the professional staff group may interfere with therapeutic aims. One observation is that adults deprived of appropriate care in infancy may seek to provide this to others as adults in their professional lives, a phenomenon that Bowlby (1988) described as 'compulsive caregiving'. One possible consequence of this problem is that the compulsively caregiving professional may need patients to remain sick in order to maintain their dependency upon the professional. At another level, these types of emotional needs in the professional may instigate a pattern of invasive, inappropriate care that might ultimately culminate in serious boundary violations. By contrast, a dismissing adult carer who may have experienced various forms of abuse in infancy and has, therefore, learnt that it is safer to remain disengaged from others may remain pathologically disengaged from patients.

Adshead (1998; 2004) suggests that forensic institutions can provide a positive, secure base-type experience for the insecurely attached patient through the provision of consistency, support and emotional containment. Adshead (2002; p. 38) comments that, however painful it might be to acknowledge, for many offender patients 'the forensic institution is the first enduring attachment that they have made in adulthood and the only place where they may feel accepted and not out of place'. By contrast, the institution may replicate early, abnormal attachment experiences in a number of ways. Institutional settings which infantilise and disempower may induce a feeling of fused, enmeshed specialness in patients. Specialness is attained at the cost of feeling helpless and, as with the preoccupied individuals, inability to function independently of the caregiving institution. In contrast to this, institutions may re-create a psychological environment which is cold, neglectful and depriving, and which mirrors the early world of the dismissive patient. Environments such as this augment the already established expectation that it is safer to settle for emotional self-sufficiency than risk seeking a difficult to establish form of emotional intimacy.

CAT, parallel behaviours, and the child sexual offender

Is it around an understanding of the interface of attachment issues, the patient, the therapist and the treating institution that CAT has a role to play in facilitating the treatment of the child sexual offender?

Attachment ideas have been developed within the CAT world largely through the work of Jellema (1999; 2000; 2001). The idea of attachment states as internal working models that predict future, interactive patterns bears many similarities to CAT theory, and Jellema (1999) has attempted to illustrate how attachment theory might inform CAT theory and practice. A central feature of her argument is that attachment states can be equated with Ryle's concepts of self-states and reciprocal roles. Jellema argues that modern attachment theory regards attachment as a form of active, internalised, aim-driven strategy to regulate intersubjectivity. 'Although patterns of attachment can be described as "states", increasingly working models of attachment have been conceptualized as structured processes or active strategies, rather than as static representations' (Jellema, 2000; p. 143).

Drawing upon her own clinical work, Jellema (2000) argues that the nature of the attachment style may determine the characteristics of the RRPs. For example, predominantly dismissing patients, who exhibit a 'think, not feel' attachment style, may enact reciprocal roles that provoke relatively little emotion. By contrast, the 'feel, not think' style of the ambivalent, preoccupied patient may be associated with RRPs too full of emotion. According to Jellema (2001), this has significant implications for therapeutic action. Firstly, dismissing patients need the opportunity in therapy to access warded-off affect or what in CAT theory has been variously described as either chronically endured or core pain. By contrast, the preoccupied patient requires a psychological structure, provided in CAT by an elaboration of the procedural sequence, as an escape from feeling too much but thinking too little.

Integrating these ideas with some of the concepts that we considered earlier, we will proceed to argue the following. Firstly, child sexual offenders admitted to secure institutions may exhibit particular attachment styles that can be represented by CAT tools such as sequential diagrammatic reformulation (SDR) and the self-states sequential diagram (SSSD). Secondly, the attachment strategies of the offender interact with the aspects or characteristics of the institution in potentially negative as well as positive ways. For example, cold, rejecting institutions may exacerbate avoidant, dismissive behaviour, whereas an institution that provides containment has the potential to act as the secure base that helps repair insecure styles of attachment. Thirdly, the offence patterns of child sexual offenders can be considered, *inter alia*, as serving an interpsychic, attachment-related function, and while, in most cases, the secure institution may remove the means of directly repeating the offence, there may be 'parallel behaviours' that can be identified and mapped with the SDR. Finally, the identification and accurate mapping of such processes may help both the offender and professional staff. The following case example illustrates these points.

Case study 1: Martin

Martin, aged 48, had spent 10 years in secure psychiatric hospitals. He was originally sentenced to 8 years in prison for indecent assault of his 9-year-old niece, pleading guilty to a specimen charge. Six years before the offences against his niece, Martin had served 4 years in prison for the attempted abduction of a 10-year-old girl. A passer-by had prevented Martin from dragging her into his car. Martin's interest in young girls had made him known to the police, and he was arrested soon after from the passer-by's description.

Martin had had little to do with his sister, the victim's mother, until he re-established contact with her on his release from prison. As a single parent, she had been grateful for Martin's help with raising her daughter. Often he would mind the child and take her out for the day. His sister described him as 'like a father to her . . . generous and devoted'. His readiness to spend evenings minding her daughter and the occasional sleepovers at his flat and overnight trips to the seaside allowed her some freedom in her social life. Later in hospital, in the early stages of a sex offender treatment programme, Martin described this time in his life. He spoke about his love for his niece and how meeting her was 'a dream come true for me . . . I'd always dreamed of meeting someone like that'. The language he used to describe their contact was significant; always benign, it contained much of the vocabulary associated with adult romantic and sexual relationships. He spoke of, 'attraction', 'beauty', 'dates', 'lovemaking' and of 'planning our lives together'.

Martin's abuse of his niece came to light abruptly. She was picked up by a police patrol car in the early hours of the morning near a seaside bed-and-breakfast where Martin had booked them in as father and daughter. She was highly distressed and had injuries that were consistent with sexual assault, binding of her wrists and whipping with a belt. Over the next 2 weeks, the child described her contact with Martin, using the same language and connotations as he later did, and also describing the collusive sense of secrecy he engendered with her. Her description of her final contact with him was different. During their evening meal, in a restaurant, she had talked about a boy in her class at school whom she liked and how her friends had been teasing her about his being her 'boyfriend'. She described how Martin's mood had changed at that moment. He looked 'fierce', and she described how they left the restaurant without finishing their meal. The child described the walk back to the bed-and-breakfast with Martin dragging her, hurting her and saying things, only a fraction of which she understood. He called her names and accused her of 'betraying their love'. This continued back at their room. The hotel owner had knocked at their room door but had been reassured by Martin's apologies and excuses. The girl had asked to be taken home, but this again intensified Martin's anger and violence toward her, resulting in the further injuries found. The girl had waited until Martin fell asleep, and then slipped out into the street.

During the course of Martin's stay in secure hospitals, a number of issues from his own childhood came to light. His parents had been emotionally cold and rejecting of him. He recalled frequent, violent arguments, his father often accusing his mother of infidelity. Martin would frequently cling to his younger sister at these distressing times and recalled being reassured by fantasies of their running away and being adopted into a 'happy' family. Eventually, his mother did leave, taking his sister, to live with another man. Martin remained with his father for several years until he was arrested for breaking into a neighbour's home via their 8-year-old daughter's bedroom window. This was his second similar offence of 'burglary', and he was put into Social Services secure care until he was 19. He described being sexually abused by adult carers and engaging in sexual activity with peers during this time.

In hospital, a number of events came to light that were seen as relevant to Martin's overall psychopathology and offending behaviour patterns. Many staff found him affable, usually polite and unlikely to display antiauthoritarian attitudes or behaviour. Partly because of this, his peers, among whom he had few close friends, generally disliked him. Staff would often chat with him. Some felt uneasy about his interest in their family lives while others saw his interest as benign, being also impressed by his memory of details that they had 'let slip'. Several staff would gratefully borrow the latest video releases of children's movies from him, as he always ensured that he received an early, preordered copy. This all came to an abrupt end one day when a rather embarrassed staff member brought one of these tapes to the attention of the clinical team. Martin had managed to record a 'personal' audio message onto the end of the videotape. It addressed the staff member's 7-year-old daughter by name and suggested that she might write to him in the hospital, since they 'both liked the same things . . . and would get on really well'.

There was an internal investigation into the matter. Martin cooperated fully, detailing the small gifts he had given staff for their children and revealing a considerable knowledge of the ages, likes and dislikes of several of the children, although he continued to describe those staff as 'the proper nurses . . . ones that know how to care'. This was a theme that emerged as Martin began to express resentment of the hospital often in respect of his no longer having contact with those staff whose boundaries had been breached. From then on, most staff, particularly those with small children, became wary of Martin. However, his old behaviours occasionally re-emerged. Although a question such as 'Your daughter likes horses, doesn't she?' was now likely to prompt a room search, checking of his videotapes and lengthy interviews about his knowledge of that and other staff's private lives. There were three such incidences in a 2-year period. In two of those cases, Martin also made complaints about the staff concerned; one complaint alleged that the staff member was sexually abusing his child. Martin's keen interest in the staff also led to his learning of other aspects of their personal lives. He became fixated on one young woman nurse, having learnt that her marriage had broken up and that she was now living with a male nurse who had reported one of Martin's attempts to glean information. Martin could barely contain his contempt for her, derogatory notices placed on public noticeboards were attributed to him, and over 4 months he made three formal complaints, in one instance accusing her of sleeping with 'all the male staff'.

During this time of his patient career, Martin had found it difficult to engage in any form of therapy. There had been little evidence of his being able to engage in a straightforward and open therapeutic alliance. Two dominant patterns emerged. In the first pattern, particularly in the early stages of therapy, many therapists reported encountering an affable side of Martin that also appeared to be linked to a suspicion that he wished either to push or cross boundaries. As with nursing staff, this process was reflected in Martin's inquisitiveness about the therapist's private life. The second pattern was enacted with professionals who sought to maintain those boundaries. Here, Martin would invariably seek to terminate therapy, citing a 'lack of trust' or clash of personalities. Not being able to work with him for more than a few sessions became something of an accepted fact for Martin's clinical team. Therefore, Martin ran the risk of being regarded as an 'untreatable psychopath', somebody to be endured and about whom professional staff must be very wary.

A CAT perspective informed by attachment theory offers a number of possible ways of thinking about Martin. In Jellema's (2000) idea of attachment style as a strategy or dimension, rather than a category, Martin appears to fall somewhere within the ambivalent or preoccupied dimension. This is illustrated by his apparent desire to form an overly close or fused relationship with an attachment figure (e.g. his victim, certain nurses and certain therapists). He gains a sense of equilibrium through the attainment of this closeness. However, this always seems to be precarious, so that he must either be highly controlling with the attachment object or hold in abeyance weapons that he can use upon those who he anticipates will betray him (e.g. the list of nurses who have received gifts from him). Furthermore, when the attachment relationship is directly threatened or blocked, he responds with rage (e.g. the attack on his child victim after her comments about a boyfriend, his dismissal of therapists who would not disclose personal details to him, his feelings regarding the cohabiting female nurse).

Initially, one response from the staff group – 'the proper nurses' – is to enter unwittingly into a collusive, entangled, ideal-care-type relationship in which there is erosion of the professional boundaries. The lending and borrowing of the children's videos best illustrate this pattern. When this need for perfect care is not requited, Martin angrily rejects those clinicians that refuse to engage with him in a more personalised way. Here Martin justifies his rejection of the more boundaried therapists on the grounds of lack of trust. In turn, this pattern of rejection becomes rigidified into a particular attitude toward him, so that it becomes 'accepted' or 'natural' to think of Martin as a patient who will not or cannot engage in psychological therapy.

Ultimately, Martin's attachment strategies are self-defeating: incarcerated in a secure hospital, he finds himself a pariah among his peer group and avoided by professional staff, a pattern that reconnects him with the primary experience of abandonment. The staff response to Martin – unboundaried closeness followed by a pattern of withdrawal and distancing – suggests an unwitting collusion with these patterns. Some of these processes can be represented in his SDR (Fig. 4.1)

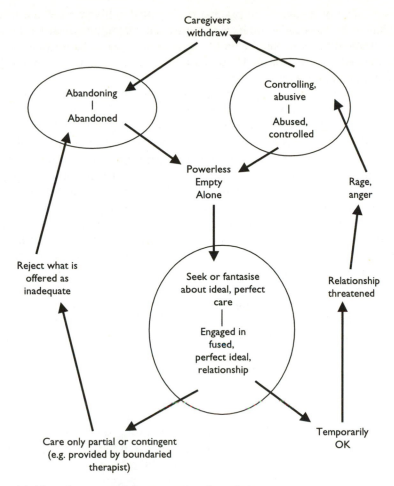

Figure 4.1 Martin's sequential diagrammatic reformulation.

Case study 2: Tom

At the age of 28, Tom had been convicted of two sexual offences against two male children, neither of whom was known to him at the time. The offences took place 6 months apart. On each occasion, he had offered money and sweets to the boys, whom he had met in amusement arcades, and persuaded them to go with him to a deserted piece of land some distance from the arcade. During the sexual assault, he beat the boys severely with a large piece of wood. In the second offence, he was disturbed by a passer-by, and the police reported that he would probably have killed the child had the interruption not taken place. He was later identified by both of his victims and given an 8-year sentence. After 10 months in prison, he began to cut his arms, and an assessment by a consultant psychiatrist resulted in his transfer to a special hospital, as he was deemed to have an antisocial personality disorder. During his 11 years at the hospital, he had been compliant with the hospital regime and attended work regularly. He had attended a social skills group and had been in individual therapy for 2 years.

Reports of his commitment and motivation to 'move on' were supported by the clinical team, who were largely in favour of his transfer to conditions of less security. It was reported that he was engaging well with staff on the ward and in the workshop, and he had been given extra responsibility by being placed in positions of trust. For Tom's transfer to be facilitated, it was agreed that he should engage in an offence-focused group treatment programme. This process included the administration of a number of formal assessments and clinical interviews. Tom's scores on one of the assessments indicated that he was overcontrolled and lacking in insight, had considerable difficulty in admitting to personal weakness and wished to present himself in a positive light. His unwillingness to admit to normal sexual interests suggested that he wished to portray himself as asexual and was 'faking good'.

His participation in one group treatment programme alerted the therapists to his continued avoidance of responsibility for his offending. Specifically, he spent much of the group sessions discussing matters relating to the hospital rather than his offending. On a number of occasions, he 'lost' or 'forgot' materials provided during the treatment programme. He continued to 'perform' well outside the group and was always polite and courteous to other members and staff in the treatment setting. His apparent motivation to ensure that what he said was socially acceptable led the group facilitators to conclude that he was unable to engage in the group sex offender treatment programme. Significantly, the clinical team appeared 'disappointed' with this setback, as he had appeared to be such a 'model' patient.

A vital clue to the origins of his apparent acquiescence lay in his relationship with his father. After his parents' separation when he was aged 4, Tom had been brought up by his father. His father had parented Tom rather erratically: his provision of care and attention was inconsistent and was punctuated by bouts of violence provoked by Tom's failure to meet his father's unrealistic expectations of how a young boy should behave. This seemed to contribute to Tom's trying to placate his father while privately suppressing the rage and humiliation for the neglect and abuse that he had suffered. These difficulties were further compounded by the clear disregard for Tom's needs. Tom reported that he had been sexually abused by his father's brother and endeavoured to stop the abuse by informing his father. His father responded by severely beating him and accusing him of attention-seeking behaviour. These experiences, together with the attendant feelings of insecurity, seemed to increase the likelihood that Tom would develop problems in learning the appropriate expression of emotion.

Overall, Tom's pattern of interpersonal behaviour was indicative of an insecure-avoidant or dismissing style of attachment. His internalised, early reciprocal roles were characterised by abusive, unacknowledging adults in relation to a child who is abused, victimised and overlooked. Tom appeared partially to dissociate himself from the adverse emotional consequences of these roles by developing subsequent self-states characterised by, on the one hand, suppression and emotional blankness and, on the other hand, by placation and compliance. These latter states represent an attempt to reduce pain and disappointment by keeping others at a safe distance.

Within the special hospital, Tom appeared to get by predominantly on the basis of being the compliant 'model' patient. This allowed some contact with other people but always in a way that Tom could control. Crucially, Tom's more difficult feelings of hatred and humiliation were kept separate, perhaps for fear that he would be unable or unwilling to contain those feelings. This pattern of avoidance is also illustrated by the way in which Tom refrained, whenever possible, from discussing elements of his history, which, he anticipated, would inevitably arouse strong feelings. An aspect of his behaviour which did alert staff to some underlying aggression was the discovery that he had been interfering with other people's belongings on the ward and damaging them. This covert expression of anger highlighted his inability to express feelings in a direct way.

It seems likely that Tom's response to the sex offender treatment group was largely influenced by these avoidant, dismissing strategies. His transference to the group was that of a potentially vulnerable, unacknowledged child to a potentially abusive and un-containing parent. In response to the threat posed by the abusive, rejecting, 'parent', group, he seemed to have sought refuge in the cut-off and compliant states. These patterns are represented in diagram form in Fig. 4.2.

CAT and the 'hard-to-help' child sexual offender

While we acknowledge the value of cognitive-behavioural group approaches in the treatment of the child sexual offender, it does appear that the format of the group in which Tom participated did not allow for a comprehensive analysis of his behaviour in the group and the institution as a whole. Nor did it allow for an analysis of the responses of staff to Tom and how they might be reinforcing his position of 'faking good' through their recognition of his conforming behaviour on the ward. Perhaps there is a role for CAT formulation as a means of mapping out the types of interpersonal patterns of behaviour that interfere with the patient's capacity to engage in offence-focused treatment. In the cases of both Martin and Tom, the diagram may have provided a communicable means of establishing a more frank consideration of the split between their earlier abused, neglected states and the subsequent, defensively derived, either enmeshed or avoidant states. Perhaps the

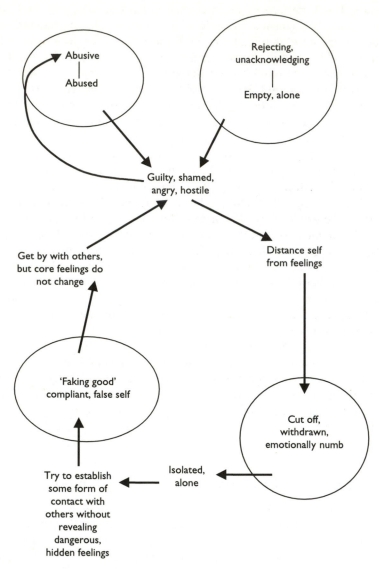

Figure 4.2 Tom's sequential diagrammatic reformulation.

potential for collusive involvement in the reenactment of these states within the institution might be reduced if all parties – the patient, and nursing, medical and therapy staff – could have been engaged, firstly, in thinking about and recognising what was happening; secondly, in thinking about the consequences of what was happening; and, thirdly, in jointly exploring alternative courses of action.

The absence of statistical data means that it is difficult to argue emphatic-ally that these case studies described are representative of a particular type of child sexual offender within secure forensic settings within the UK. In our experience, however, these people do seem to form a significant proportion of offenders who are admitted but then drift to the margins of forensic hos-pitals, often attracting such terms of opprobrium as 'untreatable psycho-path'. We would argue that, to some extent, the characteristics of this group are similar to those that Gorsuch (1999) described in a small-scale study of women who had found difficulty in gaining access to NHS secure facilities. By combining analysis of case histories and psychometric assessment, Gorsuch identified an interpersonal style dominated by a conflict between the desire for and the avoidance of intimacy and caregiving. Elsewhere, Ryle & Kerr (2002) and Dunn & Parry (1997) have all identified this pattern of both wanting and either rejecting or attacking help as being characteristic of a hard-to-help group of patients who arouse powerful and complementary reactions on the part of professional staff.

In the cases that we have discussed, we have argued that these conflicts take shape in the context of attachment difficulties. Taking into account both the potential which admission to a secure hospital has for activating attachment systems and the apparent prevalence of attachment difficulties within the child sexual offender population, we should not be surprised at the enactment of toxic forms of attachment. Knowledge of how the work task can be affected by the difficult dynamics that may prevail within the hospital environment in general (Menzies Lyth, 1988) and within secure forensic hospitals in particu-lar (Cox, 1996) should further diminish our sense of surprise when these enactments occur.

We would not wish to argue that problems encountered in the institutional treatment and management of the hard-to-help child sexual offender are always entirely predictable. However, taking into account the patient's attachment history and the idea of attachment style as relatively enduring, internal work-ing models that predict future, interactive patterns, perhaps an educated guess could be made at an early stage in the patient's hospital career as to some of the broad possibilities of future interpersonal conduct. With greater understanding of the patient, this could then be refined and formalised into an SDR or SSSD that might, in turn, form the basis of a process-oriented care plan.

Kerr (1999) has argued that, when implemented within a therapeutic com-munity, the CAT model has the potential to provide the conceptual frame-work and 'common house-language' to help frame and contain high levels of psychological disturbance. The application of CAT, which we have described here, proposes something similar. More specifically, we have suggested that the diagrammatic reformulation of the child sexual offender, informed by an understanding of attachment theory, might be used to predict the potential for problematic forms of interpersonal behaviour; that an understanding of this behaviour reduces the possibility of a collusive or inappropriate professional response and may eventually lead to a more secure, engaged relationship between the offender and the institution; and that this approach has further salience, as it helps develop or repair deficits in secure, interpersonal relating.

References

Abel, G. G., Becker, J. V. & Skinner, L. (1983). Behavioural approaches to the treatment of the violent person. In L. Roth (Ed.), *Clinical treatment of the violent offender* (pp. 46–63). Washington, DC: NIMH Monograph Series.

Abel, G. G., Blanchard, E. B. & Becker, J. V. (1978). An integrated treatment programme for rapists. In R. Rada (Ed.), *Clinical aspects of the rapist* (pp. 161–214). New York: Grune & Stratton.

Abel, G. G., Osborn, C. A., Anthony, D. & Gardos, P. (1992). Current treatment of paraphiliacs. *Annual Review of Sex Research, 3*, 255–290.

Adshead, G. (1998). Psychiatric staff as attachment figures. *British Journal of Psychiatry, 172*, 64–69.

Adshead, G. (2004). Three degrees of security: attachment and forensic institutions. In F. Pfäfflin & G. Adshead (Eds), *A matter of security: The application of attachment theory to forensic psychiatry and psychotherapy*. London: Jessica Kingsley.

Ainsworth, M., Blehar, M., Waters, E. & Wall, S. (1978). *Patterns of attachment: Assessed in the strange situation and at home*. Hillsdale, NJ: Erlbaum.

Bowlby, J. (1969). *Attachment and loss* (vol. 1). London: Hogarth Press.

Bowlby, J. (1988). *A secure base: Clinical applications of attachment theory*. London: Routledge.

Bumby, K. M. & Hansen, D. J. (1997). Intimacy deficits, fear of intimacy and loneliness among sex offenders. *Criminal Justice and Behaviour, 24*, 315–331.

Coid, J. (1992). DSM-III diagnoses in criminal psychopaths. *Criminal Behaviour and Mental Health, 2*, 78–95.

Cordess, C., Riley, W., Welldon, E. (1994). Psychodynamic forensic psychotherapy: An account of a day-release course. *Psychiatric Bulletin, 18*, 88–90.

Cordess, C. & Cox, M. (Eds) (1996). *Forensic psychiatry: Crime, psychodynamics and the offender patient*. London: Jessica Kingsley.

Cox, M. (1996). *Psychodynamics and the Special Hospital: 'Road blocks and thought blocks'*. In C. Cordess & M. Cox (Eds), *Forensic psychotherapy: Crime, psychodynamics and the offender patient*. London: Jessica Kingsley.

Dalenberg, C. J. (2000). *Countertransference and the treatment of trauma*. Washington, DC: American Psychological Association.

Dunn, M. & Parry, G. D. (1997). A formulated care plan approach to caring for borderline personality disorder in a community mental health team. *Clinical Psychology Forum, 104*, 19–22.

Figley, C. R. (1999). Compassion fatigue: Toward a new understanding of the costs of caring. In B. H. Stamm (Ed.), *Secondary traumatic stress. Self-care issues for clinicians, researchers and educators* (2nd edn). Baltimore, MD: Sidran Press.

Finkelhor, D. (1984). *Child sexual abuse: New theory and research*. New York: Free Press.

Freud, S. (1957). Some character types met in psychoanalytical work. *Standard edition* (vol. 14). London: Hogarth Press.

Freudenberger, H. & Robbins, A. (1979). The hazard of being a psychoanalyst. *Psychoanalytic Review, 66*, 275–296.

Glasser, M. (1979). Some aspects of the role of aggression in the perversions. In I. Rosen (Ed.), *Sexual deviations*. Oxford: Oxford University Press.

Glasser, M. (1988). Psychodynamic aspects of paedophilia. *Psychoanalytic Psychotherapy, 3*, 121–135.

Glasser, M. (1990). Paedophilia. In R. Bluglass & M. Bowden (Eds), *Principles and practice of forensic psychiatry*. Edinburgh: Churchill Livingstone.

Gorsuch, N. (1999). Disturbed female offenders: Helping the 'untreatable'. *Journal of Forensic Psychiatry, 10*, 98–118.

Hall, G. C. N. (1995). Sexual offender recidivism revisited: A meta-analysis of recent treatment studies. *Journal of Consulting and Clinical Psychology, 63*, 802–809.

Hall, G. C. N. & Hirschman, R. (1991). Toward a theory of sexual aggression: A quadripartite model. *Journal of Consulting and Clinical Psychology, 59*, 662–669.

Harlow, H. (1958). The nature of love. *American Psychologist, 13*, 673–685.

Holmes, J. (1993). Attachment theory: A biological basis for psychotherapy? *British Journal of Psychiatry, 163*, 430–438.

Holmes, J. & Lindley, R. (1989). *The values of psychotherapy*. Oxford: Oxford University Press.

Jellema, A. (1999). Cognitive Analytic Therapy: Developing its theory and practice via attachment theory. *Clinical Psychology and Psychotherapy, 6*, 16–28.

Jellema, A. (2000). Insecure attachment states: Their relationship to borderline and narcissistic personality disorder and treatment process in Cognitive Analytic Therapy. *Clinical Psychology and Psychotherapy, 7*, 138–154.

Jellema, A. (2001). Dismissing and preoccupied insecure attachment and procedures in CAT: Some implications for CAT practice. *Clinical Psychology and Psychotherapy, 9*, 225–241.

Kerr, I. (1999). Cognitive Analytic Therapy for borderline personality disorder in the context of a community mental health team: Individual and organisational psychodynamic implications. *British Journal of Psychotherapy, 15*, 425–438.

Laws, D. R. & Marshall, W. L. (2003). A brief history of cognitive behavioural approaches to sexual offender treatment: Part 1. *Sexual Abuse: Journal of Research and Treatment, 15*, 75–92.

Main, M. & Goldwyn, R. (1994). Adult attachment scoring and classification systems. Version 6.0 (unpublished). London: University College London.

Malamuth, N., Heavey, C. & Linz, D. (1993). Predicting men's antisocial behavior against women: The interaction model of sexual aggression. In G. Hall, R. Hirschman, J. Graham & M. Zaragoza (Eds), *Sexual aggression: Issues in etiology and assessment, treatment and policy* (pp. 63–97). New York: Hemisphere.

Malamuth, N., Sockloskie, R., Koss, M. & Tanaka, J. (1991). The characteristics of aggressors against women: Testing a model using a national sample of college students. *Journal of Consulting and Clinical Psychology, 59*, 670–681.

Marques, J. K. (1982). Relapse prevention: A self-control model for the treatment of sex offenders. Paper presented at the 7th Annual Forensic Mental Health Conference, Asilomar, CA, March.

Marques, J. K. (1984). *An innovative treatment program for sex offenders: Report to the legislature*. Sacramento, CA: California Department of Mental Health.

Marshall, W. L. (1993). The role of attachments, intimacy and loneliness in the etiology and maintenance of sexual offending. *Sexual and Marital Therapy*, 8, 109–121.

Marshall, W. L. & Barbaree, H. E. (1990). An integrated theory of the etiology of sexual offending. In W. L. Marshall, D. R. Laws & H. E. Barbaree (Eds), *Handbook of sexual assault: Issues, theories, and treatment of the offender*. New York: Plenum.

Marshall, W. L., Champagne, F., Brown, C. & Miller, S. (1997). Empathy, intimacy, loneliness and self-esteem in non-familial child molesters. *Journal of Child Sexual Abuse*, 6, 87–97.

McCann, I. L. & Pearlman, L. A. (1990). Vicarious traumatization: A framework for understanding the psychological effects of working with victims. *Journal of Traumatic Stress*, 3, 131–149.

McConaghy, N. (1989). Validity and ethics of penile circumference measures of sexual arousal: A critical review. *Archives of Sexual Behavior*, 18, 357–367.

Menzies Lyth, I. (1988). *Containing anxiety in institutions: Selected essays, Volume 1*. London: Free Association Books.

Noffsinger, S. G. & Resnick, P. J. (2000). Sexual predator laws and offenders with addictions. *Psychiatric Annals*, 30, 602–608.

Ragsdale, I. B. (2002). Assessing treatment completion of adult male sex offenders: One approach. *Dissertation Abstracts International: Section B: The Sciences and Engineering*. Vol. 63(5-B).

Ryle, A. & Kerr, I. B. (2002). *Introducing Cognitive Analytic Therapy: Principles and practice*. Chichester: Wiley.

Schaap, C., Bennun, I., Schindler, L. & Hoodguin, K. (1993). *The therapeutic relationship in behavioural psychotherapy*. New York: Wiley.

Stoller, I. (1986). *Perversion: The erotic form of hatred*. London: Maresfield.

Van Ijzendoorn, M., Feldbrugge, J., Derks, F., De Ruiter, C., Verhagen, M., Philipse, M., van der Staak, C. & Riksen Walraven, J. (1997). Attachment representations of personality disordered criminal offenders. *American Journal of Orthopsychiatry*, 67, 449–459.

Ward, T. & Siegert, R. (2002). Toward a comprehensive theory of child sexual abuse: A theory knitting perspective. *Psychology, Crime, and Law*, 9, 319–351.

Welldon, E. (1998). The practical approach. In E. Welldon & C. Van Velsen (Eds), *A practical guide to forensic psychotherapy*. London: Jessica Kingsley.

Welldon, E. & Van Velsen, C. (Eds) (1998). *A practical guide to forensic psychotherapy*. London: Jessica Kingsley.

Wood, H. (2003). Psychoanalytic theories of perversion reformulated. *Reformulation*, 19, 26–32.

Chapter 5

Stifled fantasies and the stalker's obsessions:

Cognitive Analytic Therapy for a misguided lover

Philip H. Pollock

Dan was genuinely perplexed and exasperated at the events of the past few hours. Police had arrived at his suburban, upper-class home and arrested him for the harassment of a female work colleague, transporting him to the police station for questioning. The public ignominy of the arrest at his home served only to compound the ludicrous nature of the alleged charges for Dan. He felt angry indignation and appeared outwardly shocked to the arresting police officers. Dan was interviewed in a holding cell by the assessing clinical psychologist because of police concerns about his mental state, muddled and incoherent answers to questions and transient temper outbursts, during which he expressed his disgust about his treatment and claimed to be the victim of a sectarian conspiracy by the state. He presented to the police as a clean-shaven, immaculately dressed, verbally articulate man whose dramatic and histrionic outbursts were very convincing as responses of a man who felt wrongly accused. He had an injury to his left forehead and eye, suggesting that had been physically assaulted recently. Dan was bailed that evening after psychological assessment and three, short police interviews, during which he repeatedly declared his innocence and vexation at the nature of the charges against him. The charges were pursued because of the strength of the evidence against Dan. He was not permitted to enter his workplace as condition of bail or to approach the alleged victim.

Dan had been referred for court report as a plea in mitigation to the harassment and stalking charges made by a married, 42-year-old female work colleague, who claimed that he had instigated a determined, persistent and frightening campaign of harassment over a 1-year period. The campaign consisted of unwanted following after work, circumstantial encounters at the local gymnasium, intrusive messaging (leaving apparently graphically sexual, written messages at the victim's workstation, and sending e-mails with sexual content) and 'gossip' within the workplace that Dan and the victim had an intense sexual relationship. The police had become involved after a confrontation between the alleged victim's husband and Dan at a shop near the victim's home. An altercation had developed when the victim spotted Dan in the shop and informed her husband of Dan's presence. The husband had confronted Dan, grappled with him and punched him several times, causing the facial injuries. Dan had run away from the situation without returning any defensive blows. The police arrested him 2 hours later.

Four weeks later, the meeting with Dan revealed a dishevelled, unkempt man who sat at a sideways angle to the assessor with poor eye contact. He slumped in the chair with minimal interaction and little verbal exchange. Dan commented about paintings on the consulting room walls, deflecting any conversation about the charges, and exhibiting facial tics and excessive blinking. The assessor was concerned about Dan's reality testing, his evasive, incoherent thinking, and his repeated distraction to irrelevant topics in vague and disjointed conversation. At interview, he displayed a number of mannerisms and whistles which did not conform to his work persona. At this time, he was non-compliant with medication prescribed by his general practitioner and during the weeks after his arrest, Dan's psychological state and functioning had deteriorated significantly. Dan's general practitioner had debated admission to psychiatric hospital but put off this decision until the psycholegal consultation. Dan was hospitalised at the assessor's request in view of his presentation and mental state. He was evaluated 10 days later in a much improved state and subsequently discharged.

Dan held a prominent position in a sales company and supervised over 20 staff and a central process in production at a local factory. He was known for his respect for others, self-discipline and dedication to work, and for his introversion, which was occasionally misconstrued as arrogance and aloofness. Dan lived alone in a respectable area of the city and had not come to the attention of the police or courts for criminal activities before this offence. Dan's views of the incidents were at variance with the victim's accounts. He claimed that he and the victim had had an affair during a work-initiated, team-building weekend. Their encounter was described by Dan as a romantic 'dream' for him during the 3 days they spent together. He claimed that his memories of their encounter were of a perfect fusion and 'being in a romantic haze, all sex and bliss'. Dan portrayed them as having been entwined in a sexual romance, which was idealised and cherished by him ever since it had occurred many months previously. On return from the weekend, Dan recalled being 'stung' by his colleague's matter-of-fact, cold and distanced attitude to their encounter. She refused to discuss the weekend or their future relationship with Dan except to state, 'You caught me at a bad time – I feel you took advantage of my vulnerability.' Dan felt rejected, confused, angry, embittered, shocked and baffled. Dan believed that 'we had a wonderful time. She sort of stained it by her attitudes afterwards. We were locked together for 3 whole days, and then she broke my heart by being so callous. She pulled the rug from under my feet. I got dropped like a bad habit from a real height.' Dan's hurt and confusion transformed into anger against his colleague for her disengagement, her dismissal of the importance of their encounter and her implication that he had taken advantage of her. Dan's emotional investment in the relationship was significant, and he reported feeling that she had 'stolen something from me. It wasn't justified what she did, I felt she owed me. There was a debt of love there. I thought that she had been brainwashed by someone into thinking differently about us – she just cut me off.' Dan felt his thinking about his colleague becoming more and more preoccupied, and he developed ideas that she had been 'taken away' from him. He did not want to believe she was conniving and calculating, or that she may have used him. Dan spoke of her as 'angelic, the way she looked at me, she could've been in the movies. She had a special something that I was privy to, I was privileged to be allowed to experience it.' It was felt that Dan continued to sustain a romantic vision of the relationship, despite the unfolding realities of his arrest and its consequences.

Case history

Dan was the only child of an emotionally absent father, a police detective, and an overinvolved mother who appeared to have overindulged him throughout his development. His earliest memories were of being in the presence of his mother and maternal grandmother, recalling the fondness and sense of security he felt with them. Dan offered that he had been a timid child and had found it difficult to initiate and maintain friendships, being viewed at school as an 'odd child' by teachers. He was dependent upon these two 'strong' women for company and remembered instances where he felt 'stupid because of the things I couldn't do. We'd go swimming at school, and I didn't know even how to tie my shoelaces. I had to ask the teacher. I remember teachers calling me names and being annoyed at me.' Dan experienced nervous tics and his mannerisms were the brunt of other children's jokes, Dan feeling ostracised and alone. He stated, 'I didn't fit in – I was a mummy's boy, I suppose.' His father was a 'man's man' and was disappointed in his son's lack of masculine assertiveness. Dan felt ill-equipped for life outside the family home and reflected on his father's disgust that his son was weak, not interested in sports and clinging to his mother.

Sexual interests or development were taboo topics within the household and never discussed openly. Dan recalled that his first sexual encounter had been at 14 with his similarly aged female cousin, which he described as 'occasional fumblings when I saw her. It was an unspoken kind of thing. We'd get to be alone, say, in the family caravan, and do things. I don't think we really knew what we were doing.' After episodic contact over 2 years, his cousin refused to continue these encounters, which Dan would anticipate with excitement and fantasise about for days beforehand. Dan referred to his sense of disappointment and 'empty rage in my stomach – I felt physically sick' after her rejection of his advances the last time they met. He stated, 'that was the first time I was ever really angry at a woman.' Dan claimed that he controlled any sexual urges or interests thereafter as rigidly as he could because of the painful anguish and frustration he experienced at his cousin's decision.

Throughout his adolescence, Dan was afflicted with severe facial acne, and his contact with females and involvement in social encounters were restricted because of his sense of embarrassment and sensitivity to comments by others. Dan felt self-conscious, socially avoidant and victimised by the acne. He invested his energies into solitary hillwalking and study for his career. By the age of 24, Dan continued to live with his parents and grandmother and had not embarked on an independent life in any domain except the workplace, where he was considered a fastidious, conscientious, dutiful and loyal employee. Describing his personality, Dan stated, 'I'm a bit of an anorak, quiet, keep my own counsel, but I knew I was respected at work. They thought highly of me there.' As his parents aged, Dan felt more encumbered by them, his father's retirement from a distinguished police career causing the emergence of conflict within the home, temper outbursts and demanding behaviours by his father.

Dan had never married and had begun to live by himself only at the age of 35. He had not engaged in any adult long-term relationships except a 10-month partnership when he was 23 with a young woman, Sandra, whom he described as religiously devout and 'a cross between Mother Teresa and Lolita on heat'. Dan reported that they parted company in reaction to an incident when Dan had 'spat in the bath. She went crazy, said I was foul, said I was revolting, and she couldn't be with a man who did things like that.' Neither Dan nor his partner attempted to be reconciled after an incident when she 'shut the door in my face when I went to see her. I expected her to be OK about things, but I underestimated how strongly she must've felt about my habits.' He added that this partner acted in sexually provocative ways; he felt that she 'led me on. One minute she was all for it, then she'd come off with religious stuff that meant she couldn't lower herself to have sexual contact with me. I was dangling there like on a piece of string.' As Dan spoke about the sexual aspects of the relationship, he became visibly angry. He commented, 'I was like a puppet for her. She teased me with sex, got me going then shut down. I was frustrated and flaking out.' He did openly declare that he had taken an overdose in a public bar about 1 year after the break-up of the relationship, triggered by being told by a work colleague that Sandra had commenced a relationship with a new partner. Dan left his workplace without informing his colleagues, traced Sandra to the public bar and declared his love for her in front of everyone. He then threatened to take an overdose of analgesic tablets if she did not speak with him. Sandra refused, and Dan felt that he had to make a gesture after his protestations. He swallowed the tablets with alcohol and then contacted the hospital. Dan remarked, 'I felt like a fool, but I would've died for her, for love, if I had to.' He admitted further that, the following year, he had intentionally overdosed on alcohol and his mother's hypertension tablets on Valentine's Day, posting a card to himself beforehand. Dan had not established a relationship or friendship with another woman until the recent sexual harassment.

Dan had no criminal history. He was physically fit without any medical complaints. An electroencephalogram and computerised tomography scan were normal. He had no history of substance abuse and did not consume alcohol or drugs as part of his lifestyle.

When asked about his subjective experiences before the encounter with the victim, Dan stated, 'Things were just going on as normal. I was painfully lonely, I felt that each day I was becoming more and more removed from the world. I couldn't talk to people for about a year, like I was in a bubble. I made a fool of myself when I talked to people, the way they looked at me, as if there was something wrong with me. I knew people didn't like me. If they tried, I'd try; then after a while, it all went sour. I was like a leper.' His contact with his parents had diminished over the past 2 years since their joint entrance into a nursing home (which prompted him to secure his own home). When Dan's father was accused of sexually inappropriate comments and touching nursing staff in the home, Dan claimed to feel confused and sorry that 'a man who put hard-line terrorists in jail as a policeman [was] resorting to that type of thing'. The death of his grandmother several years before had affected his mother's mental health, and he spoke at length about the trauma of his grandmother's sudden death, being found dead in bed. This represented a significant loss for Dan.

Psychological assessment for court

Psychological testing and diagnostic assessment followed, and Dan's profile on the Millon Clinical Multiaxial Inventory–third edition (MCMI–3) (Millon, Millon & Davis, 1994) showed a pattern of schizoid, avoidant, dependent and masochistic scale elevations. His Psychopathy Checklist–Revised (PCL–R) (Hare, 1991) score was minimal. The Thematic Apperception Test (TAT) and Rorschach revealed evidence of constrained emotions with confusion when stressed, a tendency to introspection and a preference for fantasy. Primitive idealisation of others was evident, associated with fantasies of dependency and regression mingled with perceptions of self as weak, vulnerable and exposed to attack. A theme of anticipated disappointment and sadness as the predominant outcome of narratives was noted on TAT stories whereby one character experienced a consuming infatuation with another, suggestive of overfocus on entangled, enmeshed relations. Dan was considered intellectually resourceful, and capable of problem solving with a full-scale IQ in the superior range. Dan was viewed as vulnerable to decompensation in his mental state when stressed.

Dan's offences consisted of the persistent and intrusive harassment and stalking of the victim over an extended period of time. Violence was never threatened and physical assault did not occur.

Types and psychotherapy of stalkers

Dan's case satisfies the criteria of Mullen, Pathé & Purcell (2000) for a type of stalker termed the 'intimacy seeker', given that his intentions were to establish a loving relationship with the object (victim), whom he believed to be uniquely placed to meet his needs and desires, and onto whom he projected special qualities. Dan's actions amounted to pursuit and privacy violations, and not threat or violence (Nicastro & Cousins, 2000), and were mostly indicative of instrumental pursuit and being an 'invader' (Hargreaves, in press) rather than expressive violence. His self-reported fantasies consisted of a dyadic, idealised love for the victim, and he acknowledged an intensity of fantasy verging on preoccupation and obsession about the imagined relationship. One-third of stalkers fulfil Mullen *et al.*'s criteria for intimacy seeking and are thought to represent the most persistent type. The relationship sought is perceived as the 'solution to the central dilemma of their life: that of loneliness and a lack of either emotional or physical closeness to another person. The persistence of their pursuit reflected the centrality that the longed-for relationship had come to occupy in their lives' (Mullen *et al.*, 2000; p. 117). Mullen *et al.* observe that 'the borderline between the banalities of broken hearts and the realms of the pathological is approached when fantasy and self-deception begin to substitute for a lack of response from the beloved' (p. 135). Dan's harassment appeared to be motivated by an intense need to be party to a consuming, loving, idealised relationship, and no signs of aggression or threat toward the victim were expressed in his outward behaviours. His stifled fantasies of blissful love motivated his pursuit of the victim, and his misconstruing of the relationship was evident in his criminal actions.

Literature on the psychotherapy of stalkers, of whatever type, is virtually non-existent. Research reports describing the classification and characteristics of stalkers have proliferated, and cogent systems to define stalkers have been devised. Much of the interest of professionals and law enforcement agencies is on the threat management of these offenders and the effects of their behaviours upon victims. According to Long (1994), when considering the gloomy prognosis of these cases, courts and social policy makers 'should not place much emphasis on psychiatry and other mental health disciplines'. He refers here principally to offenders who exhibit erotomanic delusions. Mentally ill stalkers appear to demonstrate better outcomes, and a variable outcome is noted for pure, personality-based disorders (Mullen & Pathé, 1994). Obviously, questions about insight and motivation to enter treatment and achieve change are significant factors when one contemplates offering intervention. Judgement regarding the value and effectiveness of psychotherapies requires proof.

CAT, attachment and stalking

In terms of treatment, the attachment pathology of stalking cases is a relevant starting point when conceptualising the behaviours of these offenders. Jellema (2002) reviewed the relationship between CAT and attachment theory, highlighting how the expression of anger and the narrative expression of distress differed depending on the attachment pattern detected. The preoccupied attachments of many patients were shown to be associated with certain maladaptive procedures, difficulties in ordering thoughts into narrative accounts, being cut off from the 'true self' with closed or limited dialogue, and difficulties with termination of relationships (i.e. therapy dependency). These features of an insecure attachment pattern were identified in Dan's presentation and history. CAT permits an idiosyncratic appreciation of the attachment exhibited by an individual without imposing classifications upon a case. CAT applies a descriptive explanation of the nature of the RRPs, ways of relating and unrevised cyclical procedures that occur in these types of offences. The persistent and intrusive nature of stalking behaviours requires an analysis of the offender's perceptions of self and others (victims) that account for the self-perpetuating, disordered patterns of relating in these cases.

A study of criminal stalking by Keinlan, Birmingham, Solberg, O'Regan & Meloy (1997) determined that a preoccupied attachment pattern fuelled the obsessional following and harassment seen in many stalkers who had histories of disrupted caregiving backgrounds, childhood loss and traumatic abuse. The pursuit of the victim was conceptualised as inability to resolve and manage grief, and the tendency to vent anger toward victims when relationships were unrequited. It is apparent that attachment disruptions are typical sensitivities in the histories of those who stalk and harass where the behaviours are manifestations of personality dysfunction rather than mental illness.

Only one case of harassment and stalking has been reported to date which applies CAT (Pollock, 2001). This case was that of a female patient who attempted to kill her therapist, and who was successfully treated despite exhibiting borderline erotomania (Meloy, 1989), which is 'an extreme disorder of attachment . . . apparent in the pursuit of, and the potential for violence toward, the unrequited love object' (p. 477). The CAT reformulation identified an underlying preoccupied attachment pattern (Bartholomew & Horowitz, 1991), borderline personality disorder and contrasting RRPs, such as *neglecting/rejecting-to-needly/rejected* and *idealising/saving-to-rescued/dependent*, for the patient. Despite the patient's attempts to kill the therapist, the transference within the therapeutic relationship was managed without irreparable rupture or injury to the therapist. A positive outcome was achieved in this reported case study.

It may be argued that attachment disorder forms the necessary substrate for stalking and obsessional following or persistent pursuit of a victim. Dan exhibited a preoccupied attachment pattern, problems in managing loss of relationships, distorted perceptions of relationships and failure to resolve anger and frustration within these attachments. His self-reflective capacities were limited, and Dan expressed his confusion and bewilderment about his repetitive failures in achieving relationship stability without rejection and his engaging in stalking behaviours. It was decided that CAT would be offered as the therapy of choice for these problems in Dan's case.

CAT with Dan

Dan was given a community disposal by the court and directed to engage in 24 sessions of CAT. At first, Dan voiced his anger that he had been forced to enter therapy and felt that 'you have all got this wrong, I'm the victim in all this'. He did, however, recognise that this offence was only one of several incidents when his attempts to enter a relationship had 'gone badly wrong', and that such events had occurred repetitively with many victims. Dan did state, 'I do want to sort out this confusion, and hopefully I'll get what I want.' Dan appeared, initially, motivated by a desire to understand and modify the self-perpetuating, cyclical patterns of failed encounters with females in order to improve his chances of obtaining the loving relationship he fantasised about, yet had never obtained.

Dan was provided with the Reformulation Letter after completion of the Psychotherapy File, including the self-states grid (Fig. 5.1). The Reformulation Letter provided for Dan was offered as a tentative narrative account of the important events in his life, highlighting what were considered to be important therapy-relevant procedures and patterns which had resulted in his entrance into therapy for the crimes.

The letter was as follows:

Dear Dan,

Here is the letter I said I would provide, describing how you have reached this point and how we can work to move on toward resolving difficulties which have emerged for you lately.

I appreciate that you have not sought therapy by yourself and that, in many respects, you feel that you have been forced to examine your own behaviours and to work with someone because of the recent crimes. You have spoken about your embarrassment, shame and confusion in coming to therapy and for the crimes themselves. I hope that we can work jointly toward identifying and addressing underlying problems that have led to this point. Most of this letter is formed by the discussions we have had about things and my own observations about what we need to focus on within therapy.

You have mentioned that your early years within the family did not equip you for

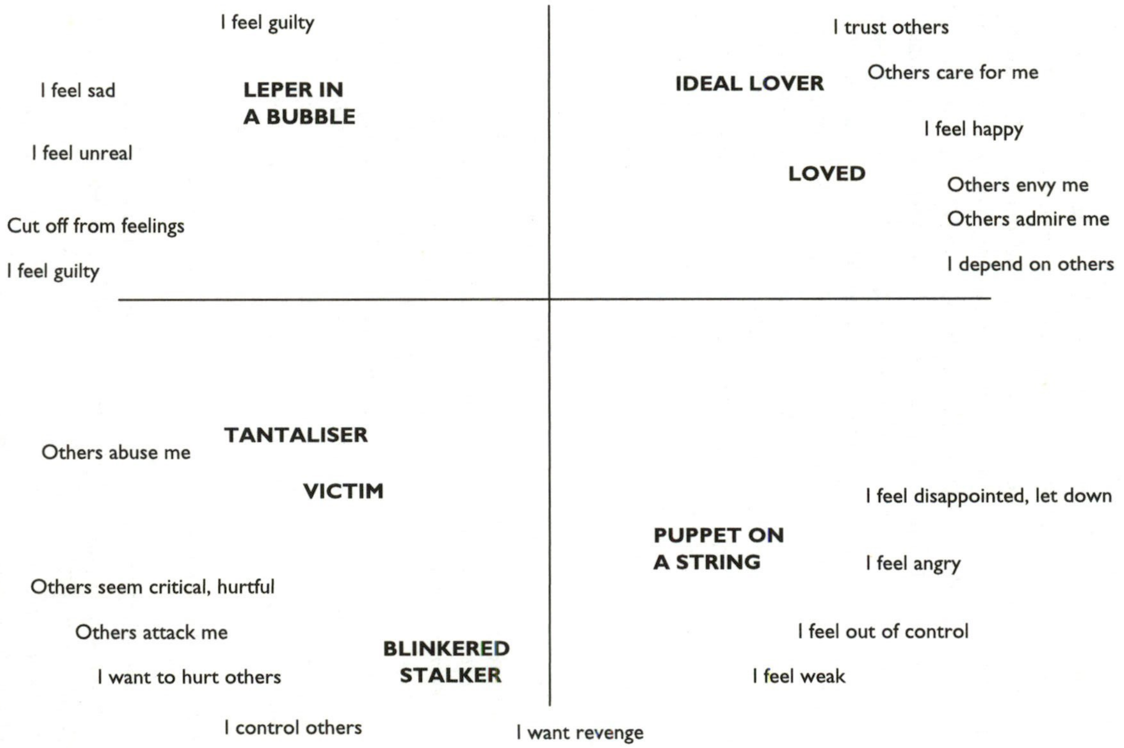

Figure 5.1 Dan's self-states grid.

dealing with the disappointments of the outside world, your mother and grand-mother cosseting you from any harshness or 'falls'. Your father frequently expressed his disappointment at your sensitivity and tender-mindedness, prefer-ring you to be masculine and 'butch'. You felt odd at school and found it difficult to establish peer relationships, describing yourself as left out, isolated and rejected. You believe that depression and loneliness set in during your late adolescence, mostly because of the way acne blighted your self-confidence and caused you to withdraw. You coped through solitary activities and education. These feelings of lacking confidence, inadequacy and being 'ugly' made you more sensitive to rejection, and you recall fantasies of being part of a loving, sexual and engulfing relationship which would 'fix everything'. Your relation-ship with your cousin was your first sexual experience, and you can remember the intense anticipation of contact with her. It appears that her rejection of your advances caused feelings of emptiness, disappointment, loss and depriv-ation. You describe her as 'a tease', and you are able to talk about yet feel scared of the anger you felt toward her. The relationship with Sandra was somewhat similar, and you resented her mixed messages about intimacy, sex and whether you were acceptable. How she acted toward you brought about a way of seeing women as 'teasers' and 'tantalisers', and you felt 'like a puppet on a string'. Driven by the fantasy of a perfect relationship, you have sought contact with women but felt that they have repeatedly taunted and tantalised you for fun. Through these contacts, you have felt used and betrayed, angry and empty once again. You have said that on many occasions you have thought that women who acted as if they liked you would then suddenly rebuff your advances, leaving you confused, empty and angry. You have felt that these rebuffs were 'tests' of your love, and you have followed, pursued and harassed them. When eventually you withdraw from this pursuit, you enter what you called the state of 'being like a leper in a bubble', isolated from others, emotion-ally needy, in grief and loss, angry and depressed. You have coped through investment in work, which has helped your career, yet not substituted for your longings for an ideal partner. After some time, your needs intensify and you begin to fantasise once again about your ideal lover, setting in motion the same, unchanging sequences.

I suggest that we should consider focusing on the following points:

- *exploring the inappropriate pursuit of females that has led to crimes, and helping you to understand the patterns of thinking, feeling and acting which precede these pursuits*
- *your unhelpful ways of seeking the idealised lover and relationship you long for and how these attempts victimise these women; why these attempts 'go wrong' for you*
- *the sequence of changes in the way you perceive women and their teasing and betrayal, the feelings of anger and disappointment which are associated*

with rejections, and how you think about these women and deal with these reactions

- *developing empathy for the victim of the crimes*
- *dealing with past hurt and mourning losses*
- *meeting your needs through more appropriate methods of interacting and developing relationships with women; helping you to avoid either being socially isolated and depressed or inappropriately pursuing women and getting into trouble again.*

The short duration of our therapy time might cause you some anxiety, given that you acknowledge that you have 'high hopes' for therapy and you have felt that you become dependent on and involved with people quickly. We must be aware of the need to explore your feelings about endings and losses in both past relationships and therapy itself.

Dan's self-states grid is shown in Fig. 5.1. The grid does show that Dan's core pain can be located in the 'leper in a bubble' state, whereby he feels guilty, sad, alone and isolated with his needs frustrated. The 'puppet on a string' state is indicative of an angry, disappointed, weak and denigrated self-image with the 'blinkered stalker' wanting revenge, controlling and wanting to hurt others (e.g. the 'victim'). The draft sequential diagrammatic reformulation (SDR) (Fig. 5.2) was presented to Dan and he responded with curiosity. Dan expressed his interest in the offender–victim RRPs and the self-state that he labelled 'puppet on a string' (*betrayed/rejected/used/provoked* pole) in relation to 'tantaliser' (SS1; *deceiving/using/teasing* pole). Dan perceived himself, as the offender, to be a passive, helpless recipient of the victim's connivance, suggesting that he perceived himself to be victimised in the first instance and only retaliating in anger and protest. Dan felt that his own distress was paramount when in the 'puppet on a string' position, and he could not recognise the victim's concerns. He did recognise that his approaches would often be rebuffed, that he would feel spurned and angry (position D, SS1), and that he would then transform this anger by rationalising that the rejection was a test, causing him to believe that he was required to persist in his advances to prove his love (position E, SS2).

In terms of transference issues, dependency and idealisation within the therapeutic relationship were anticipated, and Dan's possible anxieties about abandonment, rejection and dismissal were pre-empted.

Dialogical sequence analysis was conducted after the diagram was agreed. The sequential connection between SS3 and SS1 in the SDR was explored to elucidate the perceptions of self and others shown by Dan within the offender-to-victim RRPs (SS2). Dan stated that the 'puppet on a string' RRP position of SS1 consisted of feelings of betrayal, being used and rejection. He expressed difficulty in thinking about the victim's portrayal in the 'tantaliser' position, but could link this state with past incidents of rejection by women,

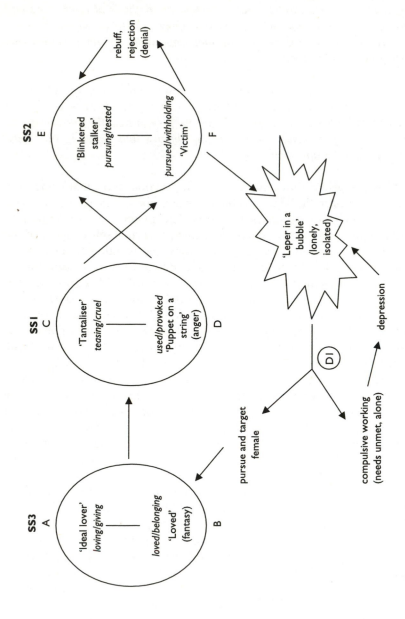

Figure 5.2 Dan's sequential diagrammatic reformulation.

particularly his girlfriend Sandra. It was evident that this relationship had forged a perception of women as teasing, self-righteous and mocking. He was helped to consider the feelings associated with this sense of being 'puppeted'. Dan spoke of the 'voice' he would couple with this position and RRP state, asking, 'How could you do this to me? What's wrong with me? Am I not lovable? Don't I get my needs met?' Dan perceived himself as wounded, inferior and 'left dangling'. The emotional reactions that emanated from inducement into this state consisted of anger, denial and rationalisation that the woman was 'playing hard to get, wanting me to prove myself, like a test, testing my determination'.

This interpretation of events by Dan prompted repeated pursuit of the victim. Dan tended to switch to SS2 ('blinkered stalker'), whereby he became intrusive, controlling and more persistent with each rebuff, causing the victim to feel invaded and fearful. Time was spent formulating the reciprocal states of mind related to each RRP and position of SS1 and SS2 because of their relevance to the offences. Dan noted the loneliness, desperation, unmet needs for affiliation and emptiness that developed after repeatedly being spurned by women. For Dan, because of the intensity of his affiliation needs and fantasies of being loved and blissfully fused with a partner (SS3), these snubs were painfully received and caused a collapse into anger, loss, grief, protestation and hopelessness. Dan mentioned the introspective preoccupation he experienced about the desired woman and the hunger he felt for human contact and union within a relationship. Dan could not detach himself from the imagined relationship and became preoccupied, transforming his angry protestation into a distorted, defensive fantasy that motivated his pursuit of the victim.

His insight improved into the sequential shifts in terms of his self–other RRPs within these self-states (as reported on the Target Problem Rating Sheet). At times of deep distress, and after repeated failures and rebuffs, Dan would divert his energies into his work duties in a compulsive, frenetic manner or would withdraw and remain in bed for days on end (survival/coping strategies). Neither of these coping strategies actively addressed his unmet human needs, and, after a period of time, Dan began to fantasise about meeting his ideal partner and the love they would share. This dilemma (D1) and the procedural loops formed the most critical issue for Dan. In many respects, it was acknowledged that Dan's intentions were acceptable and understandable, indicative of his human need for affiliation and love. The dialogical sequence transitions of a potential partner from 'ideal lover' (SS3) to 'tantaliser' (SS1) to 'victim' (SS2) were traced with Dan, and his complementary shifts in perceptions of himself were explored ('loved' [position B] to 'puppet on a string' [position D] to 'blinkered stalker' [position E]). The offender-to-victim RRPs and positions showed Dan that his acceptable desires were corrupted by the developing sequence of self and other perceptions and his actions toward the woman.

The anger Dan felt toward the victims of his advances was linked to its earliest origins when he felt teased and deprived by his cousin, the confusing views he held about his girlfriend and the actions of the recent victim. Dan spoke of the negative effects of the acne he suffered and its impact on his need for acceptance by and contact with women during his adolescence. Dan stated, 'I never knew what to do with the feelings I had. I knew I was angry about being afflicted by acne, and I felt blighted, but I wanted a girlfriend so much. I remember waking up each day with a blind hope that all the acne would be just gone, and I'd have my life back.' In many respects, Dan conveyed a sense that the acne was punishing and maliciously depriving, hoping that a magical solution would occur. His deep frustration and longings were discussed, and he expressed his resentment of 'obstacles to happiness' and how he felt that his fantasies were stifled and frustrated (e.g. women's rejections, acne). Dan had never expressed his anger openly within a trusting relationship and had not felt able to acknowledge the influence of the acne upon his feelings of deprivation. The anger and frustration he felt about his relationship with his cousin and girlfriend had exacerbated and hardened his impression of being denied.

The self–other RRP (offender-to-victim) of SS2 was a prominent focus of therapy. Dan expressed the view that his victim had, on reflection, deserved the ill effects of his stalking. Dan argued that the fact that his victim had engaged in an extramarital affair supported this view. He commented that he believed that 'people do things without any thought for my feelings. I have so much I could give someone.' He was able to talk about his sensitivity to rejection and his reactions of emptiness, loneliness and deflation when rebuffed by teasing, indifferent women. Dan's empathy for his victim was complicated by these beliefs. Dan vacillated in his perceptions about who warranted designation as a victim, often confusing his anger about being victimised throughout his life with that of the actual victim of his offence. He had difficulty in appreciating that he had victimised her and that she probably harboured anger toward him, Dan arguing, 'I know how she feels!'

Dan's dilemma and the associated procedural loops about whether either to (1) seek intimacy or (2) avoid approaching women and remain detached with unmet needs were directly addressed in CAT. The development of this dilemma was traced to its origins. After rejection, Dan would typically cope through diligent involvement in his work or through withdrawal that caused depression ('leper in a bubble'). After a period of time, Dan would engage in introspective fantasy, watching romantic films and reading novels about unrequited love. Dan's fantasising motivated him to pursue a relationship and prompted the targeting of a woman (the fantasy underlying SS3). His methods of approach to women on most occasions were half-hearted, ineffectual and lacking in confidence. Dan's lack of social skills and assertive confidence usually resulted in tactical withdrawal to preserve his self-esteem. On other occasions, the sequence which became manifest in stalking behaviours occurred when Dan felt particularly exasperated and lonely, or when the targeted woman showed any inclination to make positive responses. Further self-absorbed fantasising about the relationship would follow, and Dan would plan his approaches to this woman. These relatively normal, psychological processes transformed into stalking behaviours when Dan experienced rejection or rebuff, his anger and disappointment emerging, accompanied by the rationalisation that he was being 'tested' or that 'to win her over means I have to persist'. He revealed that he believed that his stalking was really a 'secret game between me and her – others wouldn't understand'. Dan admitted that he had exhibited this type of behaviour toward several women over a number of years prior to the known offences. Each instance was analysed jointly within the CAT framework to facilitate an improved recognition of these self-perpetuating, cyclical, damaging procedures.

Dialogic work with Dan consisted of helping Dan identify the 'voices' associated with each RRP and naming the feelings and motivations which emerged. This was accomplished through imagery work, whereby Dan was asked to imagine a scenario during which he had approached a victim. During imagery work, Dan reported that the 'loved' RRP was romantic, declaring everlasting devotion to the woman. He visualised a past incident when a victim had flirted with him for a few weeks. He decided to send her flowers at work and waited for her to leave her work address. He followed this victim on many occasions, bombarding her with anonymous poems, cards and presents at work. Dan fantasised that 'this was the one' and appeared gleeful and excited during the imagery task. The subsequent rejection of his overtures occurred when he announced his identity to this woman in a local bar while she was talking with friends. He could visualise the facial expression of the victim, who in response to this advance, called him 'a sad creep'. Dan recalled being hurt and dismissed. He remembered the feeling of being laughed at, and, during imagery, his expression was glum, serious and angry (the 'puppet on a string', position D). Dan recalled that his anger transformed into a determination to 'win her over against all the odds', and this martyr-like pursuit continued for several months ('the blinkered stalker', position E) until the victim confronted him in the street and launched a tirade of abuse and threats against him. Dan, once again, felt humiliated and rejected, withdrawing into depression ('leper in a bubble' state). Dan was helped to trace the sequence of changes in self–other RRPs across these events and to recognise the height of his risk potential within SS2. In later imagery work, a new self-state, termed 'the wiser Dan', was used at each juncture of the dialogical sequence to enter into a dialogue with each position and discuss (in a conversational exchange between each state's 'voice') the perceptions, feelings and motivations of each state and how Dan could and should act in his own interests for a better outcome. This inner dialogue created an integrated, revised internal dialogue that permitted Dan to expand his recognition of the pattern of self-defeating procedures and self–other interactions. Dan was encouraged to use this dialogue as a tool to reflect on the new ways he could perceive, feel and act when encountering women and when the sequence which inflated his risk potential began to emerge.

Dan was encouraged to discuss his thoughts about himself within differing self-states and the self-management strategies he employed to cope with difficult emotional states (e.g. withdrawal, compulsive work). He perceived himself as unworthy of love and despicable. His tactics of approach to initiating relationships were explored and their inappropriate and unhelpful consequences considered. Dan acknowledged that his self-worth and esteem were poor and that he viewed himself as inferior and defective, worthy only of rejection (SS1, position D). His social isolation was identified as a specific problem which contributed to Dan's distance from meaningful relationships and activities. Expansion of Dan's network of social contacts was addressed, and he was encouraged to enter contacts with women gradually in a more open-minded, and less desperate and intense manner.

The Goodbye Letter for Dan was considered an essential part of managing the termination of therapy, given the dependency that had become evident throughout sessions. This letter was presented to him four sessions prior to the agreed ending, and it acknowledged that loss had always been painful for him and that he had often experienced difficulty in expressing his resentment and anger about endings, which had been traumatic and distressing for him. In response to the letter, Dan commented that he considered that the termination of therapy was a sad event, but not one of rupture and mourning of a lost relationship. He spoke of his deep sense of loss when his grandmother had died and how he had never felt able to ventilate or discuss his feelings. He was helped to use visual imagery of the therapist as an internalised, containing and available 'voice' (an RRP of *nurturing/caring-to-supported*). Dan could avail himself of the imaginal dialogue with the therapist as a strategy when experiencing distress or when he felt that his risk-potential states were emerging to help him make rational decisions about how to act and choices to make.

Outcome and risk prediction

Dan's progress during CAT was assessed with the self-reported Target Problem Rating Sheet for recognition and revision of each TP identified. Dan claimed that he better understood the origins and links between the states and how they resulted in criminal stalking. At no time during therapy was a rupture or stagnation apparent, and Dan presented as motivated and keen to understand the reasons for his predicament.

Dan's stalking behaviours were persistent, intrusive and invasive, causing anxiety and fear for the victims. However, he had never exhibited verbal or physical aggression toward victims or third parties. In comparison with combinations of factors associated with violent conduct against a victim, Dan was not judged to represent a significant risk of future harm (Rosenfeld & Harmon, 2002; Sheridan & Davies, 2001). Dan's reality testing tended to become compromised when the victim's responses failed to match his fantasies, causing him to feel stressed, confused and angry. It was apparent that, prior to this arrest, Dan had offended serially in a repetitive, unrevised pattern against several victims of his pursuits.

In response to therapy, Dan was considered to have developed a degree of insight into the relationship between his personality functioning and his stalking behaviours. He was deemed capable of adequate self-monitoring and self-management. Dan was made aware that his risk potential, located within the dialogical sequence of RRPs (SS2, position E), would become manifest at times when he experienced feelings of emotional loneliness and emptiness and began to fantasise about blissful fusion with a partner. When he entered therapy, it was made explicitly clear to Dan that his advances to women (and the importance of both sides of the intimacy dilemma, D1) would represent the crux issue of therapy and test his progress. He decided not to attempt to pursue a relationship until therapy was completed, and, after 24 sessions of CAT, it was agreed that sufficient progress had been made to reduce the frequency of sessions to one each month. Dan's expanded lifestyle and social network had permitted application of therapy insights, self-knowledge and skills to real-life situations. Dan reported that he did, on one occasion, endeavour to form a relationship with a woman he had met at a local night-class at college, but he decided to extract himself from this situation because he felt that she was 'a flirt with lots of other guys in the class. I wanted to be careful, not to get her and me hurt by getting it wrong. It didn't feel right.' It was felt that this decision was indicative of Dan's recognition of the sequential shifts in self-states, the pathway to offending and a degree of victim empathy. He further exhibited an awareness of the RRPs, positions of self–other relations and emotional responses which had emerged during this incident.

References

Bartholomew, K. & Horowitz, L. M. (1991). Attachment styles among young adults: A test of a four category model. *Journal of Personality and Social Psychology, 61*, 226–244.

Hare, R. D. (1991). *The manual for the Psychopathy Checklist-Revised*. Toronto: Multi-Health Systems.

Hargreaves, J. (in press). Stalking behaviour. In D. Canter & L. Alison (Eds), *Profiling rape and murder* (vol. 5). Aldershot: Ashgate.

Jellema, A. (2002). Dismissing and preoccupied insecure attachment and procedures in CAT: Some implications for CAT practice. *Clinical Psychology and Psychotherapy, 9*, 225–241.

Keinlen, K. K., Birmingham, D. L., Solberg, K. B., O'Regan, J. T. & Meloy, J. R. (1997). A comparative study of psychotic and non-psychotic stalking. *Journal of the American Academy of Psychiatry and Law, 25*, 317–334.

Long, B. L. (1994). Psychiatric diagnoses in sexual harassment cases. *Bulletin of the American Academy of Psychiatry and Law, 22,* 195–203.

Meloy, J. R. (1989). Unrequited love and the wish to kill: Diagnosis and treatment of borderline erotomania. *Bulletin of the Menninger Clinic, 53,* 477–492.

Millon, T., Millon, C. & Davis, R. (1994). *The manual for the Millon Clinical Multi-axial Inventory* (3rd edn) (MCMI–3). Minneapolis, MN: National Computer Systems.

Mullen, P. E. & Pathé, M. (1994). Stalking and the pathologies of love. *Australian and New Zealand Journal of Psychiatry, 28,* 469–477.

Mullen, P. E., Pathé, M. & Purcell, R. (2000). *Stalkers and their victims.* Cambridge: Cambridge University Press.

Nicastro, A. M. & Cousins, A. V. (2000). The tactical face of stalking. *Journal of Criminal Justice, 28,* 69–82.

Pollock, P. H. (2001). Cognitive analytic therapy for borderline erotomania: Forensic romances and violence in the therapy room. *Clinical Psychology and Psychotherapy, 8,* 214–229.

Rosenfeld, B. & Harmon, R. (2002). Factors associated with violence in stalking and obsessional harassment. *Criminal Justice and Behaviour, 29,* 671–691.

Sheridan, L. & Davies, G. M. (2001). Violence and the prior victim-stalker relationship. *Criminal Behaviour and Mental Health, 11,* 102–116.

Chapter 6

The use of Cognitive Analytic Therapy with women in secure settings

Gill Aitken & Kirsten McDonnell

In the UK, women form a significant minority (6–15%) in prison and psychiatric secure settings. Current UK policy guidance recommends that service design, assessment and therapeutic interventions pay attention to the differential needs and risks associated with women's entry into, experience of, and pathways out of such settings (Department of Health, 2003). Specifically highlighted is the role of social inequalities and trauma associated with processes of subordination, and women's survival experiences of serious abuses of power, including sexual abuse and domestic violence (Williams, Scott & Bressington, 2003).

A recent study of women across prison and secure hospital settings identified similarities in the mental health and related needs of women across the settings (Dolan, Danks, Aitken, Davenport & Burke, 2004). Recommendations included the need to increase the range of psychological assessment and therapeutic interventions available.

However, some authors caution that people in power who typically define reality have developed the psychological theory and practice on which models are based. Men have done this for women, majority white people for black and minority ethnic people, and mental health professionals for service users – all of whom are variously gendered and racialised (Dennis & Aitken, 2003). Thus, simply providing more of the existing psychological assessment and therapeutic approaches inherently will not meet women offenders' needs (Chesler, 1972; Blanchette, 2004).

Given the individualising tendency of psychological theory in understanding the origins and solutions to distress, mental health and offending, therapy can become a 'powerful tool enabling correctional workers to negotiate, uphold and obscure the paradoxes and dominant power relations [within the prison]' (Kendall, 2000; p. 83). Cognitive Analytic Therapy (CAT) has been criticised for privileging the individual or family of origin, usually mother, sometimes father, as the site and source of a person's identified psychopathology, and for ignoring the impact of social inequalities arising out of sexism and racism (Bell, 1995).

In CAT, the identification of reciprocal roles such as the other exploiting-abusing (male parent) to self: exploited-violated (child) may enable patients to understand their coping strategies. These may include self-injurious behaviour, misuse of alcohol or drugs, and symbolic or actual with-drawal in the context of their development when in the relatively powerless child role. CAT can be experienced as promoting the empowerment of patients and self-agency, thus enabling them to develop more 'healthy', adult ways of being, including not self-injuring. However, rarely do we see in CAT diagrams and formulations reference to the legacy of social contexts, or the 'here and now' effect of the institutional systems in which a woman may find herself. For example, a woman may self-injure as a survival strategy, yet institutional policy may mean that she is placed under 5-minute observations day and night, possibly by male staff. In this, the woman re-experiences violation of psychological and physical boundaries as the system re-enacts abusive, controlling reciprocal role procedures (RRPs). These enactments have been recognised: 'We conclude that the current regime for women in [high-secure setting] is infantilising, demeaning and anti-therapeutic' (HMSO, 1992). More recently, in 2004, a women's high-secure prison in which therapeutic provision was provided was closed.

In secure settings, therapies underpinned by concepts of therapeutic risk taking may pose at least a challenge to the functioning of hierarchical set-tings, and at most an irresolvable tension in these settings, which aim to establish 'safe certainty' through risk-management strategies (Byrne, 2001). 'Safe certainty' is premised on experts' knowledge 'about the condition to be treated and the means of doing this' (p. 109). This has been translated into the application of evidenced-based prescribed medication or physical inter-ventions to stabilise illness (medical model), and the application of 'universal and standardised packages' of cognitive-behavioural approaches across mental health or offence-reduction programmes. These approaches are par-ticularly suited to randomised, controlled trial method from which scientific evidence is derived.

CAT has been applied in working with people who present with complex needs and risk. This includes in diagnoses of personality disorder (Ryle, 1998) and adult survivors of childhood abuse (Pollock, 2001), as well as in secure settings (as the production of this book evidences). In the rest of this chapter, we reflect on the ways in which we try to build into our use of CAT an appreciation of the existence and impact of social and sexual inequalities and power relations on women's lives and in the therapeutic encounters (Williams, Scott & Waterhouse, 2001). Furthermore, we reflect on how we practise therapy when working within a wider system that may be inherently antitherapeutic (Byrne, 2001; Scott, 2004).

We briefly outline the evidence for differential needs and the risks posed by and to women in forensic settings, and provide an illustrative case example of using CAT with women in prison. We highlight the need to take account of the cultural and social context of women's lives before their entry into, as well as throughout their contact with, services. In conclusion, we argue for a flexible application of CAT as a therapy model and its tools when working with women in secure settings.

Women's differential needs, risks and pathways

Up to 50% of women offenders have had some form of contact with the mental health and psychiatric system before entering secure settings, but few have had access to *sustained* counselling or psychotherapy (Scott, 2004).

The majority of women in secure settings have histories of chronic sexual, physical and emotional abuse; instability of care relations in child and adult-hood; multiple contacts with a range of statutory agencies; and poverty associated with low income, unpaid employment and being lone parents (HM Chief Inspectorate of Prisons, 1997; Stafford, 1999; Rutherford, 2003; Dolan *et al.*, 2004).

Women's offending patterns and the context of their offending are different from men's. Men are significantly more likely than women to present a danger to the public, and to women and children. In 2003, women comprised 4% (547) of sentenced prisoners for violence against the person. While 5475 men were sentenced for sexual offences, no women were sentenced (Prison Reform Trust, 2004), and 74% of all violent incidents were perpetrated by men, with the majority (32%) of women's violent incidents related to domestic violence situations (Smith & Allen, 2004).

Women enter the secure psychiatric system under the Mental Health Act 1983 from three main sources: prison, the wider secure psychiatric care system and general hospitals. Women are more likely than men to be detained under a civil section of the Mental Health Act and to be spiralled up the levels of the secure psychiatric system because of self-injurious behaviour and threats or acts against their mental health carers and property (Stafford, 1999). Where there is a history of violence (although a number of risk assessments count self-injurious behaviour as violence, see Aitken & Logan, 2004), this is often an isolated offence, linked to women's abusive pasts, or is an index offence of arson, with no intent to endanger others' lives (Stafford, 1999). Women transferred from prison are likely to be diagnosed with severe mental illness and/or personality disorder, with 35% in secure settings receiving three or more personality diagnoses (Logan, 2002). Transfers are often prompted by persistent self-injury, setting fire to bedding and threats to harm others, particularly prison and Social Services staff (Gorsuch, 1998). Once in high-secure psychiatric care, women stay longer than their male peers and up to four times longer than women peers in prison (Logan, 2002).

Women are often constructed as *differently dangerous but more so* than men – to services and to themselves. It is common to hear women talked about as having *particularly* complex needs, being *particularly* challenging and *especially* vulnerable to overt forms of abuse, and being *especially* 'toxic to the system'. On the other hand, women are sometimes constructed as 'too fragile' to be referred for therapies which explore the emotional and relational aspects of being.

Application of CAT

The illustrative case study is drawn from our work with women in secure prison and psychiatric settings. We draw on our collective experience in working with women, and for this reason we move between using 'we' and (unspecified) 'I'.

Making visible institutional positions

Although practising with a 'captive' client group, we bring into the 'closed' system the forms of communication and relating that are practised externally. These include letters to *named* individual women outlining the reason for referral and an appointment time and place for the first meeting, together with details of how to contact the therapist if they have any questions prior to the first meeting. The inclusion of, and greater transparency with, the women is to provide them with a concrete resource and to communicate their value as women and individuals. For some, this can be the first time they have been informed that they have been referred for a therapy assessment.

Negotiating systems

For therapy to take place, one needs the successful integration of, and cooperation between, a number of systems. Crisis issues, such as lack of trained escort staff to facilitate attendance, pressures on bed spaces, and the system's response to 'acts of self-injury and threats', may result in non-attendance at therapy. This includes women being moved from one (part of an) institution to another or being in seclusion or segregation. Sometimes, to establish or maintain therapeutic contact, a therapist has to agree to have up to four escorts present in an individual therapy session. Such 'risk' issues and arrangements will have been decided without negotiation between therapist and client in relation to risk issues that may present in session. At other times, therapy rooms have been reallocated to other functions, for example, visiting solicitors and assessments by other services, without prior notice. In CAT terms, the factors which mitigate against therapy taking place risk: (i) communicating strong messages about the role and status of therapy within the institution, with the institution potentially occupying depriving, devaluing, controlling, restrictive roles and (ii) the projection or experience of confusion and mixed messages between therapist and woman client which potentially re-enact earlier traumagenics. Thus, in cases of non-attendance, rather than automatically assuming a woman is not engaging, a therapist needs to check whether organisational or risk-management issues are involved.

Collaboration

In applying the basic tenet of a CAT approach as a collaborative relationship, we tentatively acknowledge the therapist's differential (power) positions in the system in relation to a woman client. Thus, we state that the therapist is able to leave the institution at the end of the day and is not subject to the same assessment processes over the years (Aitken, 2000). We also make an explicit commitment to share with a woman the contents of any formal reports and to incorporate her views before wider dissemination. At the end of any session, space is created to agree on what will be disclosed to the wider service, as well as the types of support the woman might want or need. This does not necessarily mean consensus. Differences are named and the therapist is accountable for her reasons in such cases, both viewpoints being documented. Where there is consensus, we stay alert to the different ways in which women can be silenced.

Pacing and timing of assessments and therapy

CAT is typically practised as a 50-minute structured therapy with three separate yet interrelated phases: assessment, active therapy and ending. A range of tools is identified with each phase. For example, 16-session CAT is structured as follows:

- sessions 1–3 – gathering data and preliminary reformulation – involves history taking, recognition of target problems and procedures, Psychotherapy File, diary keeping
- session 4 – prose reformulation
- sessions 5–15 – therapeutic change – active therapy
- session 16 – Goodbye Letter.

(Ryle, 1995)

In using CAT, we are mindful that many women have histories of lack of trust of authority figures and disrupted attachments. In our experience, women have not always been able to tolerate the traditional 50 minutes of 'assessment or therapy'. Reasons include difficulties with concentration, medication side effects (afternoon, rather than morning sessions are often negotiated), testing out the therapist's trustworthiness and testing out the therapist's commitments. We state that we will commit to a protected therapy space and time for 3–6 weeks for a woman to decide whether she can work with us. When a woman decides she does not want to engage, we explore the possible consequences, frame her decision as not yet being ready for engagement, and outline in writing to her and the referrer potential re-referral options. This explicitness aims to avoid re-enactment of possible earlier controlling/abusive or rejecting/abandoning reciprocal roles.

Many women's accounts are of involuntarily being in a hierarchical and authoritative environment. CAT tools, such as the Psychotherapy File, may contribute to a focus on the negatives or deficits of her as a woman. For this reason, we feel the administration of CAT tools, and the phases of therapy, need to take into account the development of a sufficient therapeutic alliance, as our 'trustworthiness' or non-misuse of our institutional power is often tested. Timing and pacing vary according to the individual needs of the woman, her experiences of the secure system, and the impact of cultural, class and gender dimensions.

Case study

Lisa, a white woman in her mid-20s, the mother of two children, was diagnosed with borderline personality disorder (BPD) in her late teens. She was remanded to prison for setting fires and subsequently sentenced to 2 years' imprisonment for arson. In the first year, she was transferred several times between the remand wing, mental health and segregation units. She was referred for assessment for therapy after 13 months because of self-injury, social isolation, 'psychotic' behaviours and threats of violence against health and prison staff.

Over a 10-month period, 24 individual sessions were held, ranging from 5 to 45 minutes. In the first five sessions, she left after a few minutes, not returning. By session 6, she started to return after initially leaving. At this stage, I started a tentative process to name and explore what was happening for her and between us (Fig. 6.1: SDR, TPP 2 and 3).

By session 8, I felt a sufficient therapeutic alliance had been established to work through the Psychotherapy File. She endorsed all the extremes, commenting, 'I did not realise how many problems I have . . . I thought I had strategies . . . was coping'. I reflected to Lisa that she looked sad, upon which she ended the session. In session 9, she brought a letter she had written and asked that I take it away to read, unable to tolerate its being read either by her or by me in session. In her letter, she stated that she felt it safer to write than to speak, as she had so often experienced being silenced (SDR, TPP 1). This was referred to in subsequent sessions, as she tested both her verbal voice and my responses as she began to talk about her feelings, experiences of how others treated her, and the range of ways she coped.

Lisa's story

She described a history of physical assault by her mother from early childhood, until she was aged 7 years, when her mother left the family home. With her siblings, she moved with her father to live with his new woman partner, and was physically and sexually abused by her stepmother. She then experienced the onset of 'voices' urging her to harm her stepmother and the family home. She coped with the voices and abuse through self-injury, initially focusing on parts of her body that could be hidden from public view. Over the years, her self-injurious acts intensified and her scars and distress became public. She disclosed the abuse to teachers and professionals involved in child services, but reported being disbelieved, unheard, and rejected. She was always returned to the family home. When a teenager, she violently attacked her stepmother and was placed in a secure adolescent service. A year later, she was discharged into temporary accommodation on state benefits and began committing burglary to support herself. She served a number of short prison sentences. Between her late teens and early 20s, she presented at Accident and Emergency on numerous occasions after suicide attempts. She was sometimes admitted as a psychiatric in-patient and described being discharged because she continued to self-injure and disrupted the functioning of the ward(s). During one in-patient admission, she received a formal diagnosis of BPD.

By her early 20s, she had given birth to two daughters. After both births, she re-experienced voices, visions and flashbacks relating to her past abuse. With both a toddler and baby to look after, and a restricted social network, she struggled to cope. She contacted Social Services for support after hitting her baby, and both children were put on the at-risk register and placed in foster care. She decided to use the 'respite from full-time childcare' positively to try to 'sort self out'. She found low-paid work in the service sector, and supported herself independently while maintaining regular contact with her children. After several months, Social Services proposed that both children be adopted, which she contested. Lisa subsequently set fire to a waste bin outside a Social Services building and was remanded to her current prison placement.

Although she was the survivor of male and female sexualised violence, she focused in therapy on her anger toward adult women figures, as opposed to males, who misused their adult or institutional positions of power, and who contravened particular gendered role expectations as sometimes impotent protectors and carers of children. Others were constructed as either controlling, attacking and abusing her or rejecting and neglecting her. This placed her in the reciprocal roles of feeling controlled, abused, trapped or (too) needy. These connected with her understanding of the victimised ways in which women are constructed, and might be expected to act, in the wider society. Lisa reflected that her disclosures about women as perpetrators were significant factors in her being disbelieved by others, often hearing 'a woman couldn't do that', as such abusive actions countered societal expectations of women and mothers.

Lisa understood her restrictive access to power resources as a child in relation to adults and described how from childhood she coped by withdrawing (Fig. 6.1: SDR, TPP 3) and at times trying to have a voice (fight back) (SDR, TPP 1). She frequently experienced her voice not being heard and, feeling powerless, sought out other indirect sources of power. These included having sex to seek care and feel loved, and self-injuring to have control over her body, communicate her distress and relieve feelings. Over time, she tried to make more public and visible her voice and express her feelings of frustration and impotency through threats to hurt others and setting fires (SDR, TPP 1a).

Despite Lisa's attempts to keep her own children safe through her self-disclosure to Social Services, she was constructed as an 'unfit' mother, rather than a mother with support needs. This angered her, as she felt positioned in similar ways to her own maternal figures who had sexually and violently abused her. Lisa self-identified as 'all bad' and 'evil' because she had hit her baby, and as an 'abnormal' woman and mother because her children were removed from her care.

Reformulation

My Reformulation Letter responded both to Lisa's letter and the content of sessions, and was read in session 11. The letter attempted to reflect Lisa's story, to accept and validate her experiences, and to name and stay with her pain. The aim was not to re-enact dismissive, silencing responses, but rather to emphasise that she was an expert in her life. The letter was to give voice to the unacknowledged hurt, abused girl-child and woman whom others, including me, could silence and ignore:

You shared how, as a girl, you tried to keep 'the burning' in the head and you always tried to do what was right, but never knew what the rules were . . . this has continued into your adulthood . . . and you've risked sharing with me what has happened to you in your life. . . . You shared when you were in [part of prison], you coped by trying not to show distress and keeping your anger hidden, and started cutting yourself – at times to release your pressure, at times to have a sense of control and at other times to punish the girl within, whom you blame for being evil and all bad. You've shared when you were then transferred to [part of prison] how you felt stripped of being a person (through having clothes and personal possessions taken away) and felt like an animal, but when you screamed and shouted, no one came and no one seemed to care. And now . . . you've taken the step again of risking letting me know what has happened to you in your life and the pain and anger you feel. You've shared that you are worried I will not believe you . . . and find it hard when I say I do believe, and you question your own sense of reality. We've explored how perhaps at times cutting yourself gives you a sense of groundedness, particularly when you've spent long periods with no one to talk to, no belongings which connect you with the wider world when you feel all alone. . . .

Diagrammatic reformulation

From session 12 onward, we started to build up a diagrammatic reformulation. This also informed the potential dynamics in the woman–woman therapy relationship. Here I, as a woman therapist, was in an institutional position of power and could influence her future life course. At the same time, I was experiencing restrictions in a wider system in which power dynamics were played out in professional and institutional hierarchies. This was explored in discussions about power relations, including how a child's experience of being abused and controlled may be re-enacted in the ways our society constructs and relates to adult women. Holding Lisa's experiences from childhood of adult women (outside herself) in mind, my task was to recognise the potential for misuses of power with the therapy encounter.

In session 16, Lisa talked about her hopelessness – whatever she attempted, 'things never change' as people see 'me as bad, dangerous', never 'the whole of me'. I reflected that Lisa looked sad. Her response was that I 'hadn't helped' but 'had made [Lisa] worse', and she left the room. Over the next 3 weeks, Lisa neither attended therapy nor sent any communication. For me as a therapist, the dilemma was either to listen and hear Lisa's voice, and thus not offer further meetings – but this could re-enact a neglecting, abandoning (woman) reciprocal role – or to continue to offer the space but be experienced as a controlling, humiliating and abusive (woman), leaving her unheard and disbelieved as in the past. To try to avoid reciprocation of the roles Lisa might be inducing, I wrote to her. In the letter, I stated my sadness and disappointment that I had not helped, thus aiming to validate and reflect her voice, while emphasising Lisa's strength in saying this directly when possibly anticipating an attack or rejection by me both as a woman and as a therapist. Alongside this, I was able to work with the system, and in discussion with another professional shared the frame of the work and themes in the SDR, linking these to Lisa's placement in seclusion/segregation. By this time, she had spent over 4 months in seclusion because of self-injurious behaviour. This facilitated a discussion with representatives of the wider system about the impact of such a depriving social and physical environment on Lisa's capacity to develop her personal and social resources. It was agreed to move her to a 'safe enough' health-care environment.

After this move, Lisa wrote, asking to meet me again. She shared that she had felt confused by my letter. She believed it would be under my control as to whether she would attend sessions or not, and had anticipated I would take the choice away from her. Discussing this, alongside the change in environment, triggered a shift in our relationship. Lisa had 'tested it' and found I had remained available after being verbally attacked and rejected (Fig. 6.1: SDR, TPP 2). This enabled exploration of Lisa's belief, as named in the reformulation, that another could not look past 'the labels' (BPD, self-harm, arsonist, threats) and see other parts of her. We explored how at times Lisa felt she

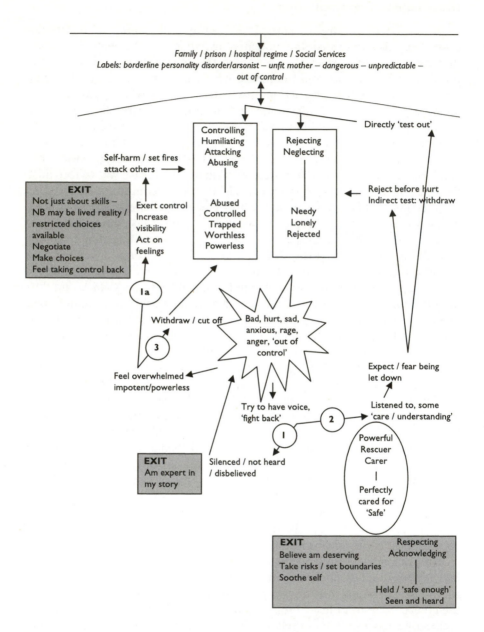

Figure 6.1 Lisa's sequential diagrammatic reformulation. Societal assumptions: women will be victims and be vulnerable; women should be 'good mothers, understanding, able to cope, put others' needs first; women are not expected to be abusers, or to hurt children.

might as well act in the ways that others communicated were expected of her. From this session, Lisa started to test taking responsibility for choices about meeting in the context of her emotional and psychological state, thus developing a more adult woman to adult woman relationship (SDR, exits).

Ending

Lisa was referred by the wider system to a high-secure psychiatric service a month prior to her release date from prison because of her continuing threats to harm professionals involved in her childcare case, and risk issues identified because of the lack of appropriate women-only supported accommodation in her local area. It seemed Lisa's case presented a challenge for services to disentangle her legitimate anger at the loss of her children from embodied actions. That is, the difference between articulating her feelings of anger and rage, and acting on those threats. During her life, despite numerous threats, Lisa had made three 'assaults' on others. In our experience, the social and emotional gendered context and understanding of assaults are often not considered. As a child, Lisa had attacked the female parental perpetrator of her abuse after many attempts at disclosure and being returned by statutory authorities to the parental home; as a young woman and lone parent who experienced herself struggling to cope, she had hit her child (and self-reported to Social Services); and while in prison she had hit a woman member of health-care staff (during an internal physical examination).

Given her imminent release from prison, assessment and agreement of the suitability for transfer to high-secure care were undertaken rapidly. The decision was made without reference to any assessment of risk and need identified in the therapeutic work Lisa had undertaken in the prison. In parallel, Lisa and I attempted to work through the suddenness of the ending of therapy through the Goodbye Letter. This named the shifts and changes as well as issues she was still working with. The letter emphasised her strengths and resources and the exits she could also draw on to manage the transition process: 'Although [therapy has been] challenging, as you feel others make decisions about you, you have run with this and have made decisions that have felt best for you at the time. This is about remaining on the steps of your journey, finding out what is helpful for you, taking some control back and recognising your strength.'

In agreement with Lisa, I negotiated follow-up sessions with the receiving service to take place 3 weeks and 3 months after transfer, which would also allow for continuity and planned handover of care. However, the second follow-up did not happen, as the receiving service communicated that Lisa had chosen not to engage in therapeutic work.

I was aware from the initial follow-up that Lisa had been attempting to use her exits. She shared that she had risked telling staff about her difficulties and some of her story. In this, she had attempted to let others know when she was feeling overwhelmed and what she needed as support, requesting quiet space with a staff member to be alongside or to talk with and off-ward access to some activities. She had also tried to negotiate a reduction in medication, as she reported dampening of feelings and difficulty in wakening in the morning. Despite experiencing a sense of not being heard and feeling powerless, as she was repeatedly informed that 'they [the system] needed [unspecified] time to get to know her/assess her', Lisa shared that she had tried to use her exits several times.

This circumstance highlights the reality of restricted resources and choices. In therapy, we may talk about choices and ways of negotiating; however, the lived reality may be more restrictive than we as therapists recognise. In moving from one system to another, Lisa experienced the receiving service as using standardised admission policies and procedures that were not interfaced with the referring service. Such universal policies could not flexibly take account of 'where she was at', and how she might have legitimacy in identifying aspects of her own needs and risks. The receiving service could be experienced as re-enacting earlier dismissing, rejecting and neglecting reciprocal roles, and Lisa's withdrawal from engaging understood as a return to (earlier) ways of surviving (Fig. 6.1: SDR, TPP 3).

Mindful of not wanting to enact the rejecting and neglecting role, I wrote to Lisa stating these possibilities and restated my commitment that no report would be circulated without her having access to it first. I also liaised with the receiving service, discussed potential dynamics and similarities with the initial stages of therapy, and named ways of working that had appeared to enable Lisa to take risks to engage.

Summary

This chapter aimed to raise a number of possibilities and tensions in applying CAT in individual therapy with women in the context of secure settings. Underpinning our approach is the conviction that we need to be accountable to, and transparent with, the women we work with, and relate to them at all times as adult women. Furthermore, we hold that index offences can usefully be understood and worked with as part of a wider holistic approach to a person's development and ways of relating. Here, we reflect on key issues that in our experience it is important to be alert to.

The *timing and pacing* of the application of CAT as a structured and time-limited model, both within and across sessions, need to be flexibly adapted according to where 'the woman is at' in relation to her own history of experiences. These may reflect gendered experiences of disempowerment in relation to both the wider society as well as statutory services; disrupted and multiple attachments over her life course; a history of understandable mistrust when she may have been variously disbelieved, and removed from, or returned to, her family of origin after disclosures of abuse. Additionally, they may reflect the loss of actual or potential meaningful roles (parental, sexual, familial, economic) through adverse or restricted stereotypical assumptions associated with femaleness, psychiatric diagnoses and offending profile. Furthermore, because of cognitive needs arising out of trauma, specific learning disability, education and medication side effects, a woman may not be able to engage in the standard 50-minute sessions. The dimension of time may also be embodied differently, particularly if a woman has spent periods in seclusion. All these factors can affect how long a woman feels able to stay in session, or the thought of long-term therapy may be experienced as too overwhelming.

As therapists, we may hold a 16–32-session equivalent CAT framework in mind, but often negotiate this in six-session equivalent blocks with built-in reviews for two reasons. The first reason is the fact of unplanned transfers. Secondly, the review process offers the woman a sense of control and involvement in the whole therapy process, something she may not have previously experienced, as well as providing her with tangible resources, as named shifts and changes are recognised. The importance of developing a working therapeutic alliance is key and, in this, the timing of the administration and development of the CAT tools should reflect the above factors.

Bell (1995) has already reviewed the *psychotherapy tool* for its lack of gender and racial specificities. Furthermore, in our experience, the tool reveals little differentiation among women, many endorsing all items. Some women experience its completion as marking out 'I've failed' and that any strengths and resources are masked, making them feel 'I'm crap . . . can't do anything right.' It is important to frame the woman's coping (survival) strategies as reflecting the resources she had access to at particular times and in particular circumstances, and understand how the use of direct and indirect strategies in accessing power resources is shaped by gender. For other women, the Psychotherapy File is used as a resource to identify her legitimate needs. For others, as in the case of Lisa, we might speculate that she drew on the tool as a resource to generate and test her own voice through the writing of a letter. Additionally, many women have used diaries, poetry and art to express their feelings for themselves and others, which can also be important shared resources in therapy.

Reformulation Letters are one of the most powerful CAT tools, in our experience. Often, this is the first time a woman has her voice validated and presented in tangible ways, such as seeing it written down and hearing it read. We try to create the conditions for women to reflect on what it was like growing up as a girl into womanhood and her journey, including her offences, to her present situation. This includes her understandings of societal, familial and personal expectations in relation to her culture, class and sexual orientation, as well as her offences, which are all named in the letter.

The sharing of these letters often evokes strong emotions of hurt, sadness, realisation of loss of potential, and key relationships and roles, as well as anger and rage in relation to the misuses of power the women have been subjected to. Therefore, framing the range of coping strategies, including offences, and emotions as understandable at the time is important. As therapists, we attempt to act as a container of coexisting aspects of the subject, which she may not be able to tolerate at this particular time. Thus, in the letters, we may tentatively name the contradictory constructions and associated feelings she may have named, or refer in more general terms to what has not yet been talked about. We are also mindful of this when constructing the SDR, because naming particular offences, such as a woman's killing her child, or her subjection to sexual abuse, can be experienced as too unbearable for her to see on paper. Thus, we may place these on separate pieces of paper, or 'cover' them in various ways, until she is ready for them to be more consciously brought into the session to coexist with other aspects.

For some women, there is the issue of whether a letter can be kept safely if they were to take it back to their part of the service. At these times, a nominated, trusted person in the service usually holds the letter for the woman and agrees to be alongside her if she wants to access it. For others, the weight of their life experiences feels too heavy to carry and hold in a letter, when they are returning to more isolated or unsupported living environments. For still others, the letter is important to hold to revalidate their experiences.

The possible impact of societal expectations and labelling the woman has experienced can also be made explicit in the *diagrammatic reformulations* – as 'outer or second skins' (Fig. 6.1). This then feeds into the identified reciprocal roles and mapping out of particular procedures and exits. Throughout this chapter, we have highlighted the impact of systems on the quality of a woman's experience, as well as the importance of continuity and joined-up approaches to care, support and rehabilitation, in a system that often operates in fragmented ways. It has been estimated that during 1 year in a secure system a woman has to negotiate and manage up to 180 staff relationships. In this context, the sharing of an SDR with key staff involved in her care is fundamental to a wider understanding of the women in context. These key staff and teams can include multidisciplinary care teams, reception services for a transferred woman, and specific staff in segregation units or wards who are tasked with her support, care and risk needs on a daily basis. In Lisa's case, key staff shifted in their perception of her from 'psychiatric patient' and 'arsonist' to a more holistic view, including that of a woman with children.

The aim of a women-centred and holistic approach is not to position women as 'victims', nor to say that women are not accountable for their actions. Rather, it is to enhance a woman's being worked with, and supported as a whole human being, and also to work alongside her to process and make sense of her internal and external emotional and life experiences, which include the potential for disrupting psychiatric and offending careers.

Transference and counter-transference issues are central to the CAT therapist, and the therapy encounter is constructed as a micro-context in which a client's identified self-limiting ways of relating (procedures) are potentially (re-) enacted. Part of the therapist's responsibility is to work with the client to recognise, understand and disrupt the re-enactment of problematic interactions (reciprocal role relations), and not to collude in such patterns (Ryle, 1998). Transference and counter-transference processes are explicitly identified and brought into consciousness through the tools of written and diagrammatic reformulation. These also help therapists keep alert to the reciprocal roles they themselves may be enacting and reproducing. These can be based on potential internalisation or sharing of wider societal norms in relation to therapists themselves as women (or men), the woman client, and the impact of different systems, such as a particular institution and care team.

When meeting a client, we assume we are working with an individual and consider how we might represent either external or internal figures or voices in relation to a client's intrapsychic or interpersonal world (Ryle, 1997). The notion of different selves and self-states has been particularly developed in relation to clients diagnosed with BPD (e.g. Ryle, 1995; 1998). However, other concepts, including the concept that we are all gendered and racialised, are not typically acknowledged as affecting clinical or clinical supervision encounters (Dennis & Aitken, 2003). For any therapist working with women in (often emotionally, relationally and materially deprived and 'controlling') secure settings, it is important to be alert to the impact of wider gendered social relations, as well as the institutional and interpersonal gendered contexts of therapeutic encounters. These contexts can heighten a range of role enactments initiated, or reproduced, by the therapist, including the risk of enmeshment and overidentification, becoming the heroine or hero, or becoming a distancing and controlling figure, rather than working in empowering ways.

In the case of Lisa, the woman therapist found herself wanting to extend sessions beyond the agreed time, as Lisa would disclose more about her past at the end of a session (flagging up abuse issues). The therapist knew Lisa would be alone in segregation and that the once-weekly session was the key relationship Lisa had access to. The role of socialisation of women as expected primary emotional carers of others was reflected upon in supervision. This was in conjunction with an acknowledgement of the feelings of relative powerlessness as a therapist and as a woman, and felt pressures to take responsibility for the wider inadequacies of the system, often at the cost of the therapist's own emotional well-being. These reflections enabled wider consideration of how to acknowledge the restrictive reality of Lisa's environment, as well as how to identify where the system could be influenced better to meet her needs and risks. This included sharing the framework of the SDR with key personnel and working to have Lisa accommodated in a health-care rather than a segregation setting.

In our experience, CAT provides a range of important theoretical and practical tools to work therapeutically with women individually and in groups. However, these need to be further informed by understanding of the impact of wider social inequalities on women's lived experiences and our own socialisation as gendered therapists. The benefit of using CAT is to facilitate the development of a sense of relational security, which women in secure settings may not have previously experienced, and also to help women process previously unresolved issues, as a way to develop and extend their range of personal and social resources and identify practical strategies.

Therapy encounters are embedded in wider 'closed yet fragmented and destabilising' systems. These systems are driven by external physical and procedural security directives, which can undermine and 'sabotage' therapy. Therapists who call into question the potential adverse impact of the wider system can be pathologised, thus paralleling the very position of the forensic psychiatric woman client. This may be further heightened when attempting to embed women-centred approaches in secure services. These services have been identified as reflecting more traditional, Western masculine ideologies of control that privilege institutionally accredited experts and hierarchical relations (Fernando, 1998; Kendall, 2000).

In sharing women-centred CAT frameworks, such as the SDR, with systems and teams, we can support a more consistent and coherent understanding and approach to accompany a woman as she makes her journey of recovery back into the wider community.

Acknowledgements

We would like to thank the women we have worked with in assessment and therapy encounters over the years, for taking the risk of sharing aspects of their internal worlds and life experiences with us. We extend the same thanks to peers in our supervision encounters. All have informed our thinking and practice.

References

Aitken, G. (2000). Women working with women: Difference and power relations in forensic therapy encounters. *Changes: An International Journal of Psychology and Psychotherapy, 18*, 254–263.

Aitken, G. & Logan, C. (2004). Dangerous women – a UK response. In G. Aitken & C. Heenan (Eds), Women in prison and secure psychiatric settings – whose needs, whose dangerousness? *Feminism and Psychology, 14*, 262–268.

Bell, L. (1995). Cognitive Analytic Therapy: Its key strengths and some concerns. *Clinical Psychology Forum*, October, 27–30.

Blanchette, K. (2004). Revisiting effective classification strategies for women offenders in Canada. In G. Aitken & C. Heenan (Eds), Women in prison and secure psychiatric settings – whose needs, whose dangerousness? *Feminism and Psychology, 14*, 231–236.

Byrne, S. (2001). What am I doing here? Safety, certainty and expertise in a secure unit. *Family Therapy, 23*, 102–116.

Chesler, P. (1972). *Women and madness*. London: Allen Lane.

Dennis, M. & Aitken, G. (2003). *Incorporating gender issues in clinical supervision*. In I. Fleming & L. Steen (Eds), *Supervision and clinical psychology: Theory, practice and perspectives*. London: Brunner-Routledge.

Department of Health (2003). *Mainstreaming gender and women's mental health: Implementation guidance*. London: HMSO.

Dolan, M., Danks, S., Aitken, G., Davenport, S. & Burke, M. (2004). *Systematic/ multidimensional needs assessment of women with mental health problems in secure care in the North West Region*. Final Report submitted to Forensic Mental Health Research and Development Office, November 2004.

Fernando, S. (1998). Part 1: Background. In S. Fernando, D. Ndegwa & M. Wilson (Eds), *Forensic psychiatry, race and culture*. London: Routledge.

Gorsuch, N. (1998). Unmet need among disturbed female offenders. *Journal of Forensic Psychiatry*, *9*, 556–570.

HM Chief Inspectorate of Prisons for England and Wales (1997). *Women in prison: A thematic review by HM Chief Inspector of Prisons*. London: Home Office.

HM Inspectorate of Prisons for England and Wales (2001). *Report on an unannounced follow-up inspection of HMP Holloway*. London: Home Office.

HMSO (1992). *Report of the Committee of Inquiry into Complaints about Ashworth Hospital*. Cited in Fallon (Fallon Report, p. 9 (2000)).

Home Office (2003). *Home Office Prison Statistics* (May 2003). www.hmprisonservice. gov.uk.

Kendall, K. (2000). Anger management with women in coercive environments. *Issues in Forensic Psychology*, *2*, 35–41.

Logan, C. (2002). Dangerous and severe personality disorder women's services pre-assessment pilot. Unpublished Academic Report. London: Home Office and HM Prison Service.

Pollock, P. (2001). *Cognitive Analytic Therapy for adult survivors of childhood abuse: Approaches to treatment and case management*. Chichester: Wiley.

Prison Reform Trust (2004). *Briefing from Prison Reform Trust*, March 2004. www.prisonreformtrust.org.uk.

Rutherford, H. (2003). Women and offending. In N. Jeffcote & T. Watson (Eds), *Working therapeutically with women in secure settings*. London: Jessica Kingsley.

Ryle, A. (1995). *Cognitive Analytic Therapy: Developments in theory and practice*. Chichester: Wiley.

Ryle, A. (1997). Transferences and counter-transferences: The CAT perspective. *British Journal of Psychotherapy*, *14*, 303–309.

Ryle, A. (Ed.) (1997). *Cognitive analytic therapy and borderline personality disorder: The model and the method*. Chichester: Wiley.

Scott, S. (2004). Opening a can of worms? Counselling for survivors in UK women's prisons. In G. Aitken & C. Heenan (Eds), Women in prison and secure psychiatric settings – whose needs, whose dangerousness? *Feminism and Psychology*, *14*, 256–261.

Smith, C. & Allen, J. (2004). *Violent crime in England and Wales*. Home Office: London.

Stafford, P. (1999). *Defining gender issues: Redefining women's services*. Report commissioned by Women in Secure Hospitals. London: WISH.

Williams, J., Scott, S. & Bressington, C. (2003). Dangerous journeys: Women's pathways into and through secure mental health services. In N. Jeffcote & T. Watson (Eds), *Working therapeutically with women in secure settings*. London: Jessica Kingsley.

Williams, J., Scott, S. & Waterhouse, S. (2001). Mental health services for 'difficult' women. *Feminist Review, 68*, 89–104.

Chapter 7

Cognitive Analytic Therapy and parents in prison

Michael Göpfert

Preamble

This chapter focuses on the prisoner with parental responsibility. It will not deal with parents who killed their children, either because of a distorted or delusional need to protect them from harm, or because, in the parent's mind, the child had become an overpowering or persecutory and abusive force. The aim is to put the prisoner as parent on the map, illustrating how the role of prisoner and the role of parent can interact in vulnerable people who might wish to fulfil their parental role.

The author is not an expert in working with parents in prison. All case examples are fictitious but grounded in real clinical experiences, and what might appear to be extreme is real. While many more fathers are in prison than mothers, the clinical experience is dominated by mothering issues (see also Hairston, 2001). This chapter reflects this.

Parent prisoners present in a number of ways, often with unexpected scenarios. There is no average or typical picture. It is important to recognise that the needs of the child(ren) should be paramount; that is, the developmental needs and the future of both child and parent, provided the parent is motivated to fulfil the parenting role. In prison, this requires the capacity to keep the prisoner as parent in the institution's 'mind'. Usually, this needs more than one or two people able to think about aspects of parenting. Recommendations at the end of the chapter will address this.

Introduction

The forensic mental health worker encounters parenting in two ways: firstly, as a professional working with parents in a forensic context (here: prison); secondly, as a therapeutic agent, working with parents. Prison and therapy are very different agendas. It is important in both to consider parenting as an aspect of the work:

Why is it important to be concerned about parents in prison and their children?

(1) A parent's going to prison has a significant effect on the child(ren)'s development, if only because of the parent's absence (however long and whatever information the child is given). The majority of people in prison are parents.

(2) The population of prisons is characterised by high rates of significant mental health problems. Mental health problems in parents are also significantly associated with developmental problems in children. Hence, there is probably a large subgroup of parents with mental health problems affecting their children.

(3) Being a parent often is an essential part of an adult's identity. Parenting requires the capacity for preoccupation with and concern for the child's well-being (capacity to keep the child in mind). Prisons are geared toward controlling prisoners, not toward supporting parents in their role day-to-day. This can result in further loss of care for the child.

(4) Evidence indicates that reintegration into strong social role identities, such as parenting, on release from prison is associated with lower rates of reoffending.

Why is it good practice to consider the parenting role of a client as an important aspect of an assessment for forensic or any other psychotherapy?

(1) Children are substantially affected by their parents' relationships. It is important for the therapist and client to consider the effect of a therapeutic relationship on any other relationships. In my clinical experience, relationships elsewhere in patients' lives can significantly improve, as well as deteriorate, as a result of therapy, including that with children if the patient is a parent.

(2) Mental health problems can significantly affect parenting capacity (Adshead et al., 2004; Hall, 2004). A comprehensive assessment across major domains of personality functioning, including that of parenting, will help decide priorities and enable informed choice of, and consent to, treatment. Treatments may vary in their effectiveness across domains, and what works for self-harm, may not for parenting issues. Treatment results do not necessarily generalise (Linehan, 1993).

(3) Difficulty in integrating the role of parent into the identity/personality of the parent represents the developmental failure of an important life-cycle transition. This can present subtly, commonly in the context of 'parentification' dynamics (Jurkovic, 1997; Chase, 1999; Byng-Hall, 2002).

(4) Parenting is a fundamental role in life, and one's own experience of

having been parented may strongly motivate care for children. The social role of caring for children ('parent', or other relative/friend) can be a source of powerful motivation for therapeutic change. The consideration of the needs of the child(ren) can provide good signposts for organising care plans for those caring for children, especially parents, that can also help maintain treatment motivation.

(5) Particularly important in a forensic context is the association of active social engagement with low recidivism rates and better community adjustment in prisoner resettlement.

General issues

Statistics

The following statistics from the UK give a brief outline of the situation and its dimensions. In many instances, they are estimates. Some of the data are taken from a speech by Cherie Booth given at the conference 'Young mothers from custody to community' (12 May 2004), organised by the Prison Reform Trust (www.prisonreformtrust.org.uk):

- In the UK, 125 000 children currently have a parent in prison.
- At least 17 700 children have a mother in prison; other estimates suggest 22 000 children of mothers in prison in the UK.
- The population of women in prison has increased from 1800 in 1994 to over 4500 women in 2004. There is no significant increase in the number of offences that women commit that would explain this change in numbers. Overall, just over 6% of the prison population is currently female (including some 600 aged 15–21).
- In the course of a year, 13 000–16 500 women are received into custody. Approximately two-thirds of these are mothers of children under 16.
- Up to 85% of women in prison misuse drugs. Numbers vary from country to country and according to culture and methods of data collection. The estimates for men are similar, but hard data are not available. Drugs are mostly brought in by visitors, and a large and conspiratorial network of relationships keeps this state of affairs going. This network of relationships itself is abusive in nature.
- The suicide rates of women in prison are increasing (14 in 2003), and so are the rates of self-harm. Again, there are no reliable hard data, but the rates are high (although perhaps not in comparison with offenders on community service orders). Many women and men in prison have histories of abuse and traumatic and deprived childhood experiences. Of course, this includes parents in prison.
- A survey in one prison found that although 95% of women felt that family contact was extremely important, 33% of women with children

had not received any family visit at all. Women observed that over time the facilities for, staff attitudes toward, ease of booking and frequency of visits had significantly declined.

- A quarter of young offenders are fathers, and a variable proportion but usually more than half of all male prisoners are fathers.
- Over 40% of all prisoners say they have lost contact with their families since entering prison.
- Prison allocation often is far away from home because of shortage of accommodation and other resources.
- Currently, rates of recidivism are going up, especially among women prisoners.
- Secure hospitals and other forensic mental health facilities have parents among their patients. Exact numbers are difficult to come by, but in some services a significant proportion of children visit their parents (Dickinson, personal communication).

Practice

Some prisons have mother-and-baby units. They have a very different culture and may represent an island of more 'normal' relationships within an otherwise often very depressing environment, especially in women's prisons. While they seem to be of some benefit, a proper evaluation of mother and baby units is not available at present. Moreover, in the UK, the time allowed for mothers and babies in those units is usually limited to 18 months, after which other arrangements for the care of the child have to be made. The effect of this time-limited arrangement has not been evaluated.

One of the main roles of prison has often been described as 'retribution' by society for offending behaviour. It is clear from the literature that a culture of retribution may not be helpful in the context of parenting and psychological development of a small child or its parents (e.g. McCord, 1998). Probation and support services for people in the criminal justice system are not particularly geared toward supporting parents. Paradoxically, the provisions inside prison are better than support services after discharge. In a number of prisons, people can choose to take part in parent-craft classes and family relationship classes. Anger-management courses or courses aiming at reducing domestic violence in men are also available as part of probation services. On discharge, the only parenting-oriented services available are generic service provisions, which are often in short supply, resulting in a 'competition' of the needs of discharged prisoners with the needs of other parents for limited resources.

Of course, some prisons have exemplary arrangements and systems in place to facilitate family visits. There are also many and increasing numbers of initiatives in the voluntary sector that attempt to support families when a parent is inside. However, it is very clear that a prison is – like so many other public services in many countries – an institution geared toward individual adult requirements. The needs of the children are not paramount in this system.

Lastly, issues of ethnic background and race are important variables in the prison population. Proportionately, many more black people serve sentences. Other differences include the way parenting and the care of children work very differently for different people (Baunach, 1988). For example, in the USA, African-American and Hispanic women are more likely to rely on grandparents and other relatives for child placements, whereas white women rely on husbands/partners or foster carers for the care of their children while serving time (Enos, 2001). This has implications for visiting arrangements, contact and a possible reunion after release.

The issues of parents within the criminal justice system, especially prisons, tend to be complex and can be solved only by multiple partial solutions. A number of proposals have been made (e.g. Boudouris, 1996; Seymour & Hairston, 2001). One key ingredient for any attempt at helping people change the way they think and offend has to be a way that allows them to take responsibility for their own actions in a structure that enables feedback and learning (for more detailed, general proposals, see Pryor, 2001).

Mental health and prison

The prison population has a high incidence of people with mental health problems, especially personality disorder (Singleton *et al.*, 1998) although the whole spectrum of psychiatric disorder is seen. People with psychotic disorders are not always well served by time in prison. Of course, parenting issues are equally relevant for those working therapeutically with psychotic issues (for details, see Cowling *et al.*, 2004a & b; Jacobson, 2004; McClean *et al.*, 2004; Seeman, 2004). Circumstances in prison are particularly complex for parents with serious and enduring mental health problems of the psychotic type.

More differentiated facilities may achieve a better deal for society in general, and for those offenders suffering from psychological disorder in particular. A recent development in New York has been the establishment of mental health courts, in an attempt at a more differentiated response to the needs of offenders within current resources and without 'being soft on crime' ('Where Justice and Mercy Meet'; by Jennifer Gonnerman, 27 July 2004, *Village Voice*).

A Cognitive Analytic Therapy (CAT) perspective on parents in prison

Offending, prison and parenting

'Parenting', a relatively new word in the English language, is intensely culturally defined (Göpfert *et al.*, 2004). It is a role relationship involving responsibility for another; 'parenting capacity' can be defined as the capacity to be preoccupied with the child, to keep the needs of the child in mind (Hill, 1996; 2004). Responsibility is a core value in the parent–child relationship. However, there is a general issue about prison and responsibility that has been detailed by Pryor (2001). In essence, prison has a strong tendency to disempower and to take responsibility away (see also Wyner, Chapter 18 of this book).

Many parents' criminal activity leading to imprisonment may have been in direct conflict with their task as parents, either because of the particular nature of their offending behaviour patterns (e.g. drug dealing), or because they could not be available as parents for their children due to the consequences of their offending behaviour, reflecting an underlying ambivalence about their parenting role and responsibility. The arrest and imprisonment might then forcefully bring the domains of criminal activity and parenting together, often in a crisis when crime directly interferes with parenting.

Parents may cope with this by keeping the domains of crime and of family life relatively separate. This can be much more separate in the mind of the offender than in the experience of children and family. The often abusive relationship patterns of power and control prevalent in the offending behaviour can be identified in the parenting and family domain, too. Even parents who have given up their criminal career might struggle with the continuing potential for abusive behaviour, as illustrated in the following vignette:

Case example: Jerry

Jerry had a history of very severe childhood physical abuse; juvenile gangland crime; multiple drug addiction, including crack heroin; and prison sentences for robberies, aggravated violence and drug dealing. When he decided to quit his 'criminal' life, he moved to a different city and came off all drugs except diazepam, which he used to contain his impulsive anger and anxiety, and to cope with his pattern of disrupted sleep. At a psychiatric day hospital, he met a woman with whom he had a much-adored child. Because of his use of diazepam and erratic sleep patterns, he was available only intermittently as a parent, although passionately invested in the relationship with his partner and in his role as parent and protector. His parenting role was constructed in terms of the responsible 'gang leader', fighting with the hostile outside world to protect the vulnerable members of his family.

A high proportion of parents are imprisoned for violent index offences. No evidence is available that adequately illuminates the relationship between the nature of index offence and capacity to parent in general. It is the duty of the psychotherapist in each individual case to understand any such possible link.

In institutions of criminal justice, life is regimented and controlled.

Prisoners, especially new arrivals, often find their experience and their new role of prisoner very stressful. Thus, the role of responsible parent is not easily compatible with that of the 'irresponsible' (i.e. deserving of punishment) prisoner. How parenting can or cannot continue varies from prison to prison, and even more so between countries. Some basic aspects of this are captured in Fig. 7.1.

The necessarily simplistic description of role relationships in Fig. 7.1 highlights the similarity between the role of the prison authority/criminal justice apparatus and the role of parent. Practicalities apart, the system makes it more difficult to fulfil and enact the role of parent for the prisoner because of the incompatibility of the two roles. Of course, there are ways in which the roles can be combined and mutually supported, but the blueprint of the system does not foster it. One of the underlying main force fields in prison is the tension between the disempowering jail and the prisoner's need to fight for a measure of autonomy and control in order to survive psychologically. In the words of one writer, prison enacts the role of 'abusive parent' (Watterson, 1996).

In the context of deprivation and loss of social status, the parenting role can enhance social status and self-esteem, especially for women. In some instances, women have been suspected of becoming pregnant in order to access resources (e.g. mother-and-baby units in prison with their less prison-like and more 'normal' environment). More generally, the prevailing cultural assumption that mothers should be primary carers for their children is important and may even serve as justification for their criminal activity in their own mind (offending in order to 'earn' the money to keep the family fed). Enos (2001) has demonstrated how mothers in prison collectively have very clear hierarchies of (1) motherhood, (2) drug addiction and (3) criminal activity in their mind (in that order).

Men tend to feel a failure for their children and often cope by cutting off

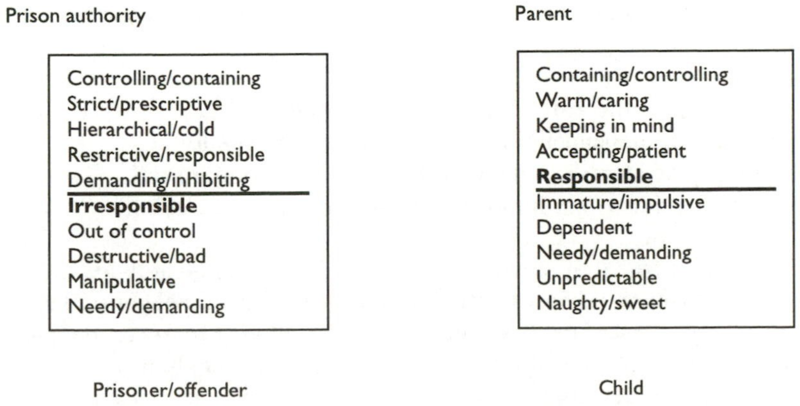

Prison authority   Parent

Controlling/containing	Containing/controlling
Strict/prescriptive	Warm/caring
Hierarchical/cold	Keeping in mind
Restrictive/responsible	Accepting/patient
Demanding/inhibiting	**Responsible**
Irresponsible	Immature/impulsive
Out of control	Dependent
Destructive/bad	Needy/demanding
Manipulative	Unpredictable
Needy/demanding	Naughty/sweet

Prisoner/offender   Child

Figure 7.1 The dynamics of prison.

emotionally from their role of father. This may reinforce a sense of being redundant, in turn increasing the risk of reoffending. In a UK study, the majority of fathers, when asked, confirmed feeling guilty or ashamed, and described an intense sense of helplessness (Boswell & Wedge, 2002). Often imprisonment is kept secret from the children. This makes it more difficult for children to process the information as they pick up the emotional issues around court hearings and imprisonment. It also makes it more difficult for fathers to accept and work through the consequences of their imprisonment, because they need to carry on as if nothing has happened in order to guard the secret.

Mental health, prisons, parenting and CAT

Mental health is associated with the patient role, prison implies a certain role behaviour for the people in it, and the role of parent also implies role behaviour: each of these terms may represent a role enactment from which a complex situation can arise. Apart from the patient role as such, a mental disorder may itself come with an array of disorder-determined role enactments, including an element of dependency defined as the 'patient role'. They may be an expression of a parent's personality disorder, such as patterns of borderline personality disorder.

Working with parents with personality disorder in prison (Fig. 7.2)

The importance of secondary gains

Becoming a father or mother may be intended to solve the issues of one's own traumatic and deprived childhood through projective processes. Beyond the general social status accorded to parents, the parenting role may be a major source of status and self-esteem in many different ways, especially to mothers:

- through parental authority and responsibility
- through the dependent affection and love of the child
- through the identification with the child as a 'good object'
- through being a very important person in someone else's life.

Therefore, it is true that parents may need children quite badly for their own personal, non-parental needs, setting the scene for emotional abuse. This does not fit very well with the 'best interests' of the child. Moreover, people who are not allowed to care fully for their children can quickly learn to talk the language of the 'best interests of the child'. The following case illustrates a number of issues with a personality-disordered parent.

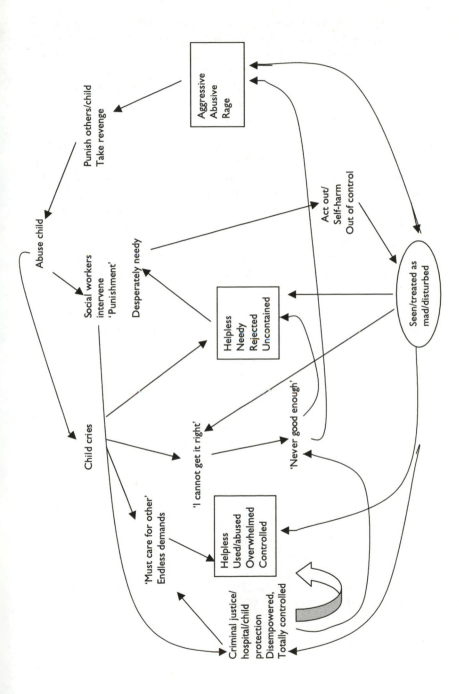

Figure 7.2 The parent with borderline personality disorder in the criminal justice system.

Tracey's case (part 1)

Tracey, aged 26, was released from a prison term imposed for giving a critical overdose of sleeping pills to her three and a half-year-old daughter. She had shown no obvious sign of remorse. A history of eating disorder and deliberate self-harm complemented her history of sexual abuse by her father. She had been diagnosed with borderline personality disorder. Her own mother was also diagnosed as personality disordered. As a young teenager, Tracey had tried to poison her mother with sleeping pills dissolved in drink.

The baby had been taken into care and was fostered by her grandmother. Tracey appeared to improve her mothering during access visits while serving her prison sentence and after release. Eventually, she was reinstated as the main carer. She had attended parent-craft classes and counselling for her abuse history as part of prerelease preparation. The counsellor's and the probation officer's report were instrumental in her reinstatement as main carer because of their experience of her as a fully cooperative client who worked on her experiences of abuse and their emotional impact. Tracey had always maintained that it was in the best interests of the child that she should resume her role as main carer.

The relationship between Tracey and her mother was strained, but the baby was developing well while being fostered by her grandmother. Two weeks after the decision about the baby's care had been implemented, a close friend of Tracey in treatment with a local counselling service disclosed to her own counsellor that Tracey had confided her anger and frustration with the child protection services and with her mother. Tracey had told this friend that she planned to abduct her child if she was not reinstated as the custodial parent. She had made detailed arrangements and preparations for this eventuality, starting with a joint outing with her mother to a place where it would be easy for her to get away with the baby.

The patterns of deception will be familiar to psychotherapists involved in providing therapeutic services to people who are referred by statutory child protection agencies. It is a very good example of how a client can deceive professionals by providing them with the precise image of the willing parent able to improve herself (see also Wright, 1976). More worryingly, the client's motivation in this case probably was less to care for the child and more the need to defeat the services which had re-enacted a pattern of criticism and emotional abuse that was already well established between Tracey and her mother.

Parentification: The effects on the child of role reversal and
emotional abuse

'Parentification' is a core variable of a relatively separate and growing body of research (e.g. Byng-Hall, 2002). It links emotional abuse and attachment perspectives. It also corresponds to the CAT concept of restricted reciprocal role repertoire. It may be particularly important to understand in the context of prison, as prison powerfully demands that the prisoner comply and satisfy the demands of the institution as represented by the prison staff. Furthermore, many people with complex mental health problems (who are numerous among prisoners) have a developmental history of significant parentification.

Caring for a parent (termed 'young carer'; see Aldridge & Becker, 1993) is normal. It is the child's way to deal with the parent's difficulty in coping. This adaptive response will have consequences for the child's psychological adjustment. Some children cope with these situations by developing task-oriented competencies, which can be a strength in their lives (Galdstone, 1965; Silver, Doublin & Lourie, 1969; Bleuler, 1974; Breznitz, 1985; Stein-hauer, 1991; Pound, 1996; Bilsborough, 2004). Sometimes, children find it difficult to develop an adaptive response, particularly if they are exposed to rigid family structures or expectations (Ryckoff, Day & Wynne, 1991).

Parentification refers to a child's feeling compelled to enact a parental role and to shoulder inappropriate responsibility (Sessions, 1987; Mika *et al.*, 1987; Valleau *et al.*, 1995; Jurkovic, 1997; Byng-Hall, 2002; Earley & Cushway, 2002; see also the title character of Dickens's *Little Dorrit*). This may be because a parent is enacting a needy and dependent role (e.g. in the case of a parent suffering from chronic fatigue), or because the parent is incapable of fulfilling the parenting role for a period of time; essentially, the child(ren)'s needs are not met (as in situations of drug addiction, but also if the parent is in prison). More generally, it has been used to describe role patterns that are an outcome or expression by the child of the emotional or concrete need of the parent, conscious or unconscious (Jurkovic, 1997), and, for some authors, include experiences of physical and sexual abuse. In the adult that has grown up with a pattern of parentification, this pattern tends to characterise much of the person's relationships, and the experience of prison can powerfully resonate as a result, often unhelpfully.

In role terms, parentification is a case of role reversal. Winnicott (1964) has provided us with an accurate description of parentification and its effect in the case of a depressed mother. According to Winnicott's observations, children of depressed mothers often live only *reactively*. Life in the 'here-and-now' is suspended in the hope that a different relationship with the parent will become possible in the future that will provide the age-appropriate parental care. Occasionally, the child may achieve what is hoped for. For many children, this never happens, turning the suspension of oneself into an internalised relationship pattern of caring for the parent and others. Most are left forever longing (sometimes desperately) for the parental care they never received. Many clinicians will be familiar with this pattern, especially in people with complex mental health needs and histories of severe deprivation and/or abuse.

In this author's experience, many, if not most, people suffering from conditions diagnosable as personality disorder display some aspect of what Jurkovic and colleagues defined as parentification (Jurkovic, 1997). While there is no comprehensive evidence yet in support of this assertion, the aetiological trauma model of personality disorder in CAT implies a combination of different abusive experiences, including experiences of emotional abuse and parentification.

Parentification dynamics may present in many different forms, which sometimes can appear inconsistent. An example is the 'gang leader' who – with contempt for any other authority – tries to create a functioning world for his gang, a not uncommon phenomenon in prison. 'Psychopathy' may be predominantly an attempt to adapt emotionally to a situation where feeling/empathy may result in increased vulnerability, be this because of an inborn error of processing emotional communication (e.g. Blair, 2001) or because of the deleterious effect of serious abuse. In some way, psychopathy can be the 'successful' resolution of the pattern, originally described by Winnicott, that restores control to the subject. Let us look at the case of Tracey again.

Tracey's case (part 2)

As a result of her friend's disclosure, a forensic psychiatric assessment of Tracey was carried out. Tracey described how she had become so murderous as a young teenager. The constant emotional and sometimes physical abuse by her mother (e.g. never being able to get it right, constantly changing goalposts in terms of what would possibly get her mother's approval, never getting any praise) left her feeling so angry that it seemed as if there was no other way out than killing her mother. When this did not work, she realised that there would not be a straightforward solution of her dilemmas.

When she had the baby, she found herself in a situation that caused very similar feelings, but now, as a parentified child, in the real role of mother. Whatever she tried, she could never completely satisfy the baby and experience herself as a 'successful' carer. The baby's behaviour made her feel exactly like she had felt with her demanding mother. Furthermore, it reactivated the situation of feeling totally criticised by her real mother both for having the baby and for the way she cared for it.

She felt in desperate need of care from anywhere or anyone. Half-impulsively, unconsciously and desperately, and half-deliberately, she gave the baby some of the same sleeping pills that some years before she had given to her mother and knew did not work. She then dropped hints with professionals that she had done so, ultimately resulting in immediate care proceedings. She herself was involuntarily received into the care of the adult mental health system for a brief period as a crisis measure, and she found herself in a world of psychosis, medication and chaos, without any capacity for understanding her particular needs.

In prison, she perfected her skill at playing the system and became the compliant, insightful, model prisoner. In short, she had learned that there was nowhere she could get the understanding and care that would make a difference to her. Manipulating the system became her defence against victimisation.

Figure 7.3 attempts to represent some essential aspects of Tracey and her context.

Tracey's case illustrates how a strong internalised parentification pattern can militate against the parent's adopting the best interests of her child because every demand situation turns the 'demanding one', be it prison, the care system, psychotherapists eager to help, or one's own child, into a representation of the demanding, needy parent. The pattern in essence is one of the perception of a demand for care coming forth from those whose task it should be to care, within the context of a power relationship linked to helplessness that leaves no recourse other than compliance. Emotionally, the deprived needy self is hidden from self-awareness under a presentation of competence (Winnicott's 'false self').

The best interests of the child are the best interests of the parent!

Frequently professionals, including psychotherapists, act as if there was a conflict between the interests of the child and the interests of their patient who is a parent (see also Weir & Douglas, 1999). There usually is the perception of a sequence in which certain needs of a patient must be met in order for progress to be possible. Commonly, the assumption is that some unresolved childhood issue needs addressing first, in order to enable the patient's parenting capacity to unfold. In Tracey's case, this was enacted by providing some counselling in prison for her childhood sexual abuse by her father in order to help her become a better mother. For Tracey, this was yet another demand interfering with her present needs.

Often, there is also a perceived conflict of interest in terms of time scales of development. Usually, the child's needs for age-appropriate development are pitched against the parents' needs to sort themselves out before being able to attend to the needs of the child. As in any polarised situation where the 'poles' are systemically bound together, the ground rule has to be that no solution will work that does not work for both poles of the perceived conflict; in other words, what is in the best interests of the child has to also be in the best interests of the parent. For this, the best interests of the parent/caregiver

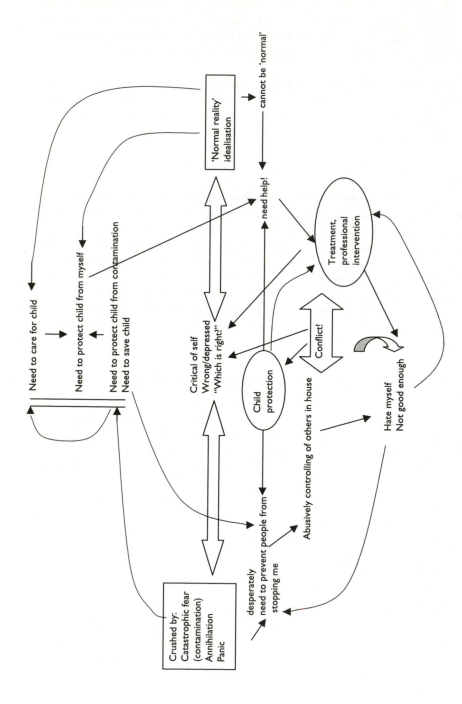

Figure 7.3 The parent with obsessive-compulsive disorder in the criminal justice system.

have to be seen as in the present and future. In order to do so, it is important to formulate possible social roles as a therapy outcome. If Tracey's main future ambition is to become a reasonable mother for her baby daughter, this ambition of hers is in conflict within herself with her need to have her child-derived needs met; that is, the conflict is not between her and the child but within herself. Alternatively, Tracey may mainly wish to develop the capacity to have adult relationships without repeating abuse patterns. This – while undoubtedly of benefit for the child – would not provide adequate care for the child. Tracey would then have to be set free from the responsibility of main carer. She would have to work out the relationship with her mother because her mother would need to become the main carer for the child without triggering battles about childcare. The guiding principle from attachment theory is that the family (or any other support system) needs to be organised in such a way that care is available to anyone when needed (Byng-Hall, 1995; 2002). In terms of attachment theory, Tracey shows all the signs of a 'dismissing' style of attachment behaviour, presenting as the model patient and prisoner, but at the same time relatively difficult to engage in therapeutic work (Adshead, 2004).

Tracy's case (part 3)

Tracey was asked what would have had to happen for her not to feel the need to develop the plan to kidnap her baby. She said very clearly that it would have helped if her relationship with her mother could be improved, and that she did not find it helpful to have to work on abuse issues with a counsellor while adapting to a prison situation that itself was abusive in her experience. The counsellor had become part of her abusive experiences. She admitted ambivalence about her role as mother and thought it helpful if she could carry on being involved with the baby, while taking care of some of her own needs. Joint work with mother and Tracey unravelled some of the background issues. Tracey's mother had herself been unable to confide in her own mother about her own, never-before-disclosed childhood sexual abuse. At the core of this was the early loss of her mother's mother due to death in childbirth, which had never been resolved. This work also focused on their joint capacity to validate each other's experience on the basis of some shared understanding.

As a result of this new information, both Tracey and her mother independently received some CAT-based counselling dealing with their relationship issues and reinforcing their capacity to give and receive validation of their emotional experiences with one another. This they had never experienced with anyone else, and it provided some of the security necessary for other change to occur. It did not resolve their conflicts but changed the way they could use conflict so that they were able to collaborate more in the care of the baby, who stayed with Tracey's mother.

Conclusion

There is a need for the routine consideration of a prisoner's role as a parent. The tools of CAT, alongside other essential tool kits such as attachment theory, offer a unique capacity to formulate the issues of parents in prison effectively and facilitate interventions that may help. The tension between the controlling, disempowering prison, in which the prisoner needs to survive both as an individual and as a parent, is key. In order to address this effectively, the prisoner needs to remain a person (see also Franciosi, 2001). This is one precondition for parenting as an issue to be 'visible' in prison so that it can be acknowledged and worked with.

Currently, raising the issue of parents in prison will potentially question the appropriateness of the institution and its task. However, unless the institution is enabled to see and embrace parenting issues effectively itself, attempts to 'get' it to do so become a demand for change from outside. It is better to enable change from within. The following are proposals for ensuring that skills within the criminal justice system are available so that parenting issues can be dealt with – they need active management, maintenance and evaluation as an integral part of the overall work of the institution:

(1)   a capacity to understand and formulate the best interests of the child and their interface with the needs of the parent.
(2)   understanding of the social role of parenting. CAT can make a particularly useful contribution here because of its capacity to link the internal with the social world through the formulation of role relationship patterns.
(3)   understanding of parenting capacity, and how to assess it meaningfully within the context of the prison system.
(4)   capacity to hold in mind the context of a child's environment – no child is ever just raised by a parent on its own. Prison is part of that environment.
(5)   ability to facilitate support for all those essentially involved in the care of the child and providing them with care or support if needed. Ideally, this can be met – with professional facilitation – mostly from within the resources of the wider family.

Acknowledgements

Keith Hyde, Julia Nelki and Tara Weeramanthri have generously and significantly contributed to this chapter. I thank them.

References

Adshead, G. (2004). Three degrees of security: Attachment and forensic institutions. In F. Pfäfflin & G. Adshead (Eds), *A matter of security: The application of attachment theory to forensic psychiatry and psychotherapy*. London: Jessica Kingsley.

Adshead, G., Falkov, A., Göpfert, M. (2004). Personality disorder in parents: Developmental perspectives and intervention. In M. Göpfert, J. Webster & M. V. Seeman (Eds), *Parental psychiatric disorder* (2nd edn). Cambridge: Cambridge University Press.

Aldridge, J. & Becker, S. (1993). *Children who care*. Loughborough: Young Carers' Research Group.

Baunach, P. J. (1988). *Mothers in prison*. New Brunswick, NJ: Transaction Books.

Bilsborough, S. (2004). What we want from psychiatrists and their colleagues: 'Telling it like it is'. In M. Göpfert, J. Webster & M. V. Seeman (Eds), *Parental psychiatric disorder* (2nd edn). Cambridge: Cambridge University Press.

Blair, R. J. R. (2001). Neuro-cognitive models of aggression, the antisocial personality disorders and psychopathy. *Journal of Neurology, Neurosurgery and Psychiatry, 71*, 727–731.

Bleuler, M. (1974). The offspring of schizophrenics. *Schizophrenia Bulletin, 1*, 93–109.

Boswell, C. & Wedge, P (2002). *Imprisoned fathers and their children*. London: Jessica Kingsley.

Boudouris, J. (1996). *Parents in prison: Addressing the needs of families*. Lanham, MD: American Correctional Association.

Breznitz, S. (1985). Chores as a buffer against risky interaction. *Schizophrenia Bulletin, 11*, 357–360.

Byng-Hall, J. (1995). *Rewriting family scripts*. New York: Guilford.

Byng-Hall, J. (2002). Relieving parentified children's burdens in families with insecure attachment patterns. *Family Process, 41*, 375–388.

Caddle, D. & Crisp, D. (1997). *Imprisoned women and mothers*. Research Study 162. London: Home Office Research and Statistics Directorate.

Chase, N. D. (1999). *Burdened children: Theory, research and treatment of parentification*. Thousand Oaks, CA: Sage.

Cowling, V. (2004a). The same as they treat everyone else. In M. Göpfert, J. Webster & M. V. Seeman (Eds), *Parental psychiatric disorder* (2nd edn). Cambridge: Cambridge University Press.

Cowling, V. (2004b). Models of service provision in three countries: Marlboro, New Haven, Sydney, Melbourne and Lewisham. In M. Göpfert, J. Webster & M. V. Seeman (Eds), *Parental psychiatric disorder* (2nd edn). Cambridge: Cambridge University Press.

Earley, L. & Cushway, D. (2002). The parentified child. *Clinical Child Psychology and Psychiatry, 7*, 163–178.

Enos, S. (2001). *Mothering from the inside*. Albany, NY: State University of New York Press.

Franciosi, P. (2001). The struggle to work with locked-up pain. In J. S. Saunders (Ed.), *Life within hidden worlds*. London: Karnac.

Galdstone, R. (1965). Observations on children who have been physically abused and their parents. *American Journal of Psychiatry, 122*, 440–443.

Göpfert, M., Webster, J. & Nelki, J. (2004). The construction of parenting and its context. In M. Göpfert, J. Webster & M. V. Seeman (Eds), *Parental psychiatric disorder* (2nd edn). Cambridge: Cambridge University Press.

Hairston, C. F. (2001). The forgotten parent: Understanding the forces that influence incarcerated fathers' relationships with their children. In C. Seymour, C. F. Hairston (Eds), *Children with parents in prison*. New Brunswick, NJ: Transaction Publishers.

Hall, A. (2004). Parental psychiatric disorder and the developing child. In M. Göpfert, J. Webster & M. V. Seeman (Eds), *Parental psychiatric disorder* (2nd edn). Cambridge: Cambridge University Press.

Hill, J. (2004). Parental psychiatric disorder and the attachment relationship. In M. Göpfert, J. Webster & M. V. Seeman (Eds), *Parental psychiatric disorder* (2nd edn). Cambridge: Cambridge University Press.

Jacobson, T. (2004). Mentally ill mothers in the parenting role. In M. Göpfert, J. Webster & M. V. Seeman (Eds), *Parental psychiatric disorder* (2nd edn). Cambridge: Cambridge University Press.

Jurkovic, G. H. (1997). *Lost childhoods: The plight of the parentified child.* New York: Brunner and Mazel.

Linehan, M. M. (1993). *Cognitive behavioral treatment of borderline personality disorder.* New York: Guilford Press.

McClean, D., Hearle, J. & McGrath, J. (2004). Are services for families with a mentally ill parent adequate? In M. Göpfert, J. Webster & M. V. Seeman (Eds), *Parental psychiatric disorder* (2nd edn). Cambridge: Cambridge University Press.

McCord, J. (1998). *Coercion and punishment in long-term perspectives.* Cambridge: Cambridge University Press.

Mika, P., Bergner, R. M. & Baum, M. C. (1987). The development of a scale for the assessment of parentification. *Family Therapy, 14*, 229–235.

Pound, A. (1996). Parental affective disorder and childhood disturbance. In M. Göpfert, J. Webster & M. V. Seeman (Eds), *Parental psychiatric disorder*. Cambridge: Cambridge University Press.

Pryor, S. (2001). *The responsible prisoner: An exploration of the extent to which imprisonment removes responsibility unnecessarily and an invitation to change.* London: Prison Service.

Ryckoff, I., Day, J. & Wynne, L. C. (1991). Maintenance of stereotyped roles in the families of schizophrenics. In J. S. Scharff (Ed.), *Foundations of object relations family therapy*. Northvale, NJ: Jason Aronson.

Ryle, A. (1990). *Cognitive Analytic therapy: Active participation in change.* Chichester: Wiley.

Seeman, M. V. (2004). Schizophrenia and motherhood. In M. Göpfert, J. Webster & M. V. Seeman (Eds), *Parental psychiatric disorder* (2nd edn). Cambridge: Cambridge University Press.

Sessions, M. (1987). Influence of parentification on professional role choice and interpersonal style. *Dissertation Abstracts International, 47*, 5066 (University Microfilms International, US).

Seymour, C. & Hairston, C. F. (2001). *Children with parents in prison: Child welfare policy, program and practice issues.* New Brunswick, NJ: Transaction Publishers.

Silver, L., Doublin, C. & Lourie, R. (1969). Does violence breed violence? Contributions from a study of the child abuse syndrome. *American Journal of Psychiatry, 20*, 152–155.

Singleton, N., Meltzer, H. & Gatward, R. (1998). *Psychiatric morbidity among prisoners in England and Wales*. London: The Stationery Office.

Steinhauer, P. D. (1991). *The least detrimental alternative: A systematic guide to case planning and decision making for children in care*. Toronto: University of Toronto Press.

Valleau, M. P., Bergner, R. M. & Horton, C. B. (1995). Parentification and caretaker syndrome: An empirical investigation. *Family Therapy, 22*, 157–164.

Watterson, K. (1996). *Women in prison*. Boston, MA: Northeastern University Press.

Weir, A. & Douglas, A. (1999). *Child protection and adult mental health: Conflict of interest?* Oxford: Butterworth and Heinemann.

Winnicott, D. W. (1964). The relationship of a mother to her baby at the beginning. In D. W. Winnicott (Ed.), *The family and individual development*. London: Tavistock.

Wright, L. (1976). The 'slick but sick' syndrome as a personality component of parents of battered children. *Journal of Clinical Psychology, 32*, 41–45.

Chapter 8

The learning disabled offender and the secure institution

Philip Clayton

This chapter describes how the theory and practice of Cognitive Analytic Therapy (CAT) can and has been used within a medium-secure setting for people with learning disabilities. An exploration of how relationship difficulties experienced within the family, society and other institutions may be replayed or re-enacted within secure settings will be described using a shared formulation. Issues of containment and power relations will be discussed, particularly taking into account perceived and actual roles, responsibilities, professional accountability and personal characteristics. I conclude the chapter with two case vignettes which will attempt to illuminate the strengths that CAT has to offer in the treatment of the learning disabled offender and perhaps help to dispel the myth that psychotherapy cannot be adequately accessed by those who have a mild to moderate learning disability.

Treating the learning disabled offender in secure provision

There appears to be a dearth of material written with a particular emphasis on the learning disabled offender, treatment approaches and the relationship between institutions and the individuals who live and work within them. There are texts that emphasise the need for further research on the treatment of individuals with an intellectual disability who have offended (Clare & Murphy, 2001; in Emerson, Hatton, Bromley and Caine), and there are more general texts that have within them accounts of treatment interventions which are focused on behaviour (Stenfert Kroese, Dagnan & Loumidis, 1999).

Sinason (1992; 1999) has written elaborately and in fine detail about the benefits of working psychotherapeutically with people who have a learning disability, including those who have offended. Crowley (2002) quite clearly states that therapeutic models, particularly modified CAT, have a part to play in the understanding and treatment of people with learning disabilities. Crowley also makes explicit the role of society and groups in the maintenance of relationship difficulties. Ryle & Kerr (2002) refer to the use of CAT in forensic settings. Pollock & Belshaw (1998) describe the use of CAT with offenders but refer to the non-applicability of the model to those who are 'intellectually impaired'. Clayton (2000; 2001) explores the use of CAT within a medium-secure setting for people who have learning disabilities while also considering the reciprocal role enactments that may occur across staff teams. Lloyd & Williams (2003) have explored the use of the contextual diagram with 'distressed' staff teams and the broader implications within the organisational context.

The treatment issue and moving on

Historically, the psychological treatment of people with a learning disability has been behaviourally focused. Many clinicians used techniques derived from early psychological theories, particularly the behavioural school, which emphasised reinforcement schedules as the means by which change in behaviour is achieved. Token economy procedures were used to change behaviour, but perhaps the personal histories of the people who the clinicians were treating were not taken into account.

It is clear from the literature that as techniques evolved, the elaboration of models followed. Cognitive-Behavioural Therapy (CBT) as a talking therapy became widely used, and the 'doing with' rather than 'doing to' became central to the therapeutic encounter. It is also apparent that at the same time Valerie Sinason (1992; 1999) from the Tavistock Clinic was concentrating her efforts on working psychotherapeutically with the emotional life experiences of people with learning disabilities as well as thinking about the effects of behaviour.

While CBT might seek to 'change overt behaviour by altering thoughts, interpretations, assumptions and strategies of responding' (Kazdin, 1980), psychotherapeutic practice seeks to work in the transference relationship in order to facilitate change. The former utilises a structured approach, driven by protocol, with psychotherapy being in the main unstructured and driven by where the patient takes it in the context of the relationship between patient and therapist.

It is the flexibility of CAT that I believe brings richness to the therapeutic encounter for both patient and therapist, particularly with those who have learning and emotional disabilities. The possibilities appear to be considerably different and perhaps advantageous with an approach that draws upon cognitive and psychotherapeutic techniques rather than being constrained to one or the other. I believe that this population is able to access this approach if the therapist is versatile and open to the possibilities of adapting the tools.

For some individuals who have a learning disability, however, the tools of CAT may seem to be inaccessible. This can be addressed by the creativity and inventiveness of the therapist. For example, I have used audiotapes to supplement patterns drawn in pictures. Indeed, one of my most memorable responses from a patient I gave a tape to was, 'Thank you for listening to me. I listened to the tape a few times and I liked the bit about my mum the best and I don't feel it was my fault any more.' This patient had unjustified, unwanted and unresolved guilt feelings, and he was able to move on from this position and achieve reconciliation with his dead mother.

As in other therapies, the therapeutic alliance is the central, if not most important, aspect of the work. The ability of the therapist to hold the patient in therapy and to contain potentially unmanageable feelings in the hope that these can be worked with is paramount. CAT tools, in particular the reformulation and SDR, in whatever form they are presented and used, are the narrative and diagrammatic (or pictorial) representations of the patient's history. They are potentially validating to the person who receives them, particularly those who have experienced negating, rejecting, abusing and minimising carers and perhaps within different contexts and groups in society. Among those curative factors that Yalom (1985) describes, 'the instillation of hope', the notion of a sense that something, somehow, will perhaps change for the better, is given to the patient whose internal narrative may have previously been 'I'm the no-hoper'.

A review of this narrative is the core objective of therapy, and CAT has the tools to enable this process to take place. It is perhaps also important to consider that other tools may be incorporated into the process.

Medium-secure provision

In considering the role of medium-secure institutional care and treatment, it is crucial to consider what psychological impact incarceration may have on any given individual, particularly taking into account personal histories and difficulties experienced during the developmental process. Many people who are admitted to such establishments have experienced trauma in many forms, such as sexual abuse, bullying, rejection, abandonment and persecution, to name but a few, and have responded in ways that have been catastrophic. Others have offended in a manner that has been viewed and understood as overtly antisocial. Often, social rules are unknown for those who have also experienced a difficult upbringing. Despite psychological assessment and formal psychiatric diagnoses, these presentations may remain misunderstood and represent a 'challenge' to services. There is often little or no concept of individuals within the service having a part to play in relationship difficulties which serve to maintain the 'antisocial' presentation (McKeown, Anderson, Bennett & Clayton, 2003). Perhaps this is where the CAT model can be instrumental in change, not only for the individual but for those who work within the institution. The shared case formulation facilitated within the model of CAT can be and has been used to inform staff about individual difficulties and the part that they may play in reciprocating the negative self to self and self to other roles.

Within medium-secure institutions, the Mental Health Act 1983 may be used flexibly in conjunction with managers and the Home Office to enable treatment and care to be provided in a secure and safe way. Security is usually a word that defines the physical features of a unit, building or complex and the numbers of staff employed within. Depending on the policies of the institution, there may be different strategies employed to deal with particular issues, such as the management of self-injurious behaviour, aggression and violence, setting fires and sexual offending. Safety is usually defined by the physical features of the environment and staffing ratio despite there being an emphasis on empowerment and personal responsibility fostered in the patient population.

Treatment programmes are often focused on reducing these high-impact behaviours, and quite often this is done through skills-based programmes such as anger management, assertiveness skills, setting fires groups and sexual offending groups. However, the personal histories of the individuals taking part in such a group may not be considered to be important for the task of the group and may indeed be lost. Reciprocal role enactments may be played out in such groups but perhaps are not addressed or understood unless it is made explicit that past ways of relating may indeed be explored, as in the psychodynamic or CAT group. Engaging patients in CAT can provide insight into potential patterns of relating that may cause difficulties in groups, or indeed be helpful in addressing different ways of relating in groups.

Reciprocal roles within the institution

It could be said that people with a learning disability are a marginalised and to a large extent patronised minority group. This immediately sets up anticipated notions of how the relationship between individuals might be conducted, placing the other person in a role which is conducive to the expected societal 'norm'. This term 'norm' is arbitrarily ascribed depending on the judges who are charged with this task (see Dreyfus & Rabinow (1982) for further discussion). Within the institution, this problem may be perpetuated by the expectations of the individuals who work, manage and live within them.

When considering the role of secure institutions, it is all too easy to locate the continuance of a given problem solely within the 'problematic' individual. Of course, in some cases, it might be that the patient is the instigator of the reciprocal role enactment, but there is always the 'other', which may be located within the self or another. This 'other' may represent for the patient all that is to be resisted, abhorred, punished, hated or humiliated. 'They' may possibly be the distillation of everything they have experienced in their lives, and this is given added intensity within the close constraints of a 'secure' environment.

Interpersonally, the 'other' persons may of course also be blind to what they represent for the patient. Unwittingly, having been affronted, they may respond in a way that confirms negative self-evaluation for the patient. Indeed, it might be that the converse occurs and that a staff member experiences a deskilling or hopeless feeling, particularly with people who seem to be throwing care back in their face. Here, the manifestation of the socially derived reciprocal role is enacted.

Relationships in terms of reciprocal roles based on power (subjugation, authority) – disempowerment could become the norm if care were not to be given to the understanding of the processes that occur between individuals. Typically and probably inevitably, power relations are a part of our daily lives, and we would consider that in the main these relationships are negotiated. When power relations are imposed, the controlling to controlled reciprocal role is in play.

Many individuals with a learning disability who are located within medium-secure provision have this role imposed upon them through the legal system and are under the responsibility of a named psychiatrist. Because there is a national shortage of psychiatrists (at the time of print) and taking into account the personal experiences of this client group in particular, it could be suggested that extreme forms of reciprocal role enactment are far more probable, such as *distant, controlling-to-dismissed, ignored*. King (2002) explores and describes common sets of reciprocal roles that have been experienced by people she has worked with, such as *abusing (bully)-to-abused (victim)*; *not being heard or understood-to-unheard, not understood*; *rejecting-to-rejected*. I have also worked with people within secure institutions and witnessed situations that have developed over time to represent familiar and similar patterns of relating such as *abusing-to-powerless victim*.

Not only is the issue of powerful individuals in the system a microcosm of what has been previously experienced in families and in society, but also the mental health system itself may represent a reinforcement of hopelessness and the inevitability of disempowerment. Symbols of power may be discreetly and unwittingly present in systems where apparent democracy is supposed to be present. Foucault (1979) has described the case file or dossier as a powerful instrument in the control of an individual. The sense that 'any' individual has 'knowledge' about another implies an imbalance in the power relationship. So the knowledge that some individuals have direct access to all pre-empts the notion of a separate autonomous and free-thinking individual and promotes the ideology of control. The discourse of the 'professionalised' individual is so written without an expression of consent.

The safe haven of the 'secure' unit

In my experience, some patients seem to have endured so many traumas in their lives that there is an almost immovable desire to remain in hospital. I have heard patients talk of the staff group as the family they never had or the hospital as the safest place they have ever lived in. The fear of leaving this safe, womb-like place has driven patients to sabotage their own progress, even to the point of displaying difficult behaviour days before planned resettlement. Subsequent anxiety is then felt by the prospective community team, who may replay the rejecting, dismissive reciprocal role. In therapy, a patient once said to me, 'If coming to therapy means that I might get better and leave, well, then, I don't want it.'

Therapy within the secure institution

Crowley (2002) writes that modified CAT can be used effectively with people who have a learning disability and King (2000; 2002) has described clinical work where modifications to the model have succeeded in bringing a rich psychotherapeutic experience into the room by using pictures, drawings and objects. This, however, is in the context of community-based services, and although I am not differentiating the use of the model from this population, I will make the distinction between differing contexts. Firstly, because medium-secure forensic services will not now (or rarely) admit people who present only with a challenging behaviour, this tends to narrow the remit to those who have offended and probably have a history of such behaviour. Furthermore, those who are referred and admitted tend to be those who have a borderline learning disability with added complications such as difficulty in relating and perhaps problematic personality traits and/or disorders. It could be argued, taking into account points made earlier, that difficulty in relating in the past is endorsed by admission to secure services, or that there is a feeling of being saved from past difficulty in relating.

The essential component of therapy is indisputably the therapeutic alliance, and the literature confirms this across all the available therapies. Within the institution, this alliance could be compromised (as described above in terms of power relations), in terms of the potential of splitting. Here, as Dunn & Parry (1997) and Kerr (1999) have described, the shared case formulation and contextual diagram come into effect. This is a shared understanding with the patient's consent of the main problem, coined in terms of the reciprocal role enactment within the context of the community team. Simple it may seem, but the knowledge base of the staff group needs to be taken into account. Kerr (1999) has begun to address this issue by offering training at a local level to enable staff groups to begin to understand what is happening at an interpersonal and organisational level with difficult-to-manage patients. Clayton (2001) also describes how helping a group of nursing staff within the institution understand a person's difficulties, and the way their response to the individual served to perpetuate the patient's problems, relieved difficulties and began to alleviate the distress experienced by both parties.

Here, obviously, ethical considerations come into play, and it is important that the permission of the patient is sought prior to sharing such sensitive material. This is, of course, common to all shared formulations, contextual diagrams (SDRs) and information that may cause the patient distress. However, there are also problems inherent in asking a patient about divulging information that might invite a response that would endanger or sabotage, and this issue is of course at the heart of the alliance.

In considering the use of CAT in a medium-secure facility, the therapist also needs to consider systemic factors which may perhaps be beyond the realm of understanding for some members of staff and which might include those who have no direct clinical involvement with particular patients. This may include staff who have a transient involvement with the patient and who have little time to understand the complexities of the personality behind the behaviour.

Gender and culture

Gender, identity and cultural issues are also variables within this population which require thought. Clarke & Llewelyn (in Pollock, 2001) explore the benefits of carefully considered therapeutic work with women who have histories of sexual abuse working with male therapists. They describe the possible benefits of experiencing a positive male role model while taking into account possible therapeutic ruptures around the abusing to abused reciprocal role (see case vignette 1). Clayton (2000) explores the application of CAT with a young Asian man with learning disabilities in medium-secure provision who had set a fire (see case vignette 2 for a similar associated cultural example).

The following case vignettes attempt to describe the process of helping the patient and staff by making the 'case note' accessible without creating an impasse or power struggle. In these case vignettes, names and possible identifying circumstances have been changed and/or omitted. SDRs have also been altered.

Case vignette I

Kathy, aged 18, was admitted to the unit by referral from a remand centre. She had been convicted of arson and was presenting with episodes of severe self-injurious behaviour, including attempted self-strangulation. Her history was peppered with episodes of sexual abuse and difficulty in relating with her siblings. She was unkempt at the assessment interview within the remand centre and uncommunicative and uncooperative with the visiting male psychologist, preferring to remain mute throughout the process. Remand staff noted Kathy's victim role and felt sorry for her and yet frustrated when she self-harmed. Her case notes reflected dramatic changes in presentation which served to confuse those she was with.

After her admission to the secure unit, Kathy continued to present as rather morose, ambivalent and cut-off. She was 'mothered' by a senior member of staff and 'fathered' by another. She continued, however, to self-harm at a rate and intensity that endangered her life.

Although Kathy was offered long-term therapy and attended for approximately 40 sessions, she remained silent. Could it be that the time wasn't right? She remained silent through a similar period of group therapy which was unstructured, but she eventually responded to a time-limited, skills group some 2 years after admission. It was interesting that staff members reported a significant change in how she related to others after this intervention. However, yet again, Kathy remained a very private self-harmer with periods of quiet, cut-off suffering. This had a profound effect on the staff group around Kathy, who found themselves both angry at her and frustrated in their desire to help her.

Kathy was referred for CAT with me, and prior to commencing therapy, it became apparent that the staff group who worked with Kathy were becoming increasingly anxious. Comments such as 'It's going to be like taking the lid off a can of worms' were common, and the anxiety from the staff group was something both myself and Kathy were to talk about. 'Why don't they let me do this now – I'm ready to take charge of myself' was a plea from her toward the end of our time together as the team around her retained an element of their caring and protective professional role. We discussed perhaps helping the staff understand what the issues were and how they could help by knowing. The concept of the shared case formulation was visible.

At the onset of therapy, Kathy was distant, evasive and reluctant to engage; however, a direct angry confrontation concerning my motivation to want to help her was a considerable shift and, from this point, the mapping out of an SDR that represented myself as a possible abuser with her attempts at keeping me away by maintaining an unkempt appearance was generated (Fig. 8.1).

As the therapy progressed and the Reformulation Letter was presented, attempts at keeping me at bay were far fewer, and she began to explore her own feelings and to realise that she was able to express herself in ways that had felt impossible prior to coming to therapy. Her ability to challenge others, including me, in a healthy manner, not enacting the victim role, was a visible change in her interactions with those with whom she came into contact. The institutional bodies, managers, ward staff and particularly those who hadn't seen Kathy for long periods of time, such as her institutional 'mother', remarked on how this different and healthy person had emerged from almost intractable early difficulties. At this point in time, our relationship had clearly changed qualitatively. Kathy was able to verbalise that all men are not horrible and began to attend her sessions with a different attitude. She was able to say that I was helping her and not abusing her as other men had done. She was, however, mindful of the motivations of others, and was accepting but wary of the attentions of male patients within the hospital.

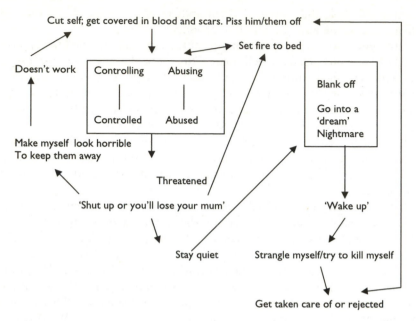

Figure 8.1 Case vignette 1.

Kathy stopped self-injuring completely. Despite having moments, particu-larly during night-time flashback phenomena which were clearly related to her abuse, she was able to manage these experiences. Sometimes she would ask a member of staff to keep her company and have a cup of tea. Toward the end of her therapy, Kathy was able to say that she wondered whether the staff understood why she felt scared of people sometimes. It was at this point that I explored the notion of sharing her diagram with the staff. With Kathy's agreement, I began the process of carefully introducing the staff to the CAT understanding of her problems. Responses to the formulation were varied from the staff group. There were understandable expressions of disgust and anger at how Kathy had been treated throughout her life. There was also an acknowledgement that nursing Kathy did not mean identifying with her. The exercise proceeded successfully. Within the following year, the authorities within the hospital responded to Kathy's new-found confidence and positive attitude toward herself and others. There was informed decision making des-pite her 37/41 Mental Health Act section (37 being a guardianship order and 41 being a restriction order). Based upon her progress and a rigorous risk assessment, Kathy was allowed to walk to the local village on her own and after a short time was allowed to carry a lighter to light her own cigarettes while out and about. Kathy was transferred to a community-based setting in her home town and is doing well.

Each 'loop' of Kathy's 'map' was colour-coded to help disentangle a potentially confusing diagram. Healthy reciprocal roles were identified throughout the course of therapy.

Case vignette 2

Tariq is a young man whose older brother died when he was 4 years of age. Although he did not know him well, as he grew up, he came to understand that he had to assume the responsibilities his brother would have been expected to accept. His father was a successful first-generation-immigrant businessman who clearly had plans for Tariq. Tariq, however, despite having a clear affinity with his cultural origins, also had tendencies toward the Western way of living and did not accept the prospect of an arranged marriage. Tariq's father became angry and resentful of his son's dissenting attitude toward him and began to exert influence over every aspect of his son's life to the point that Tariq felt powerless and ineffective. He began to endanger his life by jumping off bridges and into rivers, and cutting himself. The culmination of this chaos was his setting fire to his flat after an altercation with his father. Tariq's mother was perceptibly in the powerless role too, as were his two sisters except that they pursued a covert role of being secretly in control of their own lives, unknown to the 'head' of the family.

Prior to the commencement of therapy, the staff group were being drawn into reciprocal role enactments. They were beginning to be exasperated by and feel powerless about this determined young man who would stop at nothing to find implements to injure himself with. They also found themselves angry and resentful at his rejection of their care of him. It was clear from the onset of our 24-session CAT that Tariq was ambivalent about me, yet clearly wanting to receive help. My instinct was to think through a diagrammatic representation as soon as possible so as to contain difficult transference manifestations and to hold him in the therapeutic space. He was able to say to me that he felt understood but that he was not able to know what he could 'do' about his difficulties. He felt completely powerless in his relationship with his father and other powerful male figures, and this feeling began to be apparent in the therapeutic relationship and in relation with other male figures within the hospital. His ability to think through the diagram and to begin to trust his therapist was an emergent theme throughout the first 8 sessions to reformulation. The diagram seemed to be the central and most important tool in this therapy for both of us (Fig. 8.2).

The culmination of therapy was an ability to have himself heard by his father with all the respect that a son affords his father in keeping with cultural values and beliefs. However, the difficulties that Tariq was experiencing were not only associated with complex generational issues around expectations that his father had of him as an only son who would provide for the family as the parents grew older. Tariq's father also found the concept of learning disability very difficult to comprehend and continually referred to Tariq as

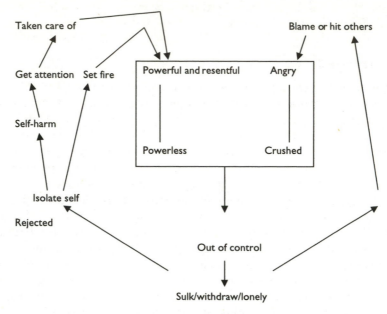

Figure 8.2 Case vignette 2.

recovering from his 'illness' in the near future and fulfilling his expected role in the family.

In both of the above cases, the initial anticipated difficulties in helping Kathy and Tariq to work through the 'relating to others' issues were soon dispelled. I found that using simple diagrams with clear examples from their lives soon brought the therapy to life. Hearing stories of such repetition in terms of damaging early styles of relating that continued for years from early childhood into adolescence and persevered into early adulthood, it was difficult to believe that healthy ways of relating might be unearthed. However, this was to be the case, and although Tariq still remains within low-secure provision and still has doubts about his ability to show his father he loves him while remaining independent, he has been able to engage in a long-term dialogue with him without feeling completely overwhelmed.

Limitations of CAT within secure institutions

Like other models of psychotherapy, CAT is a model which relies on shared understanding. Non-verbal communication is the greatest source of deriving information in any interpersonal encounter, and language is used to communicate what is happening between the two individuals. CAT uses this language and reproduces it in the form of 'the letter'. However, people with learning disabilities often have low ability to read and/or understand the spoken and written word or have other limitations in this respect.

As mentioned earlier, the intellectual ability of people referred to medium-secure facilities for learning disabled offenders is greater than in earlier times, and the use of letters and language is better received. Those individuals I have worked with who have problems with literacy often had primary emotional problems from a very early age or social and emotional deprivation that has precluded any form of educational experience. In these cases, pictures and drawings have provided a useful medium by which an alliance and shared understanding have been developed. Communication between therapist and patient may then have to rely on more imaginative methods and approaches, tools and media to enhance the therapeutic experience.

While I believe in the efficacy of CAT within such institutions, there is also the possibility of a contradiction in the power relationship of a seen 'case note' in the shared formulation unless care and inclusiveness in the treatment plan are attended to, with the patient having full knowledge of the good intention of the plan. This of course is relevant to clinical governance policies being driven in the National Health Service but clearly may also prove to be problematic with some difficult-to-work-with individuals.

I believe that the greatest problem facing the therapist and patient within institutions is the issue of knowledge. Knowledge of the processes inherent in the reciprocal relationship is potentially useful to both patient and staff group. If the therapist, the staff group and others are not aware of these processes, it is perhaps predictable that problems may continue. If, on the other hand, the therapist is aware, but the staff group are oblivious to relational issues, again, problems may persist. If the therapist and the staff group are aware but the managers are oblivious, then the fate of the therapy may be sealed, particularly as new ways of relating are attempted by the patient.

My position regarding the manager's (indeed all contact staff) awareness of the therapeutic process is not that which attributes the role to one or the other but that which promotes understanding of the overall reciprocal role process between individuals and groups. The objective is then clearer for staff members, managers, doctors and clinicians alike in order to enhance the organisational functioning. Obholzer & Roberts (1998) highlight seven needs for all members of organisations. The first three are as follows:

- clarity about the task of the organisation
- clarity about the authority structure
- the opportunity to participate and contribute.

For those in authority, there are the following four needs:

- psychologically informed management
- awareness of the risks to workers

- openness toward the consumers
- public accountability.

The shared case formulation again comes into the frame.

An example of 'joined-up' working

Some 3 years ago, I was consulted as to the difficulties an individual had presented to the service over a period of 7 years. The person in question was open to help and to involving the staff group in the process of sharing his case formulation. However, it was the nurse in charge who was instrumental in the change by approaching the manager of her ward to agree to the utilisation of staff training and in-service training. Despite the problems of 'giving little', with the issues of staff wanting to 'go further or wanting more', regular consultation on an energy-sapping weekly basis was employed. Understanding among the staff group, including the manager and the patient, was generated, and despite early problems with giving and taking, accepting and allowing, without collusion and/or 'punishment', relationships improved beyond all expectation.

Despite the apparent success of the above, such an enterprise is extremely labour-intensive and, if done properly, expensive. However, if viewed in the long term, for the prospect of 10 days' training in CAT and in-service training on a regular but limited term around the shared case formulation, I believe the cost advantage is comparable with the resources that would have been required to maintain the patient as he was presenting. The individual in question had required four-to-one physical restraint, frequently on a weekly basis, and was often given medication. Following a 1-year consultation and implementation of the shared formulation, this occurrence had reduced to once in 2 years and the patient had far greater autonomy.

Given that CAT is such a new innovation on the therapeutic menu, again resources are scarce. However, there is real, expressed interest from professionals across all disciplines in the application of CAT to people who have learning disabilities. All of the above are issues that need to be carefully considered in the planning and delivery of CAT within the institution beyond that which would normally have to be considered, given the microcosm' of the context.

Outcome measures

Currently, there are no outcome data relevant to the use of CAT with people with a learning disability and the reference standard is the randomised, controlled trial. There are clear accounts within case descriptions and follow-up outside the institution that would verify change and success in clients leading a reasonably fruitful life; however, in my opinion, these accounts have yet to be given the credibility that they deserve.

Given the lack of outcome data for this population, strategies are being developed to validate the usefulness of CAT beyond that of the single case study (Clare & Murphy, 2001). Routine assessment measures are applicable to some patients, and practising therapists are encouraged to use them as standard to build a body of data and become skilled in their use.

Notwithstanding this, I firmly believe that the single case study design has validity in itself, with follow-up contact being an indicator and instrument in the measure of change maintenance. I have followed up an individual for 3 years in the community after 24-session CAT in medium-secure provision. He had a history of imprisonment, high-secure containment and subsequent medium-secure care. It is evident to both of us that he is now able to maintain an independent lifestyle with minimal support.

The CAT special interest group (Crowley, 2002) has certainly proved motivation and commitment to the implementation of the CAT model in helping the person with learning disabilities, and the modification of CAT tools has been an innovative yet tentative attempt to deliver quality psychotherapy to people who have been denied such approaches in the past.

Developments and conclusion

Developments in the adaptation of tools used by CAT therapists include the modified Psychotherapy File and a computerised Personality Structure Questionnaire. There is also the developing creativeness of therapists working in the field in the use of ratings and techniques that help clients tell the story of their lives. It is clear from anecdotal evidence that, depending on a person's sensory preference, these stories can be told using a variety of tools beyond the conventional. As Anthony Ryle has stated, 'pushing where it moves' involves not only appropriate use of those psychotherapeutic skills required by the therapist to 'move' a therapy but also the inventive skills to create a vehicle by which the patient who has a learning disability may understand.

References

Clare, I. C. H. & Murphy, G. H. (2001). Working with offenders or alleged offenders with intellectual disabilities. In E. Emerson, C. Hatton, J. Bromley & A. Caine (Eds), *Clinical psychology and people with intellectual disabilities.* Chichester: Wiley.

Clarke, S. & Llewelyn, S. (2001). A case of borderline personality disorder. In P. H. Pollock (Ed.), Cognitive Analytic Therapy for adult survivors of childhood abuse: Case management and treatment. Chichester: Wiley.

Clayton, P. (2000). Cognitive Analytic Therapy: Learning disability and firesetting. In D. Mercer, T. Mason, M. McKeown & G. McCann (Eds), *Forensic mental health care: A case study approach.* London: Churchill Livingstone.

Clayton, P. (2001). Using Cognitive Analytic Therapy in an institution to understand

and help both client and staff. In G. Landsberg & A. Smiley (Eds), *Forensic mental health*. Kingston, NJ: Civic Research Institute.

Crowley, V. (2002). In *Introducing cognitive analytic therapy*. Chichester: John Wiley & Sons.

Dreyfus, H. L. & Rabinow, P. (1982). *Michel Foucault: Beyond structuralism and hermeneutics*. Brighton: Harvester.

Dunn, M. & Parry, G. (1997). A formulated care plan approach to caring for people with borderline personality disorder in a community mental health service setting. *Clinical Psychology Forum, 104*, 19–22.

Foucault, M. (1979). *Discipline and punish: The birth of the prison*. New York: Random House.

Kazdin, A. W. (1980). *Behavior modification in applied settings*. Homewood, IL: Dorsey Press.

Kerr, I. B. (1999). Cognitive Analytic Therapy for borderline personality disorder in the context of a community mental health team: Individual and organisational psychodynamic implications. *British Journal of Psychotherapy, 15*, 425–438.

King, R. (2000). CAT and learning disability. *ACAT News, Spring*.

King, R. (2002). An exploration of the practice of CAT with people who have learning disability from the perspective of the therapeutic relationship. Dissertation (required for UKCP accreditation, unpublished) for Inter-Regional Residential ACAT Psychotherapy Training Course.

Lloyd, J. & Williams, B. (2003). Reciprocal roles and the 'unspeakable known': Exploring CAT within services for people with learning disabilities. *Reformulation, the Newsletter for the Association for Cognitive Analytic Therapy, 19*, 19–25. London: ACAT.

McKeown, M., Anderson, J., Bennett, A., Clayton, P. (2003). Gender politics and secure services for women: Reflections on a study of staff understandings of challenging behaviour. *Journal of Psychiatric and Mental Health Nursing, 10*, 585–591.

Obholzer, A. & Roberts, V. Z. (1988). Social anxieties in public sector organisations. In A. Obholzer, V. Z. Roberts & J. Krantz (Eds), *The Unconscious at Work*. London: Routledge.

Pollock, P. H. & Belshaw, T. D. (1998). Cognitive Analytic Therapy for offenders. *Journal of Forensic Psychiatry, 9*, 629–642.

Ryle, A. & Kerr, I. B. (2002). *Introducing Cognitive Analytic Therapy*. Chichester: Wiley.

Sinason, V. (1992). *Mental handicap and the human condition: New approaches from the Tavistock*. London: Free Association Books.

Sinason, V. (1999). The learning disabled (mentally handicapped) offender. In E. V. Welldon & C. V. Velsen (Eds), *A practical guide to forensic psychotherapy*. London: Jessica Kingsley.

Stenfert Kroese, B., Dagnan, D. & Loumidis, K. (1999). *Cognitive-behaviour therapy for people with learning disabilities*. London: Routledge.

Yalom, I. D. (1985). *The theory and practice of group psychotherapy*. New York: Basic Books.

Chapter 9

A Cognitive Analytic Therapy-informed model of the therapeutic community

Implications for work in forensic settings

Ian B. Kerr & Michael Göpfert

There is a long and distinguished history within the therapeutic community (TC) tradition of working with a wide range of people with severe psychological disturbances, including those detained within the forensic system. This tradition has offered at least partially effective treatment and recovery opportunities to individuals with a range of often severe psychological problems that were beyond the means of traditional psychotherapy or mental health services. It has done so from a therapeutic viewpoint which for the most part stands in marked contradistinction to the norms and values of the custodial legal system and to the frequently paternalistic and, at times, authoritarian models employed in community-based services. However, this difference in approach has led to this powerful and challenging treatment modality being seriously neglected by both traditional community-based and forensic mental health services despite the evidence of its efficacy and cost-effectiveness (Dolan *et al.*, 1992; Gunn & Taylor, 1993; Woodward, 1999; and see comment by Allison, 2004).

A particular strength of the TC approach is the active involvement of other patients or residents in the overall therapy. They may, for example, take part in, or be responsible for, decision making about admitting or discharging fellow community members, generating a high degree of patient responsibility and participation. Since many of the community members will have experienced very similar problems and difficulties to the new arrival, this represents a further very powerful dynamic. Working in treatment with others who have 'been through it' before can offer effective support, as well as, at times, a challenge. It provides an experience of difference, and, facilitating engagement, it generates remoralisation and what Whiteley & Collis (1987) called 'affiliation'. Such engagement or affiliation is central to the recovery process, given the social nature of the self (central to the CAT model and those of group analysts – see Brown & Zinkin, 1994), and the need for social engagement and dialogue in the psychological well-being of all humans.

Models of the TC

TC models range from the democratic, permissive ('non-hierarchic') models described by Maxwell Jones (1953) to the more authoritarian ('hierarchic') 'concept' models initially developed in the USA for people with substance abuse problems (Clark, 1965; Kennard, 1999). TCs extend nowadays from time-limited, partial day treatment programmes that are largely run and operated by users themselves, and sometimes operate separately from public health-care services, to units or wards in closed institutions, such as forensic units. These may operate more as a 'therapeutic milieu' where the aim may simply be containment of the whole therapeutic system and active involvement and participation of its members. In recent years, there has been an increasing trend to see TC-based approaches as being largely applicable to individuals with severe and complex disorders, usually described as 'personality disorder'.

Given the nature of the treatment, evaluation and research evidence has inevitably tended to be naturalistic, but for those patients for whom this approach works, it has clearly been powerful and successful. However, the particular components of a TC treatment model and its essential, effective ingredients are still incompletely understood. Despite the apparent strengths and partial effectiveness of the various forms of TC, there are still major limitations at both theoretical and clinical levels, and further development at both of these levels is required. Despite the plethora of literature describing from a range of perspectives how such models operate and what their therapeutic individual consequences might be, there have been considerable gaps and, indeed, frequently contradictions between some of these therapeutic viewpoints (Kerr, 2000).

Broadly speaking, much of the earlier historic literature on the function of the TC has tended to be largely sociological, as in, for example, Rapaport's classic description of features of the TC (communalism, permissiveness, reality confrontation and democratisation) or in Maxwell Jones's well-known concept of the 'living-learning experience'. In terms of the function of the TC, Kennard (1999) has recently more usefully outlined a progression of what he calls 'defining characteristics' of the TC. Thus, he describes them initially in terms of a group of people who live together or meet to participate in a range of purposeful tasks; moves on to the existence of a culture of enquiry that is theoretically informed by a psychodynamic understanding of individual and group processes; and, finally, postulates boundary setting in which such enquiry can occur.

There is also a group analytic literature (see review by Rawlinson, 1999) which considers complex, large group processes that operate in such communities. From a theoretical point of view, these sit as an intermediary between the more sociological and individual psychodynamic models as applied to the TC. The latter have been dominated largely by the psychoanalytic literature (e.g. McGauley, 1997; Hinshelwood, 1999), which focuses on and describes, for example, severe personality disorder in terms of individual primitive defences such as splitting and projective identification. Within this tradition, however, it has also been noted by various authors that such concepts, offering rather esoteric accounts of psychopathology, are often hard to make use of clinically or in creating 'joined-up', causal accounts of experience, affects and behaviours which might be helpful to both therapists and patients (see review in Kerr, 2000).

Within the TC literature and practice, there has existed a certain tension between approaches stressing the key therapeutic role of sociotherapy (including sometimes simply befriending) and psychotherapy, although it may well be the coherent integration of the two which is likely to be most effective. Thus, there may be serious discrepancies between the values espoused within community function (such as democracy and permissiveness) and the models of individual practice which classically typify psychoanalytic practice. These latter are more traditionally characterised by a clear distinction between a superior, knowledgeable, expert therapist with access to an often complex model of psychopathology and an uninformed and often 'devious' patient whose communications and enactments may be interpreted as inherently destructive and unconsciously motivated. The patient will be expected to make use of this 'expertise', which often is expected to be mutative and helpful, lest he or she be deemed beyond help. From a CAT or Vygotskian perspective, several authors (see Ryle & Kerr, 2002) have previously argued that, in fact, such a position may not simply appear to be persecutory and demoralising to the patient, but may actually be so in reality, constituting another form of revictimisation. Unsurprisingly, many patients in such settings, whether treated by individual or group models, are unable to engage or stick with the process and drop out. When they do, the blame tends to be laid at their feet rather than being seen as an indictment of the therapeutic process or model.

There is clearly still a need for the further development of valid and effective models of TC function. In large part, this will need to be achieved by gradual, continuing dialogue and integration of ideas and practices both general and particular. For instance, the concept of motivation tends to be used as an all-or-nothing phenomenon by writers on psychotherapy in general, whether discussing willingness to stick to the therapeutic process or ultimate outcome, as for example, in forensic settings (Gunn & Taylor, 1993). From a CAT perspective, however, it would be argued (Ryle & Kerr, 2002) that this is something, along with 'psychological mindedness', which it is actually one of the tasks of therapy to help to develop. It should be noted, however, that CAT has not yet evolved or integrated ideas about the complex enactments and processes which occur at a group level, although some tentative steps have been taken in this direction. Some preliminary consideration of this area has previously been articulated (Maple &

Simpson, 1995; Stowell-Smith, Göpfert & Mitzman, 2001). This will be an important area for growth in the future in terms of the evolution of the CAT model.

The current CAT model in relation to TC function

CAT and the TC tradition share certain important fundamental features. Given that CAT was developed through an integration of both cognitive and psychoanalytic object-relations theory, there is of course also considerable overlap with various other current therapeutic approaches. However, this integration and its transformation by Vygotskian activity theory (Ryle, 1991; Leiman, 1992) and also by recent developmental infant psychology (Cox & Lightfoot, 1997; Trevarthen & Aitken, 2001; Ryle & Kerr, 2002) have created a distinctive approach which embodies many important points both of theory and practice in its model of development and psychopathology. In addition, Ryle has developed a clear, essentially trauma-related dissociative model of borderline personality disorder involving damage at different levels of the self (Ryle, 1997), whose implications, including its systemic effects, have been further explored by others (Kerr, 1999). The features of CAT include the involvement of the patient/client in active participation in the treatment and, indeed, the joint creation of an understanding of problems, their origins and ways of addressing them.

In a TC, there is the additional powerful dynamic of the engagement with a peer group who themselves have experience of similar problems. This is, in itself, of considerable therapeutic benefit (Rawlinson, 1999).

The CAT model, with its early and joint collaborative creation of a reformulation, also assists staff both in understanding and in jointly working on a patient's problems. It also helps in resisting the inevitable invitations to collude with various RRPs, a collusion which can be both blocking, self-perpetuating and demoralising for patients, and stressful for staff, as classically described by Main (1957) half a century ago in 'The ailment'.

In addition, the CAT and Vygotskian understanding of the formation of an essentially social self is important in understanding the common origins of psychopathology (possibly in conjunction with temperamental/genetic difficulties in ability to empathise, with impulse control or with the tendency to dissociate). The Vygotskian notion of internalisation of such interpersonal experience and its becoming thus intrapsychic is also of importance in conceptualising how interpersonal experience in a TC may be internalised and transformed therapeutically in the patient. Vygotsky stressed, too, the importance of working in the zone of proximal development (ZPD) of patients and of the use of psychological 'tools' (such as reformulations). Interestingly, he also stressed the power of not only an enabling adult other or caregiver but also of a peer group in enabling this to happen. Reformulations can also be seen as psychological tools of preparation, promoting engagement and therapeutic alliance. Like 'psychological-mindedness', these are not all-or-nothing phenomena.

It should also be noted that from a CAT perspective it is inevitable that any therapeutic relationship within an implicit power hierarchy carries the risk of being experienced as a re-creation of the abusive and depriving relationships with carers in early life. There then is a risk that therapy re-creates and reinforces the abusive experiences which gave rise to the issues requiring treatment in the first place. CAT attempts to reduce this risk by emphasising the collaborative relationship between therapist and patient and by generating a co-constructed holistic formulation that includes the experience of self and other.

By providing structures that allow responsibility for their own well-being to be given to people who otherwise feel helplessly stuck within their own construction of an abusive world, the TC model pushes the therapeutic boundaries a bit further. The change-inducing confrontation belongs essentially to the peer group and is informed by, and based on, everyone's experience of each other. The task of the professional is to facilitate the process; guard the rules which safeguard the democratic space within which responsibility, and with it the capacity to learn, can be given back to the individual; and provide a culture of acceptance, validation and – within limits – permissiveness. This is a complete reconstruction of therapeutic relationships.

At the core is the triangulation, as a principle, that there is always the third in any encounter with the other. The third is usually a peer or someone with a supportive role, ensuring that there are more than two views of the same situation; this can help to reduce the polarisation into 'abuser' and 'abused'. 'Truth' and 'fact' become relative, further inviting reflection rather than engagement in instant action. One of the implicit aims of a TC has been described as turning people who act into people who can think. This could be greatly aided by the role-relationship paradigm of CAT as an eminently common-sense way of externalising the 'problem' and making it accessible. In summary, the TC model provides a structure that allows responsibility for risk to be given to those who have and live the risk in the first place. And it maintains that structure by providing a multiplicity of views in the context of peer-group affiliation. This creates a setting where care tends to be more available when needed, providing a degree of security (in attachment terms) not easily available elsewhere, and an essential requirement for change to occur (Byng-Hall, 1995).

We would like also to note the special pressure on therapists and TCs in forensic settings to focus principally and inappropriately on rates of recidivism as the principal measure of therapeutic outcome (Gunn & Taylor, 1993). This can be seen to represent, in effect, an unwanted, inadvertent and anti-therapeutic collusion with authoritarian and institutional role enactments from outside.

Finally, we would like to emphasise the need for and importance of appropriate training in working with such 'difficult' patients in forensic settings and their inevitable systemic consequences, as is generally stressed in reviews of work in this field (e.g. Cordess, 1998). We suggest that CAT could make an important contribution in this area in both training psychotherapists and in training at the level of generic mental health workers (De Normanville & Kerr, 2003).

CAT and forensic psychiatry

The important contribution of CAT to work in forensic settings is described at length both in this volume and elsewhere (Pollock, 1997; Pollock & Belshaw, 1998; Ryle & Kerr, 2002; Wood, 2004). In general, CAT-based approaches have stressed a non-judgemental description (as opposed to interpretation) of the acquisition of RRPs and their enactments, many of which are comprehensible (as in psychosis) as, in a sense, coping but maladaptive or distorted enactments of roles with origins in early life. It has not been found necessary to attribute psychopathology to an autonomous and destructively motivated 'unconscious', with its risk of inherently pathologising and demoralising patients. A CAT perspective can enable a staff role of focusing on validating the patients' experience rather than providing potentially judgemental interpretations from a position of expertise.

We now present a vignette to illustrate a typical 'difficult' case in which a young man dropped out of treatment in a TC, and to reconsider and discuss this from a CAT perspective.

'Not up to it'

Jim was a young man in his early 30s who had been admitted 'voluntarily' to a residential TC of the democratic Maxwell Jones variety after a lengthy prison sentence for grievous bodily harm. He had been given a diagnosis of antisocial and borderline-type personality disorders. His treatment in the TC was part of the probation programme because of some recognition that psychological issues had contributed to his offending. He 'wanted to do better' for his son aged 6. His early life history involved parental alcoholism, violence, neglect, abuse and humiliation. He did badly at school. He had, however, been a natural sportsman and had had a trial for a well-known football club, although he had been dropped for recurrent drug abuse. His alcohol abuse and fights culminated in his prison sentence for seriously injuring a friend. Previous sentences had exacerbated his problems, and his drug abuse especially had increased after prison. He had a history of domestic violence, resulting in only occasional contact with his son. He appeared touchy, wary and paranoid, as was evident in his assessment by the other TC members and staff. However, he also had determination to try to 'get through' the treatment programme. His touchiness and wariness repeatedly led to his withdrawing grumpily although still maintaining that he was determined to finish the 'treatment' that he expected to be administered. At other times, he could be very tetchy about enquiries from others even if they were well intentioned, making it difficult for the TC to support him. On several occasions during the first few weeks, this came close to fisticuffs.

Throughout his stay, he remained reluctant about joining in the work of the meetings and work groups. He felt that work should be paid for as in prison, and that because of this attitude of his, people were picking on him or trying to make a fool out of him. Despite staff interpretations to this effect and positive and occasional negative 'feedback' from residents, he continued to struggle and on a couple of occasions went 'AWOL', smelling of alcohol on his return. He narrowly escaped being voted out. Later, he got into a violent argument with another male resident when he was again challenged about his withdrawn and at times apparently hostile attitude to others. He finished by throwing a chair across the room and storming off. He did not return but later was picked up drunk, having gone home and assaulted his mother, who had criticised him for dropping out and not sticking with it. This constituted a breach of his probation and he returned to jail. A poignant letter from there ruefully reflected on his difficulties in using the TC and his insight into and understanding of what had 'pushed his button'. Perhaps one day in the future, he hoped to give it another go. However, he was now detained for several more years at public expense and in a seriously non-therapeutic prison environment. Staff and residents were upset, but the consensus was that all that could be done had been done for him, and that in terms of sticking with the TC, Jim was simply 'not up to it' at that time.

Case conceptualisation and discussion

In discussing therapeutic approaches to such patients as Jim, it is important to bear in mind that they represent a fruitful plurality and that there are many things to be gained from a range of models. In any case, it is well recognised that 'common factors' account for a very significant amount of the variance in outcome of any therapeutic modality (Roth & Fonagy, 1996).

Although we shall approach this case essentially from a CAT perspective, given its robustness and coherence as a relational model of psychopathology, we suggest that there is still much to be learnt and integrated into this or any other model of therapy.

Within a TC, events like those surrounding Jim are often formulated within a psychoanalytic frame, and events like throwing chairs across the room may be accounted for in terms of a reified process of 'projecting feelings' literally into the community (see an account of a similar case by McGauley, 1997). From a CAT perspective, it has been elegantly demonstrated that such mysterious processes can actually and more usefully be accounted for in terms of reciprocal role enactments. Thus, the experience and behaviour of a patient are understood to represent an often extreme and intense role enactment which is responded to in a reciprocal enactment by an empathic therapist or other. Clearly, such concepts as 'projective identification' describe important phenomena, but, from a CAT perspective, do so in an unnecessarily mysterious and concretised way. Understanding Jim's act of throwing the chair across the room as a 'projection' into the community as a whole may do little to contain and comprehend his difficulties, nor does it necessarily help him work with them. Furthermore, it provides no means of conceptualising helpfully the staff group's own demoralising and divisive 'reactions' or attempts to deal with them (see McGauley, 1997). Thus, they become afflicted with what Main (1957) articulately described many years ago as an 'ailment' leading to burn-out, stress, buck passing and team splitting. It is in this area that CAT can have an important role to play in enabling a non-judgemental and empathic, integrated understanding of a patient's problems in terms of his repertoire of RRPs and their reciprocal enactments within the TC setting. It could also give an account of the systemic enactments elicited around them both in the immediate staff team and beyond, given the pressures which are brought to bear, particularly if a 'difficult' patient does not behave in a cooperative manner and get better (Kerr, 1999). This, in turn, can create further pressures on a staff team and often gets in the way of an accurate and helpful understanding of what is going on.

Such approaches may also be contrasted with more symptom-focused management of, for example, anger or self-harm (e.g. Novaco, 1989; Linehan, 1993; Linehan et al., 1993), which, while clearly effective to a point, does not aim to address or deal with underlying reciprocal roles or schemas that, unless revised, would be expected to continue to generate such maladaptive and distressing behaviour. This expectation appears to be borne out by more recent outcome studies of, for example, dialectical behaviour therapy (Verheul et al., 2003), which demonstrate reductions in self-harming behaviour, but not of underlying psychopathology.

From a CAT perspective, the apparent failure in the case of Jim could be helpfully understood as due to systemic, reciprocal enactments around the patient as well as in terms of his own role enactments. From this perspective, his historic core or primary RRPs might have been something like 'unheard, neglected, done down and abused' in relation to 'unhearing, neglecting, doing down and abusing'. There is clear evidence even from the brief description above of his enacting both these child-derived as well as parentally and culturally derived roles to others and of course to himself (e.g. 'doing down and neglecting' of self in relation to the questionable, in his mind, point of treatment). His coping or 'responsive' (Leiman, 2004) enactments would include soldiering on silently and warily, or exploding into 'abused vengeful rage'. This he might enact toward others but also indirectly or not so indirectly toward himself in his self-destructive outbursts or through his drinking (this also is arguably a seeking of a numb or zombie state). The systemic consequences of these outbursts when enacted directly to staff were that *either* they became fearful and withdrawing (unhearing and neglecting) *or* they retaliated by being angry or punitive themselves. This was also enacted by residents, and all of this compounded his sense of 'unheard' original core roles and perpetuated his coping enactments. This undermined engagement and building of a therapeutic alliance and allowed those with such views to attribute his outbursts and aggression to inherent, blameworthy and probably refractory destructiveness. Those who were sympathetic were regarded as naive by others in the staff team, who pointed out that the sympathy offered by some failed in fact to address or challenge his abusing outbursts (e.g. by explaining them with his earlier formative experiences as reflected in his repertoire of RRPs); such a challenge might have enabled some sense of 'being heard' to occur and thus engagement to happen. Overall, people were stressed and burnt-out by this man. One further important consequence of this failure was that he was deprived of a good ending and leaving from the TC, which is generally regarded as being of considerable therapeutic importance in itself (Norton, 1999; Ryle & Kerr, 2002).

These various enactments and 'reactions' are outlined in a rudimentary and speculative contextual SDR (Fig. 9.1), use of which might have helped to cut through much of this 'difficulty' and enabled some helpful work to have taken place and him to have stuck with the treatment. This framework and the CAT understandings could also help in negotiating and dealing with the outside world again in the shape of, for example, local mental health or probation services. These too would easily be drawn into reciprocal role enactments similar to those described in the diagram with staff and other residents. Reinvolvement with the outside world is well recognised to be a difficult, stressful and often relapse-provoking experience for former residents of TCs. As for the question of being 'up to it' as regards treatment in the TC, it might rather be asked whether it was the TC model itself that was perhaps 'not up to it'.

Conclusions

It is clear that TC-based approaches to working with difficult and damaged patients, particularly within the forensic system, can be effective and represent a powerful and humane treatment modality. Both the theoretical underpinnings and clinical practice of the TC could be greatly enriched by consideration and incorporation of features of the post-Vygotskian CAT model. This could help facilitate a better experience for patients, improved rates of engagement and more effective treatment for them as well as giving staff more powerful tools to work with and survive what are recognised to be at times highly stressful and undermining systemic reciprocal enactments. These would include the systemic pressures on a treatment setting from various agencies and individuals in power positions. A CAT-informed approach could also help with the erroneous assumption that all problems are located

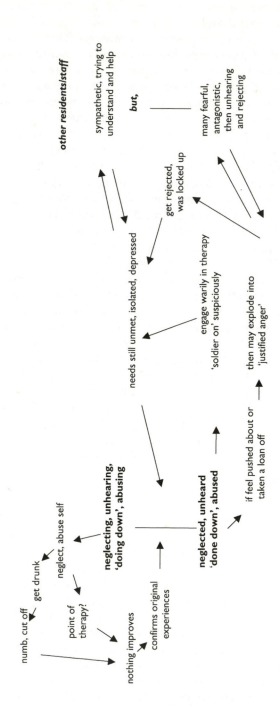

Figure 9.1 Sequential diagrammatic reformulation: Therapeutic community.

within or immediately around the patient. Such pressure comes also from line-management officers as well as other social and political agencies, including top levels of government. The tendency to individual attribution, together with functional ignorance of the systemic forces, is a property of a setting whose purpose is defined by the individual's apparent problems. Within this context, CAT could make the TC work more effectively, so reducing vulnerability to various pressures from within and without. CAT formulations could help in keeping treatment patient-centred and may assist in containing the obsession with rates of recidivism. Clearly, all therapists would want to practise in an evidence-based manner and be sure that what they are doing is effective. Similarly, these ideas and concepts will need to be evaluated further in a rigorous and formal manner, although we are fully confident that they will prove to be solid building blocks for the continuous development of therapeutic practice.

Acknowledgement

We are grateful to Dr Brigitta Bende for excellent advice.

References

Adshead, G. (1998). Psychiatric staff as attachment figures. Understanding management problems in psychiatric services in the light of attachment theory. *British Journal of Psychiatry*, *172*, 64–69.

Allison, E. (2004). Opinion, *The Guardian (Society Supplement)* 22 Sept., p. 5.

Bateman, A. & Fonagy, P. (1999). Effectiveness of partial hospitalisation in the treatment of borderline personality disorder: A randomized controlled trial. *American Journal of Psychiatry*, *156*, 1563–1569.

Brown, D & Zinkin, L. (1994). *The psyche and the social world: Developments in group analytic theory*. London: Routledge.

Byng-Hall, J. (1995). *Rewriting family scripts*. New York: Guilford.

Campling, P. (1999). Chaotic personalities: Maintaining the therapeutic alliance. In Campling, P. & Haigh, R. (Eds), *Therapeutic communities, past, present and future*. London: Jessica Kingsley.

Clark, D. H. (1965). The therapeutic community – concept, practice and future. *British Journal of Psychiatry*, *111*, 947–954.

Cordess, C. (1998). The offender. In D. Tantam (Ed.), *Clinical topics in psychotherapy*. London: Gaskell.

Cox, B. D. & Lightfoot, C. (Eds) (1997). *Sociogenetic perspectives on internalisation*. Mahwah, NJ: Lawrence Erlbaum Associates, Inc.

De Normanville, J. & Kerr, I. B. (2003). Initial experience of a CAT based skills certificate level training in a CMHT. *Reformulation (Newsletter of ACAT)*, *18*, 15–27.

Dolan, B., Evans, C. & Wilson, J. (1992). Therapeutic community treatment for personality disordered adults: Changes in neurotic symptomatology on follow up. *International Journal of Social Psychiatry*, *38*, 243–250.

Gunn, J. & Taylor, P. J. (1993). *Forensic psychiatry: Clinical, legal and ethical issues.* London: Butterworth Heinemann.

Haigh, R. (1999). The quintessence of a therapeutic environment. In P. Campling & R. Haigh (Eds), *Therapeutic communities, past, present and future.* London: Jessica Kingsley.

Hinshelwood, R. (1999). Psychoanalytic origins and today's work. In P. Campling & R. Haigh (Eds), *Therapeutic communities, past, present and future.* London: Jessica Kingsley.

Jones, M. (1953). *The therapeutic community: A new treatment method in psychiatry.* New York: Basic Books.

Kennard, D. (1999). *An introduction to therapeutic communities.* London: Jessica Kingsley.

Kerr, I. B. (1999). Cognitive Analytic Therapy for borderline personality disorder in the context of a community mental health team: Individual and organisational psychodynamic implications. *British Journal of Psychotherapy, 15,* 425–438.

Kerr, I. B. (2000). Vygotsky, activity theory and the therapeutic community: A further paradigm? *Therapeutic Communities, 21,* 151–164.

Leiman, M. (1992). The concept of sign in the work of Vygotsky, Winnicott and Bakhtin: Further integration of object relations theory and activity theory. *British Journal of Medical Psychology, 65,* 209–221.

Leiman, M. (2004). Dialogical sequence analysis. In H. Hermans & G. Dimaggio (Eds), *The dialogical self in psychotherapy.* Hove: Brunner-Routledge.

Linehan, M. M. (1993). *Cognitive behavioral treatment of borderline personality disorder.* New York: Guilford Press.

Linehan, M. M., Heard, H. & Armstrong, H. E. (1993). Naturalistic follow up of a behavioral treatment for chronically parasuicidal patients. *Archives of General Psychiatry, 50,* 971–974.

Main, T. (1957). The ailment. *British Journal of Medical Psychology, 30,* 129–145.

Maple, N. & Simpson, I. (1995). CAT in groups. In A. Ryle (Ed.), *Cognitive Analytic Therapy: Developments in theory and practice.* Chichester: John Wiley & Sons.

McGauley, G. (1997). A delinquent in the therapeutic community: Actions speak louder than words. In E. V. Welldon & C. Van Velsen (Eds), *A practical guide to forensic psychotherapy.* London: Jessica Kingsley.

Norton, K. (1999). Joining and leaving. In P. Campling & R. Haigh (Eds), *Therapeutic communities, past, present and future.* London: Jessica Kingsley.

Novaco, R. W. (1989). Anger disturbances: Cognitive mediation and clinical prescriptions. In K. Howells & C. R. Hollin (Eds), *Clinical approaches to violence.* Chichester: Wiley.

Pollock, P. H. (1997). CAT of an offender with borderline personality disorder. In A. Ryle (Ed.), *Cognitive Analytic Therapy and borderline personality disorder: The model and the method.* Chichester: Wiley.

Pollock, P. H. (2001). *Cognitive Analytic Therapy for adult survivors of childhood abuse: Approaches to treatment and case management.* Chichester: Wiley.

Pollock, P. H. & Belshaw, T. D. (1998). Cognitive Analytic Therapy for offenders. *Journal of Forensic Psychiatry, 9,* 629–642.

Rapaport, R. N. (1960). *Community as doctor.* London: Tavistock.

Rawlinson, D. (1999). Group analytic ideas: Extending the group matrix to TCs. In

P. Campling & R. Haigh (Eds), *Therapeutic communities, past, present and future*. London: Jessica Kingsley.

Roth, A. & Fonagy, P. (1996). *What works for whom?: A critical review of psychotherapy research*. New York: Guilford Press.

Ryle, A. (1991). Object relations theory and activity theory: A proposed link by way of the procedural sequence model. *British Journal of Medical Psychology, 64*, 307–316.

Ryle, A. (1997). *Cognitive Analytic Therapy and borderline personality disorder: The model and the method*. Chichester: Wiley.

Ryle, A. & Kerr, I. B. (2002). *Introducing Cognitive Analytic Therapy: Principles and practice*. Chichester: Wiley.

Stowell-Smith, M., Göpfert, M. & Mitzman, S. (2001). Group Cognitive Analytic Therapy for people with a history of sexual victimisation. In P. H. Pollock (Ed.), *Cognitive Analytic Therapy for childhood abuse: Approaches to treatment and case management*. Chichester: Wiley.

Trevarthen, C. & Aitken, K. J. (2001). Infant intersubjectivity: Research, theory and clinical applications. *Journal of Child Psychology and Psychiatry, 42*, 3–48.

Verheul, R., van den Bosch, L. M., Koeter, M. W. J., de Ridder, M. A. J., Stijnen, T. & Van den Brink, W. (2003). Dialectical behavior therapy for women with borderline personality disorder. *British Journal of Psychiatry, 182*, 135–140.

Welldon, E. V. & Van Velsen, C. (Eds.) (1997). *A practical guide to forensic psychotherapy*. London: Jessica Kingsley.

Whiteley, J. S. & Collis, M. (1987). The therapeutic factors in group psychotherapy applied to the therapeutic community. *International Journal of Therapeutic Communities, 8*, 21–32.

Wood, H. (2004). Psychoanalytic theories of perversion reformulated. In J. Hiller, W. Bolton & H. Wood (Eds), *Sex, mind and emotion: The psychological treatment of sexual disorders and trauma*. London: Karnac Books.

Woodward, R. (1999). The prison communities. In P. Campling & R. Haigh (Eds), *Therapeutic communities, past, present and future*. London: Jessica Kingsley.

Young, J., Klosko, J. S. & Weishaar, M. E. (2003). *Schema therapy: A practitioner's guide*. New York: Guilford Press.

de Zulueta, F. (1993). *From pain to violence: The traumatic roots of destructiveness*. London: Whurr.

Chapter 10

Cognitive Analytic Therapy for a rapist with psychopathic personality disorder

Philip H. Pollock

Psychotherapy for psychopathic offenders could be conceived of as perhaps the ultimate challenge for forensic psychotherapy. Offering therapy to persons who are defined by qualities such as being devoid of a capacity to connect, failure to attach and a tendency to corrupt and pervert relationships does not solicit confidence about our ability to 'humanise' these offenders' interactions. McWilliams (1994) mused about the challenges of psychotherapy for psychopathic personalities, stating that 'some are so damaged, so dangerous, so determined to destroy the therapist's objectives that psychotherapy would be an exercise in futility and naïveté' (p. 160). Strasburger comments that the psychopath is 'the least loved of patients' (2001; p. 191). Kernberg (1984) identifies the psychopath's 'malignant grandiosity' which intends to sabotage therapy and the therapist's endeavours, demeaning and devaluing efforts to help or connect with the patient. It is therefore not surprising that therapeutic pessimism reigns within the psychotherapy community about the efficacy of our effort to achieve change with these types of offenders (Meloy, 1992).

In contrast, Salekin (2002) reviewed the realities of the efficacy of psychotherapy for psychopathic personalities, arguing that the notion that they are immune to treatment may not be an entirely objective fact. He suggests that 'a considerable amount of therapeutic frustration, confusion, and pessimism to researchers and clinicians alike . . . may have blurred psychologists' perceptions of important clinical realities and stalled enthusiasm for research pursuits that would have produced and enhanced interventions for this complex clinical problem' (p. 80). The 'what works' debate regarding this disorder is likely to feature polarised opinions.

Individual psychotherapy for psychopathic personalities is limited to case studies as illustrations. For example, Schmideberg (1978) reported the successful individual treatment of a 16-year-old who maintained gains over a 10-year period. Templeman & Wollersheim (1978) used cognitive-behavioural therapy for psychopathic criminals which appealed to their 'self-interest' to motivate change. Martens (1999) reported the 3-year psychoanalytic psychotherapy of a sexually violent criminal who attained 20 years of freedom in remission. The author identified 'windows for treatment' that, if therapy is offered and these opportunities are capitalised upon, can lead to a successful outcome. Wallace, Vitale & Newman (1999) devised a cognitive-behavioural therapy for psychopathic individuals which focused upon addressing the identified impairment in response modulation which impedes self-regulation. Vaillant, Hawkins & Pottier (1998) compared cognitive-behavioural therapy for 28 psychopathic and 29 general criminals, showing that cognitive-behavioural therapy achieved poor results for the former group. Therefore, positive evidence of the advantages of individual psychotherapy is scant.

What can forensic psychotherapy offer for psychopathic personality disorder?

The concept of psychopathy has a controversial history (Blackburn, 1982). Recent theoretical and clinical developments have advanced our understanding of the differentiation between antisocial personality syndromes and the specific, superordinate designation of psychopathic personality disorder. A multitude of etiological factors have been implicated to explain the development of the condition. With the advent of Hare's formulation of Cleckley's criteria (1981) and the accumulation of cross-cultural comparative research evidence (Cooke & Michie, 2001), communication between professionals about the nature and underpinnings of the concept has improved substantially. The improvement and reliable agreement about the concept (Hare, 1996) and its measurement with the Psychopathy Checklist–Revised (PCL–R) (Hare, 1991) have encouraged research, which has confirmed that psychopathic personality disorder is relatively predictive of violence (Salekin, Rogers & Sewell, 1996; Hemphill, Hare & Wong, 1998).

The histories of those who exhibit psychopathic personality disorder are characterised by disturbed, abusive, negligent and damaging parental care (Pollock, 1999). Levy & Orlans (2000) proposed that the 'affectionless psychopath' emerges through disruption during the first 3 years of development, causing a lack of attachment capacity, chronic anger, poor impulse control and a lack of remorse and empathy for others. Smith, Gacono & Kaufman (1998) reported the absence of attachment in the responses of adolescents diagnosed as psychopathic. Frodi, Dernovik, Sepa, Philipson & Bragesjoe (2001) suggested that psychopathic individuals tend to exhibit a dismissive attachment style and an absence of secure attachments. O'Neill, Lidz & Heilbrun (2003) reported that the severity of abuse and neglect in childhood predicts psychopathic characteristics, and Widom (1978) claimed that research shows a 'clear connection' between childhood abuse and neglect and violence, with psychopathy (assessed by the PCL–R) mediating this link.

Disorder of relating (and attachment) is evident in terms of how the psychopath manages his own internal processes and also self–other relationships, tending to exhibit deficits and tendencies which imply disordered, harmful ways of interacting with the world. Pollock (1999) speculated that, on the basis of research evidence showing that primary psychopathic homicide perpetrators had endured traumatic childhood events, yet did not experience the killing of the victim as stressful, psychopathic offenders may exhibit personalities configured through the impact of abuse, neglect and poor caregiving in formative years, compromising their capacity for intimacy and attachment. A failure to internalise nurturing, caring repertoires of relating (RRPs) is compounded by the psychopathic personality's reliance on a narrow range of harmful, damaging and destructive RRPs absorbed from interactions with uncaring, abusive caregivers. Although such a thesis does not explain all of the observations made regarding the psychopath's internal and external repertoires of relating, this type of analysis does provide a model of the development of faulty, harmful ways of relating to self and others.

There are no reported case studies of Cognitive Analytic Therapy (CAT) for psychopathic personality, although the failures in internalisation (Kernberg, 1984; Meloy, 1992), the detached/dismissing attachment patterns and the deficits in empathic concern are features of the disorder that may be amenable to CAT's emphasis on reciprocal roles within relationships (e.g. self-to-self and self-to-other RRPs), dysfunctional states of mind and self-perpetuating, harmful procedures as they affect the self and others. The conceptualisation of the narcissistic, grandiose self infused with aggression must be a central facet of therapy of any type with the psychopath, and its relationship to the offender's interpersonal behaviours and perceptions of others must be understood as the core of the disorder. Meloy refers to the 'harsh' care experiences of the psychopath and how s/he internalises a *stranger self-object* as a predatory, malignant object relation in response to these events. The predator-to-prey RRPs of the psychopath guide the interpersonal relationships in terms of abuse, detachment and a lack of empathic resonance (Pollock, 1997; 2001). Psychopathic personality disorder can be viewed as a developmental process, many of its intrapersonal and interpersonal features deriving from harsh, unfacilitating parental treatment. The CAT model's focus on the derivation of self–self and self–other RRPs as identity forms marks an explanatory framework to understand some, but not all, of the psychopath's disordered and damaging action-oriented procedures.

Within psychotherapy itself, transference and counter-transference relationships with the psychopath are turbulent and require mature, firm handling. Certain counter-transference reactions have been documented. These include a real fear of assault and harm, helplessness and guilt as therapy is seen to fail, a loss of professional identity in response to narcissistic contempt and derogation, a foolhardy denial of dangers and risks, rejection of the patient, intense experiences of hatred and a rageful wish to destroy. Whether a concordant (*identifying*) or complementary (*elicited, reciprocal*) response is experienced within the transference (Racher, 1962), the therapist's task is to maintain the integrity of the therapeutic frame and alliance to avoid collusion with these potent transactions that are indicative of the psychopath's abuse of relating and the helper's investments. It is essential that clear management of these potentially harmful patterns of attachment be a core feature of therapy. CAT is well placed to decipher and facilitate management of these difficulties.

The present case describes the CAT of a 35-year-old man diagnosed with psychopathic personality disorder who was imprisoned for a series of violent rapes. The prisoner was offered individual, offence-focused forensic psychotherapy with an explicit emphasis on the link between personality and the crimes. He had refused transfer to a therapeutic community, in a different country, and no other options for therapy were available.

A psychopathic rapist: Max's history

Max proved to be a poor historian, yet Social Services documents were extensive in his case. He was the third child of his divorced mother, who had remarried 5 years later. His mother was described as alcohol-dependent, and neglectful of all of her children, and she was suspected of collusion in sexual abuse by both her first husband (until Max was aged 6) and Max's stepfather (ages 7–11). His biological father was imprisoned for sexual offences against Max, his brother and sister. The stepfather was reported to have sexually abused the three children and was later jailed for his part in a child pornography ring.

Max was received into care when aged 12, his mother's neglect escalating to unacceptable levels. Max was separated from his siblings, and his mother failed to maintain contact over the following years. He was placed in children's homes, Borstals and finally prison, when, aged 18, his crimes involving theft, motoring offences, violence, arson, criminal damage and racketeering with a known gang. No psychiatric history was documented, apart from admission to an Accident and Emergency hospital department after an incident of superficial self-harm, Max stealing medicines from the hospital before leaving. Max had a history of severe substance misuse and became addicted to injected heroin when aged 17. He had not entered any adult relationships prior to the index offences, which consisted of six rapes of women over a 15-month period. Max recalled that, during this period of crime, 'I just took everything I wanted, I didn't care. I stole money, I stole drugs, I took sex, simple as that.'

Max's offences

Max was convicted of six rapes, with three additional counts for buggery on two of the victims. Max's offences were analysed to formulate the types of interactions between offender and victims. Consistencies were noted within his actions throughout the series of offences. It was apparent that, typically, he had prior contact with all of the six victims whereby he made amorous advances to them which were rejected. For example, Max's third victim was a 19-year-old student whom he encountered at the local university library. He could not provide a reason for being in this library except to say, 'I had passed it a lot of times before. I was curious about who was in there.' He admitted that the crowds of young, female students were enticing for him and drew his attention. The preliminaries to this offence consisted of Max sidling up to the student and engaging her in conversation about her studies. The conversation, according to the victim, changed from small talk about her studies to her interests outside the university she attended and then onto topics about her sexual interests and whether she had a partner. The victim reported that Max was persistent and became agitated when she said she had a long-term relationship and was engaged to be married. She excused herself and left, making comments to her friends about Max's forceful and somewhat intrusive questioning of her about her relationship. Max followed this student for 2 days until he was sure about the location of her residence and who lived with her. Max recalled, 'I remember that she wasn't with any boyfriend – she'd only said that to make me jealous or to get me to go away. It was worse that she was rejecting me for nothing – what a bitch!'

After this rejection, Max ruminated about many past events and the wrongdoings of others against him. Max recalled feelings of 'being angry to the point where I felt sick in the stomach. I'd get a headache. I was pacing up and down. I thought, "Fuck them all". She was going to get it good for lying to me.' Max sat in his home drinking whisky and smoking cannabis, and then equipped himself with a garrotte, materials to blindfold and gag the victim, and a screwdriver to gain entry to the house. He entered the property through a kitchen window at the back of the house, and lay in wait. When the victim arrived, he made an explosively violent, blitz-type assault on her with a poker until she was overwhelmed and silent. Max tied the victim's hands and feet and blindfolded her before he sat down to compose himself. He waited and watched until the victim gained consciousness. Max's account of the crime was as follows. He played a 'game of cat and mouse, teasing her'. Max felt that he was in total control of events, and the victim was powerless, in submission and passive. He asked her what sort of sexual acts she 'wanted' and beat her if she did not name the 'things I was thinking of doing. If she got it wrong, she got hit; if she got it right, I done it to her.' The victims reported that Max would ask them to rate his sexual performance compared with their boyfriend's and also whether he was pleasing them. The language used by Max was reported by the victims to alternate from reassuring and affectionate before and after the sexual acts to debasing, derogatory and abusive with name-calling during the attacks. He spent approximately 2 hours with each victim, and at the end of the offence used the garrotte intermittently to induce loss of consciousness before reviving her with water and smelling salts. He did not ejaculate at the crime scene and, being forensically aware, wore a condom and gloves. He took several items from the victim or her home, returning to his flat and drinking alcohol until he passed out.

When asked to think about the dynamic between himself and the student victim, Max claimed that he perceived her as having 'brought it all on herself. She shouldn't have lied to me. I sort of punished her for being a stuck-up bitch, put her in her place.' He offered that she had choices and made the wrong decision when she rejected him in the library. Max watched the local news for reports of the attack, although he denied keeping press cuttings. He claimed that he usually threw away any personal items taken from the victims, remarking, 'I don't know what I took things for – it was just habit I suppose.' He noticed that he would feel less inclined to use pornography or to body-build in the weeks after each crime.

Max was caught when the final victim in the series, a young waitress, had the presence of mind to collect samples of hair and fibres from him during the assault. He was sentenced to life imprisonment. 'I suppose it brought things to a stop,' Max reflected. 'I was going crazy, the whole thing was turning into a joke. I couldn't keep up with myself. I got reckless and too confident.' At his trial, Max was diagnosed as having an antisocial personality disorder with psychopathic disorder; he was not considered to be mentally ill. Max's offences were indicative of an anger-retaliatory rapist who had prior interaction with his victims and expressed a mixture of angry and complimentary pseudo-intimate verbal interactions during the offences. There was some evidence of sadistic torturing of the victims and that he had enjoyed the violence of the offences.

CAT with Max

After 10 years of imprisonment, Max was referred for forensic psychotherapy after his engagement in a number of programmes within the prison (e.g. enhanced thinking skills, anger management, drug and alcohol awareness). He had completed the sex offender treatment programme (SOTP), which he entered while deemed to be of high risk and finished at the same level of risk. He had been manipulative, disruptive and arrogant throughout the SOTP and was described by group facilitators as derisive of other prisoners' efforts, particularly during role-plays of offence scenarios, refusing to undertake this part of the programme. Individual psychotherapy was considered necessary to address Max's risk potential, because of his refusal to enter a therapeutic community and his poor performance in group settings.

The therapist's first encounter with Max was memorable. Max displayed an arrogant, mischievous, threatening attitude, speaking condescendingly: 'You're one of society's helpers. God, you make me sick, sucking up to the government – we ought to exterminate you guys at birth. They want me to come and talk to you for an hour. How revolting is that? You're all sickly sweet. I should just kill you now for everybody's sake.' The therapist understood Max's style of engagement in terms of possible RRPs that would probably affect the developing transference and therapeutic alliance. Despite his vitriolic tirade, Max agreed to undertake all psychological testing.

Psychological testing revealed an antisocial, narcissistic and sadistic profile on the Millon Clinical Multiaxial Inventory–Third Edition (Millon, Millon & Davis, 1994), and a full IQ in the above-average range with no neuropsychological dysfunction evident. His profile on the Antisocial Personality Questionnaire (Blackburn & Fawcett, 1999) revealed a primary psychopathic pattern. Impoverished and superficial narratives were observed on the Thematic Apperception Test (TAT), and repetitive references were noted to animals killing each other within the Rorschach protocol. Max's thinking was egocentric, yet imaginative. His behaviours within the prison were bullying, manipulative, provocative and deceitful. Administration of the Hare Psychopathy Checklist–Revised (PCL-R) (Hare, 1991) indicated a score of 36.

On review of the available data, including victim reports, forensic information and his presentation and history, it was decided to offer Max 24 sessions of CAT. His initial motivation could be subsumed under the remark, 'If I have to jump through this hoop, I will – just do what you have to.' He was passively compliant, and it was felt that Max's principal drive was strategic expediency aiming at his release, and that he believed that psychotherapy was a necessary evil rather than a personal commitment.

After four sessions, his Reformulation Letter was as follows:

Dear Max,

This is the letter I said I would put together to help us summarise how you have got to this point and also to help us think about the way forward when addressing the problems in your behaviour and history. I accept that you are in two minds about whether therapy is something you 'have to do' or will be of real help for you to live a different future without crime. We can alter any part of the letter depending on your views, but it is most important that we come to a shared understanding of what problems need working at and are relevant.

Your early contacts were neglectful, abusive and damaging and have influenced the man you have become and how you see yourself, others and how the world works. Your mother was an absent, cold, unavailable woman who never showed any affection or care for you, your brother or your sister. Your father was, as you have been told, a sexual abuser who harmed you and your brother and sister. I accept that you do not remember this abuse. Your father's leaving was followed only by the entrance of an even more abusive stepfather, who targeted you for all manner of abuse over a long period of time, involving his friends at times. You have said that you cannot even think about the abuse because it generates hatred, rage and an urge to harm others (anybody). It appears that you coped with and survived these circumstances by adopting a 'dog-eat-dog' attitude, and exploiting, stealing and manipulating to get your needs met without feeling any guilt or remorse for the impact of these crimes on others. Alcohol and drug abuse have been habitual parts of this lifestyle. You appear to have developed a detached, self-sufficient and cold way of relating to the world and people, and you see people as unreliable and only of value to you sometimes. To date, your life has been destructive to many people and to yourself, and you have failed to learn from experience or punishment, continuing the same patterns of living when released from prison.

The sexual crimes you have been imprisoned for were planned and predatory, targeting young women who rejected your advances. You entered their place of residence and subjected them to angry, degrading and defiling acts of sexual violence, almost killing some of them. You have said that you cannot explain your reasoning or motivations for the crimes and do not know why you did them. You have admitted fantasising about harming women through rape for many years, and you do not feel any regret or guilt for your actions or for the harm you have caused the victims.

Across the six offences, there appear to be patterns and sequences of thinking about yourself and the victims, and in terms of your actions and decisions that emerge as you build up to and carry out the crimes. It would be helpful to explore and analyse why you do what you do in the way that you do toward certain types of victim.

I suggest we work on the following target problems:

- *your own experiences of abuse and their possible links to the expression of associated emotions during the index crimes; resolving your own memories of abuse and understanding their effects on you*
- *your lack of feelings for the victims and their suffering*
- *the sequence of ways of thinking about others and yourself; your feelings, actions and decisions that lead you to be 'primed' to commit a sexual crime; the destructive feelings expressed and how these ideas and feelings emerge; how you see yourself during the crime, how you see the victims and how you relate to them*
- *the types of fantasies you have about harming others and how these fantasies precede the crimes; these fantasies as the 'breeding ground' for your feelings of hatred, rage and wish to harm others*
- *your feelings about yourself; seeing yourself as damaged, bad and deserving of disgust; how you have coped with your own suffering and trauma as a child and survived*
- *your own emotional needs and how they never seem to get met in relationships, leading to rejection and anger; how you have failed to manage these reactions and disappointments*
- *identifying the state of mind that develops when you are 'primed' to offend; your 'risk potential', something you must take ownership of and*

learn to understand, monitor and manage to prevent future crimes from occurring.

I appreciate that you feel that you have openly stated that your background is difficult to discuss and that you are wary of the value of therapy and suspicious about 'letting your guard down' to reveal such information, fearing it may be used by someone against you or given to those who may try to harm you. I acknowledge your problems in trusting others and your suspicions about my motives within therapy. I hope that we can work in partnership to change these repeating ways of thinking, feeling and acting to end the destructive consequences for you and others.

The therapeutic alliance with Max became challenging in the early sessions. He was known within the prison as a manipulative troublemaker who exploited and bullied more vulnerable prisoners and extorted money for protection. He was also a known drug dealer and user. Max's behaviours when in contact with prison governors were almost obsequious, but he devalued and sniggered at them when they gave positive reports to hearings or multidisciplinary professional meetings. Max was considered by prison staff to be two-faced and 'one to watch'. His history of exploitation of others through his crimes, his deceptive lifestyle based on taking advantage of others, particularly the vulnerable, and theft and manipulation were markers for transference and potential corruption of the therapeutic alliance. It was doubtful that Max could derive meaningful benefit from the therapeutic relationship without exploitation or manipulation.

Problems arose quickly between the therapist and Max. After the sixth session, a prison governor asked the therapist why he had told Max not to attend work because of sessions, Max having informed the prison staff that he was provided with sessions every day. A prison probation officer also requested a meeting with the therapist to discuss the reasons for Max's decision not to engage further with her to undertake certain programmes (e.g. an anger-management group programme) because he was attending therapy sessions. The therapist felt that a barrage of accusations and misunderstandings was emerging between professionals as a result of Max's tactics. The therapist felt cornered by angry professionals and disappointed by Max's behaviours. Challenged at the next session, Max responded with gleeful, almost triumphant and childish sneering, claiming that professionals were 'just being all uppity and stupid. What's the big deal? It's only stupid courses and stuff.'

The therapist's counter-transference responses were, initially, anger and a feeling that Max was exploiting the therapy to his own advantage, intending to avoid responsibilities he disliked and incite animosity between professionals. Max had been repeatedly late for his sessions, claiming that he had been sleeping or playing cards with other prisoners for money and tobacco. Therapy was being devalued and the therapist felt manipulated. It was considered that he was displaying the RRPs enacted through manipulative cycling (Bursten, 1972), and these were tentatively incorporated into the reformulation and monitored (Fig. 10.1, SS4). The main sequence of positions and RRPs of manipulation consists of the offender engaging in a ploy or ruse designed to exploit and humiliate the recipient, who is then devalued, the offender achieving a sense of glee, triumph and narcissistic amusement or delight from this process. Initial transference and counter-transference RRPs were noted as manipulative and suggested that Max was resistant to and abusive of the therapeutic process. These types of strategies had underpinned Max's lifestyle to date and represented his habitual use of people for his own needs and tactics to influence relationships. When he was compliant, it was felt that Max was employing false cooperation to strategically serve his own ends; when manipulative, he abused relationships with disregard. The RRPs of *manipulating/exploiting-to-manipulated/exploited* were added to the reformulation with the expectation that the therapy could be corrupted because of these RRPs or that Max would engage only for self-serving purposes.

The draft SDR is shown in Fig. 10.1. The RRPs which could be extracted from his offence behaviours and self-reporting suggested that he showed a transitional sequence of self and other (victim) perceptions that culminated in the crime-specific offender-to-victim state of mind (a dialogical sequence

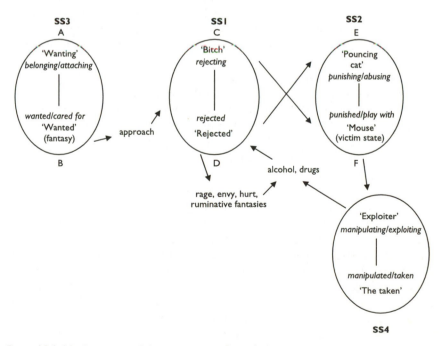

Figure 10.1 Max's sequential diagrammatic reformulation.

analysis leading to the dominant offence position of 'pouncing cat', SS2). When in this state of mind, Max was primed to commit an interpersonal offence, and this represented his highest risk potential to women. The passage through these states could be traced through three particular states of mind and RRPs of self-states as Max's drive to rape escalated (i.e. SS3 to SS1 to SS2). He moved through an initial state of idealising the woman he met, hopeful of intimacy and of obtaining a sense of idyllic connection (SS3). Max could acknowledge that being 'wanted' was relevant to him, given his experiences of failed care throughout his life and sense that he had to exploit others to survive. Typically, Max's interactions with women that he approached failed to develop further, and he felt rejected by them (SS1). The disappointment, rage and perception of himself as rejected and despicable were apparent at this juncture. Max could readily verbalise that he would become preoccupied and ruminative about the reasons for the rejection and tended to develop thoughts about the victim's preference for other men over him, inducing envious feelings and exacerbating his anger. It was apparent in his statements to the victims of each crime that Max solicited each victim's appraisal of his sexual prowess in comparison with her partner, talking about how her boyfriend would feel if he knew about the sexual acts she was enduring with Max (a reflection of his destructive envy). The crime-specific RRP consisted of punishing and degrading the victim (SS2; offender-to-victim RRP) in 'cat-and-mouse' style, almost a recapitulation of Max's own abuse by his stepfather and other men. SS4 in Fig. 10.1 depicts the survival strategies that Max used and his self-perception as a manipulative, exploiting and stealing offender who considered his victims to be 'stupid' (SS4, 'the taken').

When Max was presented with the Reformulation Letter and the draft SDR (Fig. 10.1), he studied both intensely and reflected for a long time on their relevance and accuracy. The reformulation did trigger a change in his engagement, prompting Max to reveal past memories stimulated by the process. In particular, he recalled a further incident at approximately 9 years of age when he spent 3 weeks in hospital. He was unsure about the reasons for the admission. Max remembered becoming emotionally close to a particular nurse on the ward with whom he believed he had developed a 'special relationship'. He could not name her but recalled that she was young and attractive. Max reported spending many hours with her in the hospital ward while she read to him, and cuddled and pampered him in a way that he had never been treated before, in sharp contrast to his mother's neglect and his stepfather's abuse. His memories of this nurse were idealised, Max describing her as 'the most beautiful thing I'd ever seen. I remember her smell, her warm skin and the feel of her hair when she snuggled up with me. I didn't want to leave the place ever – it was magic.' During the first weeks, Max believed that he was cocooned in a blissful haven from the abuse at home. He mentioned further that the intensity of his feelings toward the nurse were easy to recapture when he could plunge into these memories with vividness. The relevance of these memories was explored (memories associated with SS3, his first experience of genuine mothering), and Max stated his own view that the SDR should be altered to include this state of mind. At the next session, Max informed the therapist that he had entered a 'dark mood' since discussing the letter and the SDR. He had become self-absorbed, irritable and aloof from other prisoners and staff, refusing a visit from a male friend for the first time. He had maintained self-control through avoidance of others, but he felt that 'something's been triggered off in me by all this'.

At the next session, Max divulged that he had remembered more about his time in hospital and was unsure about the importance of this new information. During his stay in hospital, he claimed, 'something happened, I remember a feeling, a horrible feeling, like I'd done something wrong when I was there. It's to do with the nurse.' The fact that Max was unclear about these events was acknowledged, and he was offered time and opportunity to think about their veracity. Opportunity was given to allow Max to decipher the authenticity of these memories and their significance, without premature formulation. At the next session, Max reported that he was 'pretty clear about what happened there. I must have put the whole thing in a box.' He declared that his relationship with the nurse had become vitally important to him while in the hospital, that his feelings for the nurse were all-consuming and a new experience for him at that time of his life. Max then recalled that another patient, a child many years younger than he, had entered the hospital ward, and this event changed his relationship with the nurse.

During this session, Max observably struggled with the associated emotions when discussing this event, vacillating between modulated rage, despair, becoming tearful and hurt, and a detached, zombie-like state. His recollections were that the nurse had transferred her attention to this newly admitted child and that he felt confusion, rage, agitation and envy because of this. He disclosed that he began to exhibit attention-seeking behaviours on the ward, such as breaking toys, bed-wetting and smearing faeces on the wall on one occasion. His overtures were not successful, and he remembered an instance when the nurse he felt so much devotion for called him 'a disgusting, filthy boy' after he had smeared faeces. Max claimed that 'my whole world fell apart. I was due to go home, back to the shit there, and she [the nurse] just ignored me. I was gutted. Maybe I was trying to tell her something about how shit I felt, I don't know.'

The night before discharge, Max waited until all of the children on the ward were sleeping and the staff were absent. 'I waited and waited, then got out of bed. I went over to the wee shit [the newly admitted child] and looked in to see if he was asleep. He was in a crib thing, he must've been about three at the most. I punched him and punched him and punched him, all over him. I felt the hatred, I wanted to kill him. He woke up screaming, then I didn't know what to do. I panicked. All I could think about was the nurse being mad at me, rejecting me. I lifted him up, started to cuddle him, said it was all right.

He wouldn't calm down or shut up, so I remember hitting him again, full on the face. He just whimpered, I got off-side and waited. The nurses came and nothing much happened. I don't think they knew what happened. I left the next day.' Max was asked to reflect on the way that these events had affected his perception of others (women in particular) and himself.

An immediate link was made between the movement from being *belonging/ attached-to-wanted/cared for* to *rebuking/rejecting-to-disgusting/rejected* to *punishing* and *destructively envious* within his relationship to the nurse and little boy. It was apparent that Max had, during the offences, perceived the female victims as ideal, and then rejecting of him, and that he developed the belief that they were worthy of punishment. The dialogical sequence for Max of wishing to be wanted, to feeling rejected, to feeling a desire to punish the victim was highlighted. His preoffence state of mind consisted of indignation at rejection, hatred and envy of the victims' superiority, intolerable self-disgust that he felt was induced by the victims and a desire to punish the victims for their actions. These RRPs were further incorporated in the reformulation.

In session 10, Max was invited to discuss the traumatic abuse he had endured to clarify the victim state of SS2. Max disclosed that he had suffered repetitive, sexually sadistic abuse at the hands of his stepfather from the ages of 7 to 11. He claimed that he could not recall his biological father's abuse of him. He could remember specific instances of abuse by his stepfather and other men, and was asked to identify the most disturbing and unpleasant memories of abuse. Max recalled his stepfather's abuse of him to be beating followed by acts of oral sex and buggery, abuse that was debasing and extreme. Max was helped to disclose these memories, and it became clear that the stepfather had, in Max's mind, caused the most psychological distress and left him feeling a sense of rage and hatred. The RRPs which he identified to encompass the abusive interactions were tentatively formulated as *merciless torturing-to-toyed with* ('cat and mouse' self-state), highlighting the perpetrator and victim RRPs he felt best described his experiences. Max openly voiced his rage and hatred against the perpetrators, particularly his stepfather. He could articulate that this victim state and RRP was the most intolerable state of mind and position he had experienced, and his manner of coping with this induced state at the time of the abuse was to 'shut myself down, as if it wasn't going on. I was like a toy. I couldn't do anything to this guy, but I did feel the hate seething in me, building and building.' His anger was compounded by his mother's lack of interest in his welfare and dismissive reaction to his disclosures about the abuse. She beat him for speaking so badly about his stepfather. Max reported that he would associate a voice with this victim position saying, 'I will not let anybody ever hurt me again. I will have my payback.' He could not contemplate the motivations or state of mind of the perpetrator.

During these sessions, Max presented as emotionally detached and covertly hostile, and he acknowledged being 'filled with hate when I'm made to think about this'. Despite this reaction, he persisted with his disclosures and admitted that he felt the need to 'get it all out of me. It's been eating me up.' The majority of memories of abuse consisted of invasive, brutalising, degrading acts of physical, sexual and verbal mistreatment. Max recalled that he would sleep in parks and misuse glue to avoid being alone in the home with his stepfather. He felt that antisocial behaviours improved his feelings about himself (the advantage of exploiting others, manipulation to achieve self-esteem inflation).

Max decided through discussion with the therapist to target a specific memory of abuse that he had suffered from his stepfather through imagery rescripting and reprocessing therapy (IRRT). The objective of introducing IRRT was to permit a detailed analysis of the victim state ('the mouse', SS2) and to resolve this facet of his presentation. Max described an occasion when his stepfather had forced him to perform oral sex, and had ejaculated in his mouth and then urinated on him, calling him a 'disgusting little shit', and claiming that he enjoyed this. Max recalled that he was then physically assaulted by having his testicles pinched with tweezers and forced to consume his stepfather's faeces. Max's reaction to the reliving of this event consisted of a prolonged period of silence which lasted for almost an hour. Max could link the experiences of abuse with his survival strategy of shutting down into a zombie state, detaching from others whom he perceived as dangerous and harmful, and the emergence of intense feelings of rage and hatred. These observations helped to clarify the nature of RRPs underlying the 'cat-and-mouse' self-state, which could be conceived as a recapitulation of his own abuse experiences. Max did find it impossible at this stage to contemplate or articulate the possible states of mind of the perpetrator. The CAT reformulation permitted a concentrated focus upon the nature of the perpetrator–victim RRPs within this abuse state.

IRRT and CAT

IRRT is a cognitive-behavioural intervention devised by Smucker, Dancu, Foa & Niederee (1996) that addresses the aftermath of childhood sexual abuse and its reverberations in adult life. IRRT has been incorporated into CAT reformulations to good effect, as reported in a number of cases of adult survivors of childhood abuse (Pollock, 2001), helping to elaborate the internalised RRPs within the victim state or position, and addressing the traumatic symptoms associated without losing the overarching reformulation's relevance. A brief synopsis of IRRT is proffered here, and its integration into CAT reformulation and therapy is illustrated with Max as a case example. The ways in which IRRT and CAT complement each other in the reformulation and therapy process are described also.

Pollock (2001) proposed that other techniques and therapeutic approaches, such as IRRT and eye movement desensitization and reprocessing (EMDR) (Shapiro, 1995), could be viably introduced to resolve certain states such as the *victimised, paralysed, crushed, controlled, punished, injured* and *debased* RRPs, to name only a few, that are typically encountered in survivors of childhood abuse. EMDR resolves the state with little emphasis on the reciprocal nature of the abuse itself, dealing with the failure to process the emotional fallout of these experiences and reducing symptoms such as post-traumatic stress disorder in particular. IRRT focuses on the intrapersonal and interpersonal elements of the abuse and considers the internalised script or narrative that has been retained and incorporated by the survivor.

IRRT has a number of components. After comprehensive assessment, a process of imaginal exposure is undertaken whereby the survivor re-experiences the traumatic event or a composite of several events of abuse. The survivor is encouraged to relive the traumatic events in the 'here-and-now' and to experience fully the psychological reality of the abuse. This aspect of IRRT is an excellent opportunity for the CAT therapist to investigate the survivor's perceptions of the underlying RRPs of the abuse and to develop an understanding of the *abuser-to-victim* self-state. The experiential nature of the imaginal exposure process permits the survivor to articulate the fundamental RRPs of the dynamic between perpetrator and victim and the perceptions, thoughts, feelings and 'voice' associated with the abuse. The 'child' victim's perspective and experiences are identified during the exposure phase.

After the exposure process, the survivor is requested to re-enact and then rescript the trauma through mastery imagery whereby the traumatic scenario is imagined once again. The 'child' victim is rescued by the healthy 'adult' self or by other effective individuals (e.g. police, superheroes or the therapist), and the perpetrator is confronted and removed from the scenario. The final component of IRRT involves the survivor's developing adult-nurturing-child imagery, the intervening adult soothing or comforting the child by protective, rescuing and nurturing behaviours.

The decision was made to undertake IRRT with Max for a number of reasons. Firstly, the CAT reformulation placed core emphasis on the significance of the multiple abuses that he had endured and their relevance to his personality development. Max's configured personality was viewed as a direct response to this abuse, and his pathway to the offending was considered a fundamental developmental trajectory from the abuse. Secondly, it was anticipated that IRRT would provide a mechanism to clarify the internalised RRPs of the abuse and promote a better understanding of the link between the childhood abuse and Max's offending, particularly the offender–victim RRPs, which appeared to be re-enactments or recapitulation of childhood abuses. It should be stated that Max did not report any specific post-traumatic stress disorder symptoms as defined by DSM-IV (American Psychiatric Association, 1994), and the disorder identified in his case was assumed to indicate the detached, psychopathic response to repeated trauma often observed in male sexual abuse victims. Max could openly discuss his own behaviours as a perpetrator but could not project his thinking to contemplate the abuser's motivations, intentions or perceptions, as in a difficulty in theory-of-mind and mentalisation (Fonagy & Target, 1997; Bateman & Fonagy, 2004).

The process of IRRT with Max

IRRT was undertaken with the prior agreement of the prison authorities and medical staff, given the predicted intensity of the process, Max's propensity to act out and the obvious need to contain his behaviours throughout the IRRT. The rescripting of the abuse scenarios heralded the emergence of Max's acknowledgement and re-experiencing of disturbing, intense emotional responses. Initially, Max entered the abuse scenario as his adult self, but found that, during the imagery, he was beaten back and pushed out of the room by the perpetrator (his stepfather). Max commented that he could hear the abuse happening while outside the room and conveyed his sense of rage toward the stepfather: 'I want to kill him, he deserves it now.' This stage of IRRT required sensitive containment of Max's homicidal rage which had been activated. When asked to think about whom he could enlist to deal with the perpetrator, Max offered, 'Only someone as bad as him [the perpetrator] could do this.' Time was spent attempting to identify an individual or parties that Max believed could act accordingly. Max brought in an imaginary creature that he had seen in an occult book, a winged serpent that swooped on victims and carried them off to a lair, where it killed and ate them. He imagined this creature attacking the perpetrator, taking him out of the room and torturing him before killing him. The 'abused child-self' ran out of the room and the building. It is obvious that, in many respects, the IRRT rescripting phase incited violence in Max. He was asked to 'find' the child but stated initially, 'Why? I'm not his keeper.' He was encouraged over sessions to trace the child and to enter into a dialogue with him. He found him huddled and hiding in a cellar in a derelict house.

Max's manner of relating to the child was disconcerting for the therapist, yet revealingly diagnostic. Max reported spending time looking at the child, the child refusing to respond or make eye contact, remaining motionless, silent and huddled. Max's immediate impressions and thoughts were expressed as follows: 'Why should I care what happens to him? He's a little shit, he can look after himself now.' There was no expressed sense of empathic concern, sympathy or desire to connect emotionally with the abused child. Further attempts were made to encourage Max to make contact with the child. At the third rescripting session, Max felt that the child rejected an offer of help and reported beating the child furiously and spitting on him (similar to his stepfather's actions toward Max as a child).

After taking stock of the developments throughout IRRT, Max was asked to enter into a dialogue with the child, assuming both roles. He could articulate that the child had 'had enough of being everybody's toy. He's saying, "leave me alone, all you do is use me. I'm not going to let you any more. It'll be payback time soon." ' Max was able to engage in an inner conversation of 'voices' ('utterances' in dialogical work) that concluded that he could not look after the child and did not want to, but did not want the child harmed any further either. Max commented, 'I can't take away his pain, but I won't let him get hurt any more. You shouldn't be able to do that to a kid. People should be hung for doing that sort of stuff to kids.' This represented the first sign of any empathic resonance or protective response on Max's part during therapy.

The IRRT facilitated a number of therapeutic processes within the CAT framework. Firstly, it helped to delineate the perpetrator-to-victim positions, voices and self-state encapsulated as 'cat and mouse' (SS2). Secondly, it promoted the first opportunity for Max to achieve a sense of adult–child connection, encouraging a nurturing stance and a space to think about and empathise with the abused child's experiences as a victim. Thirdly, Max was asked to contemplate the possible link between the perpetrator's states of mind and positions and its relevance to the offender–victim position and RRPs during his own crimes. Max developed an appreciation that his experiences had engendered abuse-tainted, action-oriented procedures which influenced his self–other behaviours.

After IRRT, a list of target problems (TPs) within CAT itself were agreed with Max as follows:

(1) *Traumatic resolution* – The victim rage and hatred associated with the 'cat and mouse' self-state were clarified through IRRT and partially resolved. Max was able to articulate and label the victim rage he harboured and to accept the need to address these lingering destructive emotional states.

(2) *Develop an awareness of the destructive ways of perceiving and relating* – Max was encouraged to acknowledge that his survival strategy when a child had consisted of detachment, avoidance of meaningful relationships and feelings. The sequential shifts between self-states identifiable during the offence were noted, and the patterns of destructive relating leading to the offender–victim scenario were examined. The changes in perception of himself and the victim were traced and the projection of internal states and inducement of roles noted. Max was asked to consider the link between his identification with the perpetrator as a result of his own abuse experiences and how this translated into damaging procedures against victims.

(3) *Victim empathy* – Time was spent facilitating an examination of Max's concepts of his own victimisation and hurt and considering the anguish he had caused through his offences. Empathic concern and resonance

were markedly deficient, and Max's capacity to mentalise with others' states of mind was assessed to be minimal.

(4) *Fantasies of harm* – The RRPs which formed the fantasies of harming others were examined, and it was observed how these fantasies functioned to sustain his self-worth and to express destructive states of mind and his need to assume a powerful, dominant and punishing position toward a deserving victim.

(5) *Max's identity* – It was recognised that Max's interactions with others and patterns of relating throughout his development had soiled his sense of identity, and that he perceived himself as despicable, disgusting and rejected. His sense of envy of more worthy others was identified and linked to the offences. Max perceived others as 'fair game' and viewed manipulation to achieve his own needs as acceptable, an indication of his morally corrupt, grandiose and devaluing perceptions of himself in relation to others. His propensity to steal and to engage in other crimes was viewed as manifestations of these RRPs.

(6) *Ruminative anger and offence premeditation* – The link between Max's tendency to ruminate and incubate anger and hatred through immersing himself in past memories of abuse (e.g. when rejected by a woman), his consumption of substances and his offence planning was identified. Max's choice of victim, his methods of approach and control, and the nature and sequence of the criminal acts were noted and discussed to derive an understanding of his states of mind before, during and after the crime.

(7) *Acknowledgement of Max's needs* – Max's genuine desire for intimacy and attachment with a partner were recognised and considered. His lack of heterosexual skills was apparent, and the contribution of this problem to his offending considered. The pseudo-intimate facets of his offending behaviours were noted.

(8) *Max's risk potential and prediction of offending* – Max and the therapist agreed to explore the destructive parts of his personality and their relevance to forecasting scenarios whereby an offence was likely to occur in the future.

After reformulation and IRRT, the initial transference patterns observable in the first sessions did not significantly influence the later development of the therapeutic alliance. Max did not devalue the therapeutic work or abuse its process, remaining focused on the goals of the agreed work. His progress was positive during the initial 14 sessions of CAT, and it was considered that Max had developed personal insights into the origins, nature and functioning of the named self-states and was beginning to grasp the gravity of his offences and their impact upon his victims. Max was readily able to contemplate the behavioural aspects of his crime and the expressions of destructive elements of his personality within the offences. He acknowledged that his perceptions of himself were of a damaged personality who caused destruction for others.

He was able to appreciate that his task was to monitor, regulate and control his own risk potential and that he could manage his own distress and disturbance through alternative strategies.

On occasion, Max was asked to 'check in', using imagery with his survivor–child state, and he offered that 'we're OK, still sad and wary though'. His ratings of recognition of TPPs improved and Max felt that, subjectively, he had developed insight into the nature of the harmful procedures which had led to his crimes. Furthermore, Max claimed that he felt that some revision and resolution had been gained regarding his own abuse, stating that he felt less troubled by 'nasty thoughts and feelings of killing someone or doing hurt to them'.

A critical incident occurred outside the therapy process which disrupted the therapeutic work after 18 sessions of promising progress. Max entered the 19th session and dismissingly claimed, 'I've finished with all this. I don't want to do any more.' He explained that he had begun to write to a woman in the community, a friend of a fellow inmate. They had exchanged letters and Max was thrilled by the interaction. The therapist and the therapy were rejected with an air of grandiosity and detachment. The therapist did not see Max until 4 months later, when he requested a review.

Max entered this next session in a desolate, angry and hostile mood, visibly tense and tetchy. He eventually revealed that he had continued to write to this female friend, who had sent him sexually explicit letters, had visited him in prison four times and seemed to be shy, a 'little minx, all sex and no knickers, but innocent and like butter couldn't melt in her mouth'. Max admitted that he had become emotionally involved with her and had spoken to her about a future together. She divulged that she had borne four children to a violent man who had attacked her on many occasions, and she remained fearful of her ex-partner's actions against her. Max reported feeling protective toward her and angry that he could not 'deal with the guy and sort him out'. Unfortunately for Max, after many months of correspondence and regular visits, this woman wrote to inform him that she had decided to 'move on with her life', that Max's offences sickened her and that his intensity of feeling scared her. Max was devastated and reacted through violence within the prison, wrecking his cell and attacking a prison officer. He felt confused, rejected and homicidal (SS1).

Time was spent encouraging Max to revisit the reformulation and SDR and to use these tools to make sense of these events. Max's emotional state interfered with this process, but after two sessions he began to link this woman's actions toward him and his emotional reactions. The sessions identified the RRPs of *belonging/attached-to-idealising care* (SS3) to his initial hopes about the relationship as it blossomed. Max reported that he had felt a new-found aspiration for a loving relationship, wanting to protect and care for this woman. Her rejection of him had evoked the disgusted, hated state and had prompted Max to fantasise about punishing the woman for her dismissal (SS2). The manner of the rejection echoed Max's abuse ('the mouse' state) in that he felt toyed with. His disappointment and bemusement were acknowledged, and he was asked to think about the relevance of past RRPs which had become enacted during this failed romance.

Max's violent conduct at this time within the prison reflected his continuing capacity to harm. Max offered that he recognised that the woman had activated a sense of envy that encouraged him to fantasise about hurting her ex-partner in a similar way to the reaction he experienced when hospitalised as a child. Max was helped to acknowledge the strength and intensity of these recapitulated feelings and the associated motivations to harm others. The dialogical sequence underlying these transitions in states was explicitly discussed, and ways of managing his reactions were considered.

Several additional sessions were agreed to work on the TPs. Ratings of recognition and revision were noted, particularly resolution of Max's experiences of trauma, his awareness of the destructiveness of certain self-states, the triggers for his fantasies of harm, and the RRPs underlying his ruminative anger and offence planning. Max was able to discuss the 'crash' of being rejected and recognise how rage and destructive feelings had emerged (using the SDR). He learnt to self-monitor the sequence whereby he began to incubate rage and consciously devised plans to offend against women. Max's perceptions of women had been further soiled by his recent episode with the visiting woman. It was apparent that he perceived women as superior, rejecting, abusing and exploiting. Max acknowledged that his methods of approaching women in the past had been naive and inappropriate, and his heterosexual skills and knowledge were discussed at length. The transition from idealising a woman to wanting to punish her for rejecting his advances was explored, Max stating 'I always wanted to knock those bitches off their pedestals. I hated all that virginal, holy way they got on.' This manifestation of 'splitting' is often observable in cases of rape. His need for intimacy was explored at length, and Max was encouraged to review the sequential transitions in RRPs and positions antecedent to his raping a woman. The RRPs within his fantasies were reviewed, and Max was helped to understand the correlation between his actions during the offence and these fantasies.

The authenticity of Max's new-found appreciation of each victim's trauma and development of inhibiting empathic concern was more difficult to establish. From his position of being worthless and uncared for, Max explained that his own survival had become his main objective in life, and he expressed the view that 'other people must beware'. He was willing and adept at exploiting others for his own needs, expressing his envy at anyone who had succeeded in life and gathered material possessions or status.

Risk assessment and outcome

Max did develop improved insight into his personality and its destructive potential, and TPs showed positive changes within therapy, particularly

Max's empathic appreciation of the victims' plight. Max realised that his personal experiences of being victimised had damaged his personality and resulted in further harm to others. Max was able to demonstrate an improved intellectual recognition of this link, and his emotional remorse was assessed to have extended to a basic appreciation of the victims' suffering.

Max was released into the community, and, after 3 years of liberty, his history of reoffending has consisted of one crime of theft from an off-licence. He has not committed a sexual offence within this time. Max is in a relationship with an older woman and no difficulties are reported. He has obtained employment and not abused drugs, yet regularly uses alcohol. The theft was triggered by an argument with his employer, who claimed that Max was intoxicated on arrival at work, Max explaining that he decided to vent his anger by getting drunk but did not have the money to buy alcohol.

Max's case is presented here to illustrate that applying the CAT model focuses on the psychopathic personality's early care experiences and the internalisation of a restricted, harmful range of RRPs, which are enacted through damaging and destructive patterns of relating to others and oneself. In this disorder, it is just as important to stipulate and identify the origins of the narcissistic, aggressive self and the limited repertoire of relating that is manifest in the psychopath's behaviours. The developmental origins of the RRPs are traced to caregiving scenarios and, in Max's case, traumatic abuses and neglect. The offences evolved from sequences of interactions with others and the offender's perceptions of himself and others, culminating in damaging, unrevised procedures and serial crimes. The thrust of the therapy was not to 'reparent' the offender, but to provide him with techniques and tools to enhance his self-knowledge and insight, and enable him to make choices about his actions in the future.

References

American Psychiatric Association (1994). *Diagnostic and Statistical Manual of Mental Disorders* (4th edn) (DSM-IV). Washington, DC: American Psychiatric Association.

Bateman, A. W. & Fonagy, P. (2004). *Psychotherapy for borderline personality disorder: Mentalization-based treatment*. Oxford: Oxford University Press.

Blackburn, R. (1982). On the relevance of the concept of the psychopath. *Issues in Criminological Psychology*, 2, 12–25.

Blackburn, R. & Fawcett, D. (1999). The Antisocial Personality Questionnaire: An inventory for assessing personality deviance in offender populations. *European Journal of Personality Assessment*, 15, 14–24.

Bursten, B. (1972). The manipulative personality. *Archives of General Psychiatry*, 26, 318–321.

Cleckley, H. (1981). *The mask of sanity* (4th edn). St Louis, MO: Mosby.

Cooke, D. J. & Michie, C. (2001). An item response theory analysis of the Hare Psychopathy Checklist–Revised. *Psychological Assessment*, 9, 3–14.

Fonagy, P. & Target, M. (1997). Attachment and reflective function: Their role in self-organization. *Development and Psychopathology, 9*, 679–700.

Frodi, A., Dernovik, M., Sepa, A., Philipson, J. & Bragesjoe, M. (2001). Current attachment representations of incarcerated offenders varying in degrees of psychopathy. *Attachment and Human Development, 3*, 269–283.

Hare, R. D. (1991). *Manual for the revised Psychopathy Checklist.* Toronto: Multi-Health Systems.

Hare, R. D. (1996). Psychopathy: A clinical concept whose time has come. *Criminal Justice and Behaviour, 23*, 25–54.

Hemphill, J. F., Hare, R. D. & Wong, S. (1998). Psychopathy and recidivism: A review. *Legal and Criminological Psychology, 3*, 139–170.

Kernberg, O. F. (1984). Severe personality disorders: Psychotherapeutic strategies. New Haven, CT: Yale University Press.

Levy, T. M & Orlans, M. (2000). Attachment disorder as an antecedent to client and antisocial patterns in childhood. In T. M. Levy (Ed.), *Handbook of attachment interventions* (pp. 1–26). San Diego, CA: USA Press.

Martens, W. K. J. (1999). Marcel: A case report of a violent sexual psychopath in remission. *International Journal of Offender Therapy and Comparative Criminology, 43*, 391–399.

McWilliams, N. (1994). *Psychoanalytic diagnoses.* New York: Guilford Press.

Meloy, J. R. (1992). *The psychopathic mind: Origins, dynamics and treatment.* Hillside, NJ: Aronson.

Millon, T., Millon, C. & Davis, R. (1994). *Manual for the Millon Clinical Multiaxial Inventory* (3rd edn). Minneapolis, MN: National Computer Services.

O'Neill, M. L., Lidz, V. & Heilbrun, K. (2003). Adolescents with psychopathic characteristics in a substance abusing cohort: Treatment, process and outcome. *Law and Human Behaviour, 3*, 299–313.

Pollock, P. H. (1997). Cognitive Analytic Therapy for an offender with borderline personality disorder. In A. Ryle (Ed.), *Cognitive Analytic Therapy and borderline personality disorder: The model and the method.* Chichester: Wiley.

Pollock, P. H. (1999). When the killer suffers: Post-traumatic stress reactions following homicide. *Legal and Criminological Psychology, 4*, 185–202.

Pollock, P. H. (2001). *Cognitive Analytic Therapy for adult survivors of childhood abuse: Approaches to treatment and case management.* Chichester: Wiley.

Racher, H. (1962). *Transference and countertransference.* New York: International Universities Press.

Salekin, R. T. (2002). Psychopathy and therapeutic pessimism: Clinical lore or clinical reality. *Clinical Psychology Review, 22*, 79–112.

Salekin, R. T., Rogers, R. & Sewell, K. W. (1996). A review and meta-analysis of the PCL-R: Predictive validity of diagnosis. *Clinical Psychology: Science and Practice, 3*, 203–215.

Schmideberg, M. (1978). The treatment of a juvenile psychopath. *International Journal of Offender Therapy and Comparative Criminology, 22*, 21–28.

Shapiro, F. (1995). *Eye movement desensitisation and reprocessing.* New York: Guilford Press.

Smith, A. M., Gacono, C. & Kaufman, L. (1998). A Rorschach comparison of psychopathic and non-psychopathic conduct disordered adolescents. *Journal of Clinical Psychology, 53*, 289–300.

Smucker, M. R., Dancu, C. V., Foa, E. B. & Niederee, J. (1996). *Imagery rescripting: A treatment manual for adult survivors of childhood sexual abuse experiencing PTSD*. Milwaukee, WI: Cognitive Therapy Institute of Milwaukee.

Strasburger, L. H. (2001). The treatment of antisocial syndromes: The therapist's feelings. In W. H. Reid, D. Dorr, J. I. Walker & J. W. Bonner (Eds), *Unmasking the psychopath: Antisocial personality and related syndromes*. New York: Norton.

Templeman, T. L. & Wollersheim, J. P. (1979). A cognitive behavioural approach to the treatment of the psychopath. *Psychotherapy, Treatment and Research, 16,* 132–139.

Vaillant, P. M., Hawkins, T. J. & Pottier, D. C. (1998). Comparison of psychopathic and general offenders in cognitive behavioural therapy. *Psychological Reports, 83,* 753–754.

Wallace, J. F., Vitale, T. J. & Newman, J. P. (1999). Response modulation deficits: Implications for the diagnosis and treatment of psychopathy. *Journal of Cognitive Psychotherapy, 13,* 55–70.

Widom, C. S. (1978). *A methodology for studying non-institutionalized psychopaths*. In R. D. Hare & D. Shilling (Eds), *Psychopathic behaviour: Applications to research* (pp. 71–84). Chichester: Wiley.

Chapter 11

Community-based Cognitive Analytic Therapy with perpetrators of domestic violence

Challenges to the orthodoxy

Calvin Bell & Justin Hamill

Beyond the forensic setting, it might be assumed that clients/patients who pose a risk of serious injury to others are so rare that few clinicians will encounter them in their consulting room. However, given the high prevalence rates of domestic violence against women,[1] it is hard to imagine that CAT practitioners working with (especially personality-disordered) men will not at some time, knowingly or not, encounter a client who has been physically violent behind the closed doors of his own home. Approximately a quarter of all violent assaults known to the police (most domestic assaults are not reported) take place in the home (Morley & Mullender, 1994; Mirrlees-Black, 1999). Though crime surveys are generally regarded as under-reporting prevalence rates, the most recent British Crime Survey (BCS) (Walby & Allen, 2004) found that 45% of women respondents recalled being subject to domestic violence (abuse, threats or force, sexual victimisation or stalking) at least once in their lifetime. In regional random incidence surveys in Britain, as many as one in three women have disclosed experience of some form of domestic violence worse than being grabbed, pushed or shaken, most of which required some form of medical attention. Nearly a third of the cases reported to the 1996 BCS required medical attention, 59% involving injury and 13% resulting in broken bones. Studies reveal that some 10–13% of women have been subjected to physical violence by a current or past partner within the preceding 12-month period (McGibbon *et al.*, 1989; Mooney, 1994; Stanko, 2000; Walby & Allen, 2004). Surveys by Mooney (1994) and Painter (1991) both found that one in eight of the women interviewed alleged that they had been raped by a current or ex-partner. At their most stark, Home Office figures typically reveal that virtually half of the women murdered in England and Wales are killed by their current or ex-partners; according to the 2004 BCS, this results in one woman being killed every day.

The dominant discourse among domestic violence practitioners has emphasised the historical and cultural aetiologies of this widespread social problem, and therefore has eschewed individual interventions in favour of cultural, political and legal reform. Domestic violence has been construed as instrumental behaviour on men's part, a product of unequal power relations between the sexes, designed to secure and maintain control and access to domestic, sexual and emotional services from women (gain); this is seen as requiring a criminal justice response rather than being a product of psycho-pathology (pain) requiring treatment. The provision of programmes for domestically violent men, whatever their context or method, can therefore collude with the 'bad apple' explanation of domestic violence, whereby the public and social policy makers seek solutions to identify and treat and/or punish individual men (symptoms) rather than engage with the wider social and cultural phenomena which continue to support men's use of violence (causes). The most promising prescriptions for change seem to lie in multi-agency initiatives which acknowledge the historical and social roots of men's violence and the familial and institutional subordination of women, and which harness community resources to provide the necessary collective momentum to hold perpetrators accountable and to overhaul the cultural values and norms which maintain the status quo (Shepard & Pence, 1999).

Nevertheless, the number of perpetrators convicted by the criminal courts remains tiny (typically less than 2% of those reported). It is also clear that many women experiencing domestic violence want help for their abusers, rather than punishment (Burton *et al.*, 1998). Perpetrator treatment pro-grammes have therefore developed within both the voluntary and the statu-tory sector (though provision remains very patchy), and, influenced by the dominant profeminist way of framing the problem, have led to edu-cational groupwork as the intervention method of choice. These principles are enshrined in Respect's[2] Statement of Principles and Minimum Standards of Practice.

For its part, CAT draws heavily upon those analytic traditions which locate the roots of psychopathology in dyadic object relations, the internalisation of parent–child roles leading to internal conflict and the onset of symptoms. Traumatising experiences in infancy and skills deficits, particularly in the area of self-reflection, are also recognised as contributory factors, especially with personality-disordered clients. However, in our work with men who are vio-lent, we find these intrapsychic and individualised aetiologies, taken alone, unconvincing. While many of our clients exhibit clear mental disturbance, others do not. Many bear the physical and emotional scars of severe abuse from childhood, while others have grown up in verifiably 'good-enough' circumstances. It may be of interest to note that research[3] consistently identifies a boy having *witnessed* his father abuse his mother as a much stronger risk marker for the subsequent perpetration of violence toward an intimate partner (and therefore for transmitting violent behaviour from one generation to the next) than direct experience of family-of-origin abuse. Claims are made by some researchers that a significant proportion of domestic violence offenders had neither witnessed nor experienced violence as a child.[4] We therefore rate socio-cultural factors alongside psychological ones as key pathogens, particularly in the context of disorders which are syntonic with traditional sex roles and of the very gendered violence which is wife abuse.

Moreover, we often find that the notion of complementarity within the concept of *reciprocal roles* is construed by many practitioners as somehow bestowing equal responsibility for the violence on both perpetrator and victim (cf. the feminist critique of systemic family therapy). We regard as collusive any attempt to allocate responsibility other than to the perpetrator alone by suggesting that both parties share the pathology. To imply that the female victim somehow elicits the perpetrator's actions, or is co-responsible for her continuing victimhood, is to reinforce her abuser's justifications and to deny the contextual reality of most women's lives, where the factors that affect their options are at least as much social as they are psychological.

One size may not fit all

However, we fear that the prevailing (radical) feminist ideology and the large-scale adoption of standardised cognitive and educational group intervention approaches by probation and voluntary sector agencies to working with domestic violence offenders, both here and in the USA (see Healey *et al.*, 1998; Austin & Dankwort, 1999), have led to the loss of the psychological insights which are common currency in any psychotherapy undertaking. Outcome studies for these programmes continue to give very mixed results, and attrition rates are universally high for both court- and non-court-mandated programmes (Dobash, Dobash, Cavanagh & Lewis, 1996; Burton *et al.*, 1998; Healey *et al.*, 1998; Bennett & Williams, 2003; Puffett & Gavin, 2004). There is as yet little empirical knowledge of what works: we continue to operate at the frontier of our understanding. This suggests that the adoption of any single treatment approach is premature and begs the question of whether the current 'one-size-fits-all' model meets the needs of all perpetrators. Domestically violent perpetrators constitute a diverse and markedly heterogeneous population, and the growing typology literature (e.g. Dutton, 1988; 1995; Gondolf, 1988; 1999; Saunders, 1992; Johnston & Campbell, 1993; Dutton & Starzomski, 1994; Holtzworth-Munroe & Stuart, 1994) questions the dominant epistemological assumptions that wife abuse is a unitary phenomenon predicated *entirely* on sexism and the patriarchal domination of women. We therefore suggest that corrective programmes may show improved results if intervention modalities are fashioned to match offender characteristics (something which CAT excels at). The dearth of community-based programmes also means that *group work* is unlikely to be available in most areas.

The following vignettes may serve to illustrate the way our practice departs from the conventional use of CAT in order to address some of the particular concerns of working with men who perpetrate domestic violence.

The potential of treatment for increasing risk to victims

There are particular dangers for partner/victims associated with the adoption of traditional psychotherapeutic approaches with this group of offenders (whatever model is chosen), and if there is anything we have learned during the years we have been working for change with men who are violent to their partners, it is that therapist's overriding responsibility must be that of *primum non nocere* ('first do no harm'). In other words, the provision of psychotherapy for an abusive man must never compromise his partner/victim's safety. This is much more easily said than achieved! Referrers (as well as therapists themselves) have at times been guilty of the mistaken belief that to concentrate efforts on the perpetrator *automatically* equates to the improved safety of his (ex) partner. However, our experience suggests that the very *offer* of treatment to a perpetrator can in fact expose his partner to additional risk. Though the majority of the hundreds of domestically violent men who have .been referred to us have attended on a voluntary basis, because of shame, denial, ambivalence, embarrassment and the cultural imperative for men to be seen as self-sufficient, few do so without considerable *external* pressure. By far, the most common precipitant motivating a man to participate in treatment is his partner's ultimatum or his attempt to encourage her to return where she has already left him. Women's advocates, researchers (e.g. Gondolf, 1988) and our own experience suggest that a client's attendance is indeed likely to be the most significant factor in his partner's decision to remain with him or even to return where she has already managed to leave. Merely accepting an abusive man into treatment therefore exposes a proportion of partner/victims to risk that they would have otherwise avoided by leaving or staying away from him. Moreover, many partners feel a false sense of security from the not unreasonable assumption that acceptance of her abusive partner into treatment implies that he is safe to be treated within the community (as opposed to in prison) and that the prospects of change are reasonably good. Our 'quick-fix' culture, the growing 'therapeutic society' and the, at times, magical powers attributed to professionals can all conspire to promote unrealistic expectations (by partners and referrers) of success being either guaranteed or reasonably certain.

Limits to confidentiality

I remember speaking to one woman who had just been assaulted for the first time by her fiancé. She had broken off their engagement but had informed her abuser that she would reconsider if he sought help. When I confirmed (in line with our policy) that her partner had in fact just approached us to be assessed, she told me with relief that she could now resume their wedding arrangements. I explained that, generally, only those men who *completed* treatment showed signs of sustainable change and that many men did not attend at all despite making initial contact with the centre and that, of those who did, most dropped out during the first few weeks. We therefore regard the provision of information about programme protocols and the prospects of change in her abuser as an essential first step in considering a partner's welfare and in empowering her to make informed decisions. Knowledge, after all, is power.

While it is by no means unique to this population, the tendency for domestically violent men to represent themselves in an exculpatory manner which favours themselves and minimises their violence and abuse or projects the blame onto their victims is well known. However, the extent of the discrepancy between self-report and the accounts of their partners or of third parties is at times astonishing. Without safe access to partner corroboration, therapists can easily be seduced into believing that the incident of violence which precipitated the referral was isolated and uncharacteristic, or into attributing cause to 'dysfunctional' relationship dynamics. Invariably, however, partner contact reveals or confirms suspicions that a single assault is but part of a long litany of physical, psychological and frequently sexual and financial abuse. The best source of information as to whether a client is eligible, suitable or a safe-enough candidate for treatment is the partner/victim herself. Our assessment and therapy contracts therefore make clear that we require to consult the client's partner and to maintain contact with her throughout treatment.

Jonathan (a well-educated, white, middle-aged professional) referred himself to us, complaining that he feared that his occasional 'loss of temper' might be putting his primary relationship at risk. He denied any physical or sexual violence but admitted to 'shouting from time to time'. Our (female) colleague then carried out a home visit to interview his (teenage) partner, who described the event that precipitated his self-referral as one in which the man had come home from the office and demanded sex from her; she refused him. He then stripped and beat her; she resorted to cowering beneath a kitchen worktop to avoid his further blows. Having a fuller picture of context and risk levels (had there been children involved, we would also have had to manage the child protection concerns), we went on to work with Jonathan for over a year and, after weekly contact with his partner for some months, managed to facilitate her safe separation from him (a high-risk time for many women).

Barry (a white factory worker in his 30s) dropped out of CAT after 3 weeks. His partner had not responded to our early letters and telephone calls, but we finally managed to catch up with her. We discovered that once Barry had been accepted into treatment, she had returned to him (having left him after his most recent bout of violence). After withdrawing from treatment, he had informed her that his therapist had regarded him as such a model client that he no longer needed to attend. We were of course able to disillusion her.

Though client/counsellor confidentiality has never been absolute because of the requirements of the Children Act 1989 and the Prevention of Terrorism Act 1976, as well as some archaic statutes relating to treason, and because of the possibility of counsellors being required by the courts to disclose privileged information, the working precept of most psychotherapists is that the efficacy of the therapeutic alliance increases in proportion to the extent of confidentiality: honesty should be rewarded with privacy. In general practice, it is held that these fundamental principles will be overthrown by any disclosure, resulting in alienation of the client. However, in the context of working with domestic violence perpetrators, it is our contention that, in order to maximise partner and child safety and to minimise inadvertent collusion, therapists should ensure direct or indirect contact with current (and future) partners. While we should not lose focus on *treatment targets*, we evaluate our work by the extent to which it has enhanced or endangered the safety of the partner concerned (and any child in the home).

Cultural imperatives as competitors to parentally derived roles

As we have argued above, we find purely intrapsychic explanations for men's use of violence in the home inadequate and rate cultural and social influences, particularly traditional gender imperatives, as being at least as powerful (if not more so). This is never more obvious than in the military context. Military discipline seeks to dismantle the repertoire of *reciprocal roles* in the individual (insofar as they conflict with the mandates of the military). Personal autonomy and power-sharing are replaced with (patriarchal) hierarchy (rank) and authority (command/obey); emotional literacy is eschewed and vulnerability prohibited; and the instrumental use of force to achieve corporate ends is normalised. These are universal features among domestic violence perpetrators. Little surprise then that research reveals the considerably higher level of domestic violence perpetrated by military men than by their civilian counterparts (Shupe *et al.*, 1987; Prigerson *et al.*, 2002). Military discipline creates and reinforces a new repertoire of specifically controlling *reciprocal roles* such as the following:

controlling/ordering ⇔ controlled/obedient – *no personal choice*
dominating ⇔ subordinated – *inequality*
punishing/abusing ⇔ punished/broken – *can be rebuilt/educated to comply*
blaming ⇔ blamed – *always someone else's fault especially victim's*
rejecting ⇔ rejected – *ultimate sanction, i.e. court-martialled for failure to conform to the military family's cultural norms*

Mike, an ex-army sergeant, was referred by Social Services for therapy in relation to his physical and emotional abuse of his 6-year-old son Nick, and his controlling behaviour toward him and other family members. Mike and Nick's mother were now separated, and Mike's contact with his son had been substantially limited by court order. Mike sought further contact with Nick, who demonstrated significant attachment to his father, but his adversarial and rejecting attitude to social workers and other professionals threatened to undermine attempts to achieve any contact scenario that might meet Nick's needs.

Assessment revealed no witnessing or experience of abuse in Mike's family of origin, and no significantly controlling or abusing reciprocal roles were identified, but a rejecting role was. However, exploration of his experiences in the military identified the acquisition of typically 'military' controlling roles, and that these were enacted within the family through excessive demands for conformity and obedience, backed up by physical punishment. Threats of rejection and abandonment as coercive measures had also featured after Mike had been confronted by Social Services with demands for acknowledgement of responsibility for wrongdoing, and compliance with sanctions.

In the 24-session therapy, Mike's experience of himself as controlled and punished by the child protection system was acknowledged and related to similar experiences in the army named as reciprocal roles, and the parentally derived rejecting role was also identified. As trust developed in the therapeutic relationship, these militaristic roles were recognised by Mike within the therapeutic interaction and also as enacted within the family. Mike's frequent attempts to elicit therapist collusion with him as a victim and threats to abandon the work facilitated recognition of the rejecting role (with its punishing and controlling impact on the therapist), and this role was related to Mike's experience with Social Services, and again recognised within his family relationships.

Progressive recognition of therapist reliability in the face of rejection and rupture, alongside consistent development of positive roles such as

supporting ⇔ supported
listening ⇔ heard
understanding ⇔ understood
holding ⇔ held
trusting ⇔ trusted

were contrasted with initial perceptions of the therapist in the negative controlling and punishing roles. 'Punishing' contact constraints were thus progressively re-evaluated as expedient risk management measures. Mike, having left the army and found other work, has successfully collaborated with Social Services in trials of extended, unsupervised contact and now enjoys a level of relationship with his son that is satisfactory to both. The recognition of the parentally derived rejecting role and its enactment in therapy with consequent rupture tensions may well have provided validity to the externally (military) derived controlling and punishing roles in the client's perception. However, it was clear that exploration and re-evaluation of the applicability of these roles in the family and other social contexts had been necessary to enable the client first to identify them within himself and then to reassess their current validity.

Reciprocal roles (RRPs) in this case were as follows:

client (perpetrator) ⇔ victim
client ⇔ courts/Social Services
client (initial) ⇔ therapist
punishing/abusing ⇔ punished
blaming ⇔ blamed
controlling/ordering ⇔ controlled/obedient
rejecting ⇔ rejected

Accountability of therapeutic endeavour to child protection agencies

Geoff (white, mid-20s and unemployed) was referred for therapy in relation to risks he posed to his newborn daughter, Josie, and his partner, Helen, to whom he was strongly attached, and who had already facilitated his recovery from a heroin addiction. High risk levels had been ascertained from his record of frequent and severe (sometimes armed) violence and aggression against police, past intimates, family members, other professionals and other men. In the absence of any current custodial constraint, he was perceived as sufficiently dangerous and unpredictable to warrant keeping him within the family to reduce the risks of abduction, suicide or lethal assault that might be occasioned by excluding him (while applying at the same time a raft of risk management measures to address the child-protection concerns).

The 26-session therapy contract required routine feedback to Social Services and probation after all sessions, and regular reports to the guardian and family courts. In addition, his partner was to attend the service for support, to challenge collusion with Geoff and to monitor his behaviour through completion of both physical and psychological abuse checklists. This partner involvement, with its potential for being perceived as disloyalty, created additional concern for her safety. Both presented as extremely resistant and Geoff as an aggressive and unwilling client.

Initial sessions were devoted to the development of trust within the therapeutic relationship through compassionate exploration of his developmental trauma. This included the naming of paternal abuse; the recognition of blaming, punishing, abusing and rejecting reciprocal roles; and the development of an SDR which highlighted his experience of being made responsible and punished for adult distress. The conditionality of his paternal relationship and his tendency to placate and resentfully punish those who failed him or proved disloyal was also identified.

The near total elimination of confidentiality initially had a heavy impact on the therapeutic relationship, but gradually was used by the therapist and perceived by the client as a two-way process in which the therapists were able to advocate for Geoff and the family in the context of his 'stand-off' with statutory services and clarify misunderstandings. The negative consequences of ruptures in Geoff's relationship with Social Services and indirectly with therapy were mitigated through use of the SDR to permit more flexible and tolerant responses by both parties, and with the relationship sufficiently re-established, further insights into the enactment of rejecting and punishing reciprocal roles and their damaging consequences were facilitated. Improvements in the relationship between Geoff and statutory agencies increased as partner and health visitor feedback confirmed that safety was being adequately maintained, and where violence or aggression did occur, such transparency contributed to sufficient self-disclosure on Geoff's part to enable challenging work in therapy without premature termination through perceptions of the therapist as disloyal.

Geoff's experience of acceptance in the therapeutic relationship was extended gradually to his relationship with statutory services, where he was progressively able to leave behind expectations of reward for compliance, communicate his needs and experience assertively, and become proactive in his engagement with risk-reduction measures, this manifesting as a capacity to leave the family voluntarily for preplanned alternative accommodation when necessary. His child's name has since been taken off the child protection register, and Geoff enjoys a collaborative working relationship with his social worker.

The use of high levels of scrutiny and the sacrifice of confidentiality in this case provided sufficient child and partner safety to facilitate the use of CAT tools in the recognition of reciprocal roles and the diagrammatic identification of a placation trap. These CAT tools subsequently enabled the sufficient 'bridging' of ruptures between the client and referrer to enable therapeutic work to continue.

Summary

In our practice, we have attempted to integrate the split worlds of the private (behind closed doors) psychotherapy endeavour – which tends to psychologise violence and lead to generally very poor results with this client group – and the publicly accountable, profeminist, educational (antitherapy) perspective, through the use of CAT, informed by a macro-social analysis of gender and power. Especially where a violent client's *reciprocal role repertoire* has been derived from *both* family and cultural experience (which makes for a particularly dangerous combination), we are of the view that unidimensional approaches are unlikely to be sufficient to prioritise partner/victim and child safety and to bring about sustainable change.

Notes

1   While both gay and heterosexual men and women experience domestic violence, women form the overwhelming majority of the most heavily abused group (Walby & Allen, 2004). Women are killed by their male counterparts at far higher rates than are men by women (47% versus 8% based upon the 1997 Criminal Statistics for England and Wales, typically two women killed per week in the UK). They are physically injured to the point of needing medical attention as much as 10 times more often than men and they suffer far more damaging psychological trauma (e.g. Mirrlees-Black, 1999).

2   National Association for Domestic Violence Perpetrator Programmes and Associated Women's Services.

3   Hotaling & Sugarman (1986) through a comprehensive review of family violence literature found that 88% of studies with adequate comparison groups revealed that witnessing parental violence was a significant *predictor* of adult violence against a female partner. For their part, Straus *et al.* (1980) maintained that when compared with men from non-violent parents, men who witnessed their parents' domestic violence are three times more likely to abuse their own partners. Exposure to interparental violence also features as a strong candidate for predicting the development of attitudes that support violence against women (Stith & Farley, 1993; Silverman & Williamson, 1997). A high proportion of men had witnessed their father being violent to their mother among the population of homicide offenders studied by Dobash *et al.* (2002).

4   In her sample of domestically violent men, Caesar (1988), found that 38% had neither witnessed nor experienced violence as a child.

References

Austin, J. B. & Dankwort, J. (1999). The impact of a batterer's program on battered women. *Violence Against Women, 5*, 25–42.

Bennett, L. & Williams, O. (2003). Controversies and recent studies of battered intervention program effectiveness. Violence Against Women On-line Resources.

Burton, S., Regan, L. & Kelly, L. (1998). *Supporting women and challenging men: Lessons from the domestic violence intervention project*. London: Policy Press.

Caesar, L. P. (1988). Exposure to violence in the families of origin among wife abusers and maritally non-violent men. *Violence and Victims, 3*, 49–63.

Dobash, R. *et al.* (2002). *Homicide in Britain*. Research Bulletin. Department of Applied Social Science (DASS), University of Manchester, 1–3.

Dobash, R., Dobash, R. E., Cavanagh, K. & Lewis, R. (1996). Re-education programmes for violent men: An evaluation. *Home Office Research and Statistics Directorate, 46*.

Dutton, D. G. (1988). Profiling of wife assaulters: Preliminary evidence for a trimodel analysis. *Violence and Victims, 3*, 5–29.

Dutton, D. G. (1995). *The domestic assault of women: Psychological and criminal justice perspectives*. Vancouver: University of British Columbia Press.

Dutton, D. G. & Starzomski, A. (1994). Psychological differences between court referred and self-referred wife assaulters. *Criminal Justice and Behavior, 21*, 203–222.

Gondolf, E. W. (1988). The state of the debate: A review essay on woman battering. *Response to the Victimization of Women and Children, 11*, 3–8.

Gondolf, E. W. (1999). MCMI–III results for batterer program participants in four cities: Less 'pathological' than expected. *Journal of Family Violence, 14*, 1–17.

Healey, K. (1998). *Batterer intervention: Program approaches and criminal justice strategies*. New York: US Department of Justice.

Holtzworth-Munroe, A. & Stuart, G. L. (1994). Typologies of male batterers: Three subtypes and the differences among them. *Psychological Bulletin, 116*, 476–497.

Hotaling, G. T. & Sugarman, D. B. (1986). An analysis of risk markers in husband to wife violence. *Violence and Victims, 1*, 101–124.

Johnston, J. R. & Campbell, L. E. G. (1993). A clinical typology of interparental violence in disputed-custody divorces. *American Orthopsychiatric Association, 63*, 190–193.

McGibbon, A., Cooper, L. & Kelly, L. (1989). *What support?* London: Hammersmith and Fulham Council (Community Police Domestic Violence Project)/Polytechnic of North London.

Mirrlees-Black, C. (1999). Domestic violence: Findings from a new British Crime Survey self-completion questionnaire. *Home Office Research Studies*, 191.

Mooney, J. (1994). *The hidden figure: Domestic violence in North London*. (The findings of a survey conducted on domestic violence in the North London Borough of Islington). Islington Council.

Morley, R. & Mullender, A. (1994). Domestic violence and children: What do we know from research? In A. Mullender & R. Morley (Eds), *Children living with domestic violence: Putting men's abuse of women on the child care agenda*. London: Whiting & Birch.

O'Neil, J. M. & Harway, M. (1997). A multivariate model explaining men's violence toward women: predisposing and triggering hypotheses. *Violence Against Women, 3*, 182–203.

Painter, K. (1991). *Rape in marriage*. London: Department of Social Policy.

Prigerson, H. G. (2002). Population attributable fractions of psychiatric disorders and behavioural outcomes associated with combat exposure among US men. *American Journal of Public Health, 92*, 59–63.

Puffett, N. K. & Gavin, C. (2004). *Predictors of program outcome and recidivism at the Bronx Misdemeanor Domestic Violence Court*. New York: Center for Court Innovation. www.courtinnovation.org, April.

Saunders, D. G. (1992). Child custody decisions in families experiencing woman abuse. *Social Work, 39*, 51–59.

Shepard, M. F. & Pence, E. L. (1999). *Co-ordinating community responses to domestic violence*. London: Sage.

Shupe, A. (1987). Family violence in the military. In A. Shupe (Ed.), *Violent men, violent couples* (pp. 65–86). Lexington, MA: Lexington Books.

Silverman, J. & Williamson, G. (1997). Social ecology and entitlement involved in heterosexual battering by college males: Contributions of family and peers. *Victims and Violence, 12*, 147–164.

Stanko, B. (2000). The day to count: A snapshot of the impact of domestic violence in the United Kingdom. *Criminal Justice, 1*.

Stith, S. M. & Farley, S. C. (1993). A predictive model of male spousal abuse. *Journal of Family Violence, 8*, 183–201.

Straus, M. A. (1980). Wife-beating: How common and why? In M. A. Straus & G. T. Hotaling (Eds), *The social causes of husband–wife violence*. Minneapolis, MN: University of Minnesota Press.

Walby, S. & Allen, J. (2004). Domestic violence, sexual assault and stalking: Findings from the British Crime Survey. *Home Office Research, 276*.

Chapter 12

Cognitive Analytic Therapy for rage-type homicide

Philip H. Pollock

> How lucky the raging child who meets a person who discerningly responds, someone who senses, intuits the pain, the complaint, the demand for righting things, the need for healing.
>
> (Eigen, 2002; p. 13)

Police attend a 'kitchen-house' in a lower-working-class area of Belfast, having been contacted by neighbours worried that another domestic argument had become too disquieting to ignore, the neighbours standing at their open doors fearful of becoming too involved. As they enter the house, the drama that has been played out is blatantly apparent to the police officers. In a front room, a young mother lies dead with over 50 stab wounds randomly and indiscriminately inflicted by her husband, who is sitting on the settee, 2 feet away from the body. His eyes are glazed and staring at the wall in front of him. He is still tightly gripping the screwdriver in his hand and shaking physically. The couple's 3-year-old daughter is found locked in the adjacent kitchen and screaming.

Six months later, at a clinical interview while imprisoned, the husband and father, Alex, a 24-year-old taxi driver, shows the same glazed, zombie-like reaction as he narrates his recollections of the killing. He mentions that his recall is 'patchy, bits and pieces of stuff', his train of thought becoming derailed and disjointed as he talks about events. Alex offers, 'We had a fight, an argument. I've never hit her. I snapped, lost it altogether. Then she was dead and I sort of woke up to my senses. It was the child crying I think that clicked me out of it. . . . That wasn't the real me that did that. Who did do that? Maybe somebody else came in and I can't remember.' Alex's 6-month period of imprisonment had been punctuated by attempts at suicide by superficial cutting of his wrists. He reported sleep disturbance most nights, nightmares, lethargy, apathy and inability to function generally. He would engage in rituals of prayer to a photograph of his wife to assuage his grief. By day, he experienced intrusive images of his wife's face, imagining that he could hear a 'yelping sound' (his wife's reaction to the stabbing) and his daughter's screaming. Alex had been deemed to be unable to work or engage in any education within the prison. His family had rejected him, and he stated 'I've been disowned'. Alex's facial expression was blank, his emotional responses blunted, his eyes staring as he struggled to find words to grasp the event he had birthed and which had also collapsed his world so catastrophic-ally in one instant. Alex showed frequent bouts of inconsolable tears, interspersed with episodes of emotional shutdown and disengagement.

The history taken from Alex was telling in terms of the absence of indi-cators of psychopathology or mental disorder. Alex was a physically fit, independent, popular, sociable and hard-working young man who was con-sidered by those who knew him to have adored his daughter and family life. Soccer was his consuming passion. He was known as a loving son, and he had, despite social pressures, shrewdly avoided becoming entangled in the paramilitary violence that was rife among his friends and the local com-munity. Before the killing, he had neither been antisocial nor attended for mental health problems. Now, he was facing life imprisonment for killing his wife of 5 years.

The self-report information gleaned revealed that, on the day of the killing, Alex's wife had become aware of his litany of extramarital affairs, had chal-lenged him and had threatened to leave the family home with their child. The developing argument had been characterised by his wife's questioning of his virility, claiming that his daughter was the child of a former lover about whom Alex harboured jealousy and hatred, and threatening to cause his public humiliation and financial ruination. These statements were offered by Alex as examples of provocation and could not be verified. His loss of control and 'overkill' were clearly apparent in the offence.

The personal and family history given by Alex was corroborated through interviews with his parents and brother. Alex was the younger of two brothers born into a working-class Belfast family. His father was retired from the ship-building industry and was a respected 'hard man' and prominent figure in the local community, one of the earliest paramilitary commanders in the Loyalist areas of the city. His mother was devoted to her sons and family. The extended family were emotionally close, and Alex enjoyed many strong and significant attachments to these people. His schooling was relatively unremarkable, Alex being identified as a talented soccer player and achieving positions on regional teams. His father's pride in his son's sporting achieve-ments was obvious, and Alex was scripted by the family in the position of the special, talented son who brought recognition and esteem for the family within the community. His mother kept newspaper clippings of his soccer triumphs. On leaving school, he became a taxi driver, a job that was accept-able because his working hours fitted his soccer training and matches. Alex did not report any criminal history and had resisted entering the local para-military groups, mainly on the advice of his father. He was perceived to be 'above' this activity, and the paramilitary groups and members whom he knew colluded in this and did not place any pressure on him because of the importance of his position on one of the main soccer teams in Belfast. He accordingly received dispensation from many commitments and other favours (e.g. free alcohol in certain pubs, entrance to nightclubs, privileged treatment in restaurants, etc.). Attracting girls had never been difficult for Alex, and he enjoyed the advantages of his status as a local hero. His parents did report that he had been involved in 'fighting for girls' in his adolescence, yet these instances seemed to pre-date his attainment of status within the community. Neither alcohol nor drug misuse was apparent throughout his early history.

When aged 18, Alex met his wife, whom his family embraced as 'his child-hood sweetheart', as if the couple were destined for marriage and a successful life together. Alex, on reflection, believed that he was keen to conform to the family's expectations. A daughter was born when Alex was 21, and he recalled being teased by his friends and team-mates because she was a female child, a cultural sign of his lack of virility. Alex's wife, Megan, worshipped him, and the roles assumed within the couple's relationship could be defined in terms of RRPs such as *worshipped/adored-to-worshipping/adoring*. Megan was appeasing, placating and supportive, a quiet person, physically attractive and referred to as 'Alex's trophy'. She mirrored his fame. Alex was a dedicated father to his daughter and spent as much time as possible juggling his duties as a father and husband, his work and his soccer commitments.

However, the years preceding the killing of his wife had witnessed a decline in Alex's esteem, prestige and status. A series of events eroded his personal confidence and his standing in the community. Alex had lost his regular position on the first-team of the local soccer team, because he had been frequently injured and could not achieve consistent playing form. Many friends and newspaper writers commented that his best days were over, and that he was a disappointment and had not lived up to his promise. On one occasion, he was berated as a failure and disappointment in a public bar by a soccer fan. Alex felt that he had lost his status within the community. He recalled finding it more difficult to impress women and feeling that he needed to mature. Alex felt that he needed to regain and reclaim the limelight and devotion he once enjoyed. He began to frequent nightclubs and drink excessively, becoming involved in a litany of extramarital affairs, which, on reflection, he thought meant very little to him emotionally and were empty sexual conquests that became troublesome when the women gossiped about their involvement with him. A long-term friend had confronted Alex about his behaviour and the views of the community, many people feeling that he was acting disgracefully toward his wife and child. Alex dismissed any criticism as intrusive and unwarranted, feeling that he was driven to win over as many women for sex as he could. This flirtatious behaviour was to contribute to Alex's downfall.

In the months before the index offence, the police had been called to Alex's home on a number of occasions because of his violence against his wife. The violence was alcohol-fuelled and had prompted a Social Services investigation because of concerns of danger to Alex's daughter.

Alex's killing of his partner was an explosive, reactive form of violence, triggered by a catalysing interaction with the victim, who was stabbed in an overkill fashion. His offence was considered a rage-type homicide without evident mental or organic disorder.

Psychotherapy for rage-type killings

Several theories have explained the actions of the rage-type killer such as Alex. When one considers psychotherapeutic work for the rage-type killer, a number of target areas require consideration.

Firstly, the offenders tend to deny the fact of the offence and either cannot discuss the event because of difficulties in representational capacities to think about their actions, or display split-off, dissociated, amnesic attitudes to the offence. Self-reflection and mentalisation are limited, and the offence scenario remains unintegrated and lacking in any narrative structure or content. Post-traumatic stress symptoms are often present (Pollock, 1999). The crime is, in reality, disowned, undigested, unmetabolised and not assimilated. Alex could not think or talk about the offence in a coherent way.

Secondly, the offence is viewed as the end-product of an internal crescendo of incubated stress, often referred to as an acute or chronic catathymic crisis (Wertham, 1937; Meloy, 1992). A series of events cause a build-up of anger, tension and depression, occurring typically within a close-attachment relationship in which dependency, control and symbiosis are characteristic. The offender believes that all other options for release of this inner tension or resolving the relationship problems are exhausted or not available. The offender experiences 'too much-ness' (Wientrobe, 1985) and does not possess the mental equipment to digest and detoxify the emergent, confusing dilemmas and inner distress, resulting in explosive violence which obliterates the threatening (as perceived by the offender) victim and the internal object relation which has developed in the offender's mind about the relationship with the victim. Projective identification of inner turmoil occurs, and the victim is perceived as containing the unacceptable impulses and thoughts, and is viewed as controlling, invading, entrapping and humiliating. The offender's mental space cannot contain these feelings, and the offender cannot 'think' about the issues and distress, resulting in the discharge of violence against the victim, who is then destroyed (as is the object relationship), indicating the failure to digest these psychological contents. The offender reports feeling confused and unable to think about his own or the victim's states of mind prior to the offence. Problem solving fails and rational thinking is bypassed. The offender cannot construct a clear mental model of the RRPs underlying the offender-to-victim relationship and, after the fact, the crime itself. The catastrophic release of psychic energy during the violent act represents a total failure to contain, manage and control the inner turmoil and conflict experienced within the relationship.

Thirdly, the offender often displays what has been termed a tenuous 'narcissistic exoskeleton' (Cartwright, 2002) in the form of a self-serving, grandiose self which rigidly covers a vulnerability to threat, intrusion and control from others within relationships. Therein exists the offender's Achilles' heel. Others' failure to mirror or reflect the grandiose self exposes the offender's underbelly of inadequacy and stimulates the obliterating rage which cannot be digested (Megargee, 1966; Kohut, 1972; Meloy, 1992; Hyatt-Williams, 1998). The narcissistic injury tends to take the form of humiliation or criticism; control or entrapment within a relationship, as in a woman's teasing about sexual prowess; empathic failures by a partner to idealise the offender; activation of insecurities; and injured pride. Most offenders of this type have a rigid, defensive compliance, need for approval and admiration, emotional overcontrol and sensitivity to others' criticisms. As Cartwright (2001) stated, this narcissistic configuration is vulnerable to the impact of all manner of interpersonal devaluing and insult. For many, the offender's veneer of rigid emotional control and 'normality' belies turmoil of incubated sensitivity that can be ruptured through an escalation of events, culminating in out-of-character explosive violence. The offender lacks insight into the link between these personality sensitivities, the build-up of incubated frustrations and anger, and the form that the perceived threat takes within the ultimate offender–victim relationship. The victim is perceived to provoke the offender and blamed for initiating the violence through threatening, controlling or devaluing attitudes.

Fourthly, the problematic relationships with the victim (this is relevant even if the offence is entirely displaced onto another victim) require analysis, given the themes of conflict between marked dependency, intrusive control, narcissistic entitlement to act autonomously and the dysphoric stalemate emerging during the dangerous juggling act that culminates in homicide. The offender feels threatened by the victim who is 'inside' him/her psychologically and needs to be evacuated to remove the anxiety of the threat (to self-esteem, psychological integrity, etc.). Several theories to explain reactive violence have argued that certain relationship dynamics are fertile soil for the growth of catathymic violence.

Finally, the fact that most rage-type killings involve known parties places the offender, through his collapsed psychological control and fatal actions, in a perpetual dilemma and conflict because of killing a loved (or ambivalently loved) person. The offender experiences profound regrets, grief and guilt and mourns the lost person. Mourning is inevitably complicated (Fraser, 1988). The explosive violence displayed damages the grandiose self for ever, and the all-good self is irretrievably lost and tarnished and cannot be retrieved as all-good once again.

The referral of Alex for psychotherapy

Alex was referred for therapy after 10 years' imprisonment. He had been released on parole after 9 years, but, recently, his licence had been revoked after further offences. Alex had became involved in a relationship while in prison and had been released to live with this new partner and her two children. A relationship between this partner and a long-term male friend had caused insecurity and jealousy for Alex. When he discovered that he had contracted a sexually transmitted infection, he drank excessively and confronted his partner at a local barbeque, superficially stabbing with a kitchen knife her male friend, who threatened to have him arrested. Alex had repeatedly hit his partner on the head with a motorbike helmet in temper in this public place before stabbing her friend. This incident had prompted the prison authorities to review Alex's treatment needs on his return to prison, given that he had received no interventions before the parole release.

Assessment and reformulation

Clinical interviewing combined with the administration of psychological tests (Minnesota Multiphasic Personality Inventory–2 (MMPI–2) and Millon Clinical Multiaxial Inventory–3, Third Edition (MCMI–3)) and diagnostic assessments (Rorschach and Thematic Apperception Test (TAT)) indicated that Alex exhibited a narcissistic personality configuration with underlying feelings of vulnerability, shame and poor self-esteem, perceiving himself as flawed and damaged. His character disorder was formulated in terms of a 'narcissistic exoskeleton' which defended against an underbelly of dysphoria and inadequacy. His Personality Structure Questionnaire (PSQ) (Pollock et al., 2001) score was 9, within normal limits, suggesting that Alex did not exhibit identity disturbance. Administration of the structured interviews for post-traumatic stress disorder (PTSD) showed that, after 10 years, he continued to suffer from this disorder, which was directly caused by his own violent actions during the index offence (Pollock, 1999). Alex's violence was perceived as a reactive, ego-dystonic and explosive type, most probably representative of a crescendo of incubated frustration released in a raging attack on his wife, who had come to embody a composite, provoking target.

Alex's narrative account of the index offence showed many features of an impoverished, unformulated story. His version of events consisted of minimal sequential thinking, simply described as a rapid, confusing and traumatising flow of events. After 10 years of imprisonment, Alex could comment about the offence only as follows:

> We had a fight – it was all very fast and just happened. I had a screwdriver and she was yelling. Some things she said, I can't remember – it all just happened. She shouldn't have said what she said. I remember her

face, a scream, but that might've been my daughter. I remember the red mist coming down over me, and then 'wallop', I hit her. I think I hit her about two or three times. Then it was all blank until the police station. It's like a dream still.

Alex's narrative was poorly constructed and affected by his traumatised mental state. It was felt that the narrative function of the Reformulation Letter could be offered as a tool to help Alex to take the first steps toward reflecting upon the precursors to the offence. The Reformulation Letter was as follows:

Dear Alex,

This letter is written with the intention of trying to help you think about what has happened and to make some sense of these confusing and tragic events. It is based on all of our discussions and my observations of the case to date. We can alter any parts of the account if you consider that necessary.

I would suggest that we might best think about the times in three parts: before the crime, the crime itself and the changes that have happened as a result of the crime. Your history – and you know I have spoken to your family – indicates that you were a young man who was considered to be 'special' and talented within the community. Your family viewed you as a 'local hero' permitted special privileges because of your achievements. You recall feeling invincible, worshipped and the 'pride' of your family. Your wife worshipped you and never confronted or challenged anything you did. For you, she was the perfect 'fit'. As long as you remained in this position of 'the big boy in the big picture', you felt great about yourself and your lifestyle. Unfortunately, events conspired to undermine this 'hero' position, and you felt that, over time, you became depressed as you lost your status, privileges and talent (e.g. becoming injured, losing your place in the team, the public mocking you and calling you a 'has-been'). You coped through alcohol misuse and tried to feel better about yourself by having affairs, contacts you recall as empty, unsatisfying encounters. Your physical fitness suffered and your depression became worse. You state that you remember feelings of being useless, worthless, 'washed up' and a failure. Anger at yourself was made worse by your wife's change in her behaviour and attitudes toward you. She became nagging and confronting, calling you names (particularly a 'bad father') and demanding that you 'sort yourself out'. You can acknowledge how angry she made you feel, and you dealt with this by either assaulting her or leaving, but drinking alcohol more. Several times, domestic violence occurred, and the police were called. Your rage and depression appear to have increased in the months before the offence.

You cannot talk about the offence and what happened that night. I accept that you will probably need to 'dose' yourself when trying to discuss the offence. You have nightmares and struggle to think about the crime, feeling overwhelmed, guilty and regretful. I accept that you feel a complicated mixture of loss about your actions and their effects. We must help you understand the unfolding sequence of events that led to the offence, what the offence was about and where your rage came from, and also resolve this difficult sense of loss. After the offence, you were left with a self-inflicted sense of being damaged, bad and racked with regrets. You view yourself as having destroyed someone whom you loved deeply and having ruined your own life. Your painful loss of family and your daughter is also apparent.

I suggest we work on the following things:

- *helping you understand how your personality and behaviour before the crime caused you to become so full of rage; the decline in your feelings about yourself and how the offence 'popped out' of your personality; how your depression and anger built up and where it came from*
- *how we can understand the nature of whatever happened between you and your wife and the reasons for your explosive violence against her; the marital relationship and how you thought about women and relationships in the past; the shock you feel about what you did and how to make sense of what has happened – we may have to help you 'dose' yourself on thinking about this, given how much you have traumatised yourself by your own actions*
- *helping you deal with your sense of loss, grief and rejection by your family*
- *helping you rebuild your self-worth, given how damaged and bad you feel about your actions, without resorting to strategies that have failed in the past.*

Alex's reaction to the letter was positive, and discussion took place about the preoffence, offence and postoffence target problems, Alex claiming that he felt that the 'shock' about his actions should be addressed first because of its interference with his everyday functioning and the distress caused. A number of areas for therapy were targeted and defined within the self-states grid and draft sequential diagrammatic reformulation (SDR) (Figs. 12.1 and 12.2).

Alex completed the Psychotherapy File and identified the depression trap in particular and its link to his alcohol misuse. Alex's self-states grid (Fig. 12.1) identified a variety of healthy and pathological RRPs and positions. The named self-states were incorporated into an SDR (Fig. 12.2), which is composed of a three-part SDR with *preoffence* (SS1 and SS2) phases, an *offence* phase (SS3) and a *postoffence* (SS4) phase. The reasons for constructing the diagram in this manner are that Alex's crime emerged from his preoffence personality functioning and that the consequences of his explosive violence irreversibly corrupted his psychological status and changed him fundamentally as an individual. The SDR represented one of the tools for Alex to contemplate the links between his development, personality and

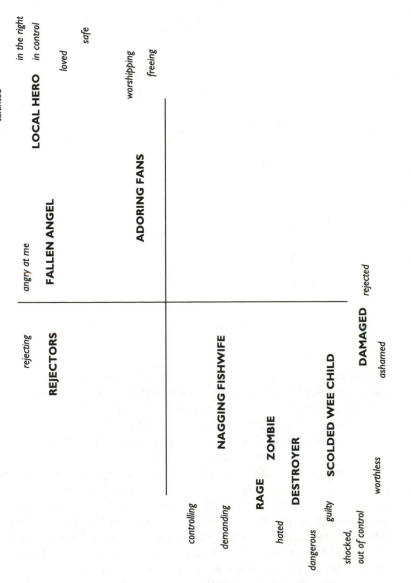

Figure 12.1 Alex's self-states grid.

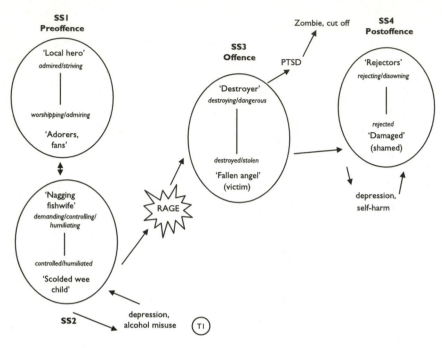

Figure 12.2 Alex's self-states sequential diagram.

the crime itself. The target problems and tasks of therapy agreed were as follows:

(1) *Understanding the nature and function of Alex's 'narcissistic exoskeleton' and the unwanted feelings beneath.* The decline of Alex's grandiose self could be observed as he lost his sense of status and entitlement. His wife's threats and challenges caused a climax of already incubated rage and despair in Alex. The offence was characterised by a projection of his own rage onto the victim, who came to represent all the people who had humiliated, criticised and infuriated Alex over many months. His failure to detoxify this building rage (which had leaked as depressive symptoms) left him 'primed' or 'kindled' to release a raging attack. The fatal violence can be viewed as the end product of the ultimate conflict experienced within the attachment between Alex and his wife (the domestic violence was a preliminary indicator of the pent-up aggression between the couple). Her comments (if she really made them) about his sexual prowess, paternity, failed status and the exposure of his failed narcissistic self provoked the type of overkill and reaction shown by Alex.

(2) *Constructing a therapeutic space to help Alex think about the symbolic nature of the violent act and the reasons for its 'overkill'.* The offence part

of the SDR served to provide a specific focus for both therapist and Alex to think about the actual RRPs and states of mind that operated at the time of the crime.

(3) *Tracing the origins within his marital relationship of the tension and distress that had culminated in an explosive climax of violence and the killing of his wife.* Alex's relationships with women had been typically flavoured with similar patterns of self-perpetuating sequences. At assessment, Alex failed to connect his past perceptions, attitudes and ways of relating within adult relationships to the killing of his wife.

(4) *Exploration of the offender–victim relations, the sequential shifts that occurred and the location of the self-state where Alex's peak risk potential emerged.* Consideration was given to the inherent weaknesses and fallibilities in his psychological armoury which resulted in the killing. The abrupt and catastrophic switch between self-states and the rage that was released was targeted to convey the link between the contextual relationship of the marriage and Alex's personality functioning and patterns of relating to his wife and past partners. Alex remained confused and shocked by his own actions and could not articulate the hidden dynamics of the offence.

(5) *Helping Alex to grieve for his wife and tease out and resolve the reality that he had destroyed a loved person and his guilt and culpability for this act.* The complicated mourning process and experience of PTSD symptoms required resolution and management.

(6) *Helping Alex to orient his perceptions to living without his family and constructively making reparation for his offence.* Alex's need for narcissistic repair was discussed and the importance of resisting a return to the type of functioning which promoted his vulnerability to aggression.

CAT for Alex

Alex was offered 24 sessions of CAT. He expressed his anxiety about what might be involved in this task, particularly any examination of the index offence itself, yet he did engage appropriately. The therapist noted that Alex was motivated to appease, placate and impress. The joint negotiation of target problems clarified the task ahead for Alex.

The Reformulation Letter was offered as a narrative scaffolding for Alex about the nature of his grandiose, special self-state (SS1; labelled by Alex 'the big boy in the big picture/local hero') and how this facet of his personality had functioned for him, sustaining his sense of self-worth and esteem. He recognised that his family and wife had colluded with the fuelling of his grandiosity and that his success in soccer had raised his status, privilege and entitlement. Alex could recognise that striving for achievement, attention and glory were pursuits that emerged from childhood fantasies (he saw himself as a 'Roy of the Rovers' comic book soccer hero adored by the public). Numerous examples could be garnered of the association between this self-state and his talents and the resulting admiration throughout his history. As Alex put it, 'I never really had to try hard for anything. I had natural talent, everything came easy.'

In many respects, it was acknowledged that this strategy of *striving* in relation to *admiring* (SS1) was a reflection of healthy narcissism and development of self-worth within his culture. Alex was helped to reflect upon how this sense of entitlement had expanded to the point whereby he expected that others would behave toward him in a worshipping, admiring manner, feeding and nourishing his self-importance and entitlement. Alex recalled that his wife Megan enjoyed being 'the trophy girl on my arm'. He acknowledged that this part of his personality had positively served to enhance his self-esteem throughout his life so far, and he continued to think that he desired and depended upon the feedback of others to feel worthy and acceptable. This was apparent within the prison, as Alex had become a 'jail-house lawyer' for other prisoners and had amassed numerous qualifications and commendations in such activities as Braille translation, theatre workshops for prisoners, defending prisoners' human rights and obtaining a degree in English. Alex offered these achievements as a measure of his success since imprisonment and how well he had progressed and become accepted and liked. It was felt by the therapist that Alex continued to strive for recognition, attention and admiration from others, a reflection of his need to feed his deflated narcissistic self-state and to shore up and repair his damaged sense of self. The function of this side of the 'narcissistic exoskeleton' was discussed, and Alex was requested to consider the vulnerability associated with dependency upon others' admiration to achieve self-worth and esteem.

When addressing the relevance of the narcissistic functions of SS1 to the index offence, Alex and the therapist examined how events accumulated to expose the 'underbelly' of this state (SS2, 'scolded wee boy') and the ways in which Alex began to react to the absence or drying up of attention, admiration and the sources which had psychologically sustained him. He could recall instances before the offence in which his narcissistic pursuits had failed and how he had experienced feelings of rejection, humiliation and inadequacy. His decline in public reputation served to motivate compensatory behaviours such as engagement in several extramarital affairs as a means of winning 'victories', but Alex could recognise that a strong dysphoria and exasperation had emerged, causing him to resort to alcohol intake. The effects of this trap (T1) were highlighted, given their cyclical and compounding exacerbation of his problems (increasing his depression, his decline in fitness as a soccer player, influence on his marriage, etc.).

Alex's failure to resolve the effects of his incubating anger and depression was noted. Documentation from the case file had recorded that several incidents of alleged domestic discord were attended by police in the 10 months prior to the index offence. Alex reported that mounting anger and stress because of the disintegration of his narcissistic procedures had become manifest in marital strain with his wife Megan. He admitted that she had confronted him about his alcohol misuse, his lack of interest in his duties as a father and rumours about his affairs with women. Alex had pushed and 'manhandled' his wife on these occasions, the couple arguing and Alex destroying furniture or leaving the home to drink in a public bar. It appeared that his actions during the index offence could be viewed as the climax of these mounting stresses.

The most difficult task in therapy for Alex was contemplating the events of the index offence itself. It was hoped that the CAT tools would promote the development of a 'do-it-yourself psychic digestion kit', giving Alex a device to think about his states of mind. When the subject was broached, Alex became dissociated and felt that he could not think about the act or its meaning. His recall was partial (his offence was not substance related), and his memories were fragmented and traumatic in quality. It was apparent that Alex could not find the psychological means to represent the act, and their narrative qualities were poor and unintegrated, causing PTSD (e.g. flashbacks of his wife's face before he stabbed her, a piercing scream, his daughter's crying, the warm sensation of blood on his hand). His sense of 'too much-ness' (Wientrobe, 1985) was acknowledged, and a number of sessions were spent discussing ways to articulate, represent and formulate the offence event and its RRPs. Alex could only 'dose' himself with episodic discussion about the offence, often dissociating into a zombie-like state of mind (SS3).

This aspect of his presentation fits the types of PTSD reactions observed as a consequence of the reactively violent killing of a known victim (Pollock, 1999). It was decided to employ eye movement desensitisation and reprocessing (EMDR) (Shapiro, 1989) for these traumatic features of Alex's experiences, given the relative success of EMDR for homicide perpetrators (Pollock, 2001). After three sessions of EMDR, Alex felt more able to cope with discussions about the offence itself with less distress evident. It was felt that the beneficial changes achieved with EMDR would facilitate developing a narrative analysis of the offence. Alex's sleep pattern settled and he reported a decrease in intrusive images, fragments of memories and nightmares.

Through dialogical sequence analysis, the therapist encouraged Alex to identify the RRPs and positions within his marital relationship, past relationships with women and their sequential changes culminating in the offence. Alex acknowledged that he had perceived women as 'toys or trophies, one or the other' before his marriage, and that he had a masculine, devaluing and disrespecting view of women. He reflected that he had married Megan because of her compliant and unchallenging adoration of him. He voiced his understanding that he was, in many respects, dependent upon his wife to sustain his self-worth and to collude with his need for mirroring and unconditional appreciation. Megan's position and RRP were noted within SS1 ('adorers'). Alex's marriage had been untroubled throughout his success, although he disclosed that he had taken opportunities to enter sexual relationships with other women on many occasions, perceiving these encounters as 'notches on my bedpost, nothing more'.

Difficulties within the marital relationship had emerged in reaction to Alex's inability to feed narcissistically through achievement, the decline in attention and the changes in others' perception of him from local hero to failed, disappointing 'has-been'. His wife's knowledge of his affairs, and her confrontation of him about his drinking and lack of purpose combined to alter Alex's perceptions of the relationship. He stated that Megan began to act in a controlling, invasive and rebuking manner, causing him to feel trapped, belittled and inadequate. He was helped to consider that the emergence of this RRP placed him into a position that reminded him of being a 'scolded wee child' (SS2). Alex recalled believing that his wife had no right to control or rebuke him. He acknowledged that his drinking and irresponsibility increased to assert his masculinity, liberty and emancipation (i.e. staying out overnight without informing his wife). The threatening behaviours of his wife in terms of the RRP of *demanding/controlling/humiliating* ('nagging fishwife') in relation to *controlled/rebuked/humiliated* ('scolded wee boy') were incorporated in the reformulation at SS2. The relationship between inducement into this position, its RRP and his incubating rage was identified. The circular nature of the trap between alcohol and depression was noted, and the procedural loop with the failure to revise this behaviour was discussed.

The articulation of the RRP and the positions which were constructed during the offence were more difficult for Alex to contemplate. Sensitive dialogical sequence analysis was undertaken, focusing on the preoffence RRPs and states (SS1 and SS2) and how his mounting rage created the *offence* part of the SDR (SS3). Alex described his sense, before the offence, of wanting to 'empty my head of the shit she'd put in, that everybody had put in'; to evacuate his mind of 'the pressure building up'; and to free himself from the controlling, oppressive humiliation he felt his wife caused him. Alex spoke of the escalation in the argument with his wife prior to the offence and her devastating comments, which, he felt, provoked his rage. In cases of rage-type killing, it is apparent that the act of killing creates a new RRP and state which cannot be assimilated and causes traumatic reactions in many cases.

In Alex's case, the evolving sequential changes in the RRPs of the relationship with his wife, who was perceived as a composite threatening object evocative of several unpleasant feelings for him, represented the context for the killing through explosive, pent-up rage as the narcissistic self-state was compromised. The preoffence self-states identified formed the substrate for the creation of new RRPs and positions during the offence. Alex was helped to formulate perpetrator-to-victim RRPs of *destroying/emancipating-to-destroyed threat*.

The loss that Alex felt for his wife was obvious, and he expressed his genuine remorse for killing a loved partner. He had, since imprisonment, had his wife's and daughter's names tattooed on his arm, and spoke of his grief and inability to mourn for them. The dilemma and conflict for Alex was addressed through a dialogue process using imagery. Alex assumed the RRP of shamed 'destroyer' and offered an intensely emotional apology to his wife, idealising her as a 'fallen/broken angel' (SS3). His emotional investment in the relationship and the catastrophic nature of the disrupted attachment proved difficult to resolve, and several sessions focused upon finding methods to help Alex disentangle his feelings about his actions and their consequences.

Alex's damaged self (SS4) proved more difficult to address in therapy. He expressed his feelings of shame, deserved punishment and self-castigation. His mood was appropriately depressed; episodically, he appeared inconsolable and withdrew from prison and other activities. These reactions were viewed as manifestations of SS4 of the *postoffence* part of the SDR. He had engaged in two incidents of superficial cutting of his arms after the assessment phase of CAT. Alex displayed strategies of either narcissistic striving for achievement and attention (return to the RRPs of SS1) or depressive withdrawal and self-disgust (SS4, 'damaged' position). This pattern was explored and Alex was helped to develop more appropriate ways of achieving acceptance from others and self-approval. Alex discussed his belief that his family's rejection of him, although understandable, generated further feelings of being a 'low-life murderer, like some piece of shit'. The transformation in self which had occurred was acknowledged, and Alex was helped to accept the need to change the ways in which he obtained psychological supply.

Analysis was undertaken with Alex to trace explicitly the sequence of events (internal and external) that would inflate his *risk potential* of offending. The significance of SS1 and SS2 is readily apparent in this case as the precursor to a magnification of this potential to harm. A relapse-prevention plan based on the SDR was devised as a portable guide for Alex. His parole failure and the circumstances surrounding his violence were further incorporated in the reformulation.

Outcome and risk prediction

In terms of the target problems agreed, CAT for Alex was relatively successful in that he developed improved insight into the functioning of those parts of his personality that led to the offence, the unfolding self–other and self–self RRPs which translated rage into murder and the sequence of events which were involved. He was able to name and reflect upon his actions and locate their origins and sources within the reformulation. Alex achieved some integration and resolution of the complicated and traumatic bereavement he had caused for himself. Post-CAT psychometric assessment showed that PTSD symptoms were minimal. CAT provided a representational space for him to think about his actions and to understand their emergence. Alex was able to talk openly about the offence without distress yet show appropriate remorse. His narcissistic strategies were acknowledged, and he was helped to address his newly self-created damaged self.

This case is indicative of an offender whose personality was configured in a manner whereby reactive, rage-type killing is context-dependent within an attachment relationship. The fact that the killing is contextually bound (it is obvious that two incidents of serious violence occurred within partnerships) permits the therapist to express a degree of confidence when making statements about Alex's immediate and longer-term risk of reoffending. Entrance into an adult partnership inflates all aspects of risk in such a case. The aim of CAT is to equip offenders with self-knowledge and insight into their own personality functioning and behaviours to enable them to self-monitor, self-regulate and self-manage without similar patterns becoming evident. On release from prison into the community, this offender has succeeded in avoiding reoffending violently for 3 years to date. Alex entered a relationship after a year of release. The supervising probation officer was advised of the SDR and the CAT work undertaken, which provided a communicative tool for both offender and professional to monitor his risk potential.

One of the advantages of CAT in such a case is that the designation of preoffence, offence and postoffence parts of the reformulation allows the sequential and sensitive analysis of the crime, which the offender himself finds difficult to tolerate and 'hold'. The containing function of the SDR encourages the identification of the RRPs within the personality from which the violence emerged. The creation of new RRPs during the actual offence can be contemplated by using the narrative within the Reformulation Letter and SDR as tools to prompt the offender's thinking. It is often difficult to articulate the nature of the underlying RRPs of the offence. The lexicon of words we can use (to verbalise the offender's experiences) do not do justice to the criminal act. Alex struggled to describe the crime, but could offer that he intended to 'wipe her out', 'scrub her', 'make her nothing', 'put her in her place', 'snuff her out and shut her up'. These statements suggest a relational facet between offender and victim in RRP terms (e.g. *obliterating-to-destroyed*) which must be explored and agreed in the offender's language.

Issues regarding victim provocation are debated through naming of the RRPs in play. In this case, victim empathy was not mixed with externalisation of blame, and complicated bereavement required resolution. It is interesting in this case that the offender's liberty had been revoked after 9 years when he committed a second offence against a partner in which similar, if not the same, RRPs were observable, and the violence was a mirror image of the index offence (e.g. repeatedly hitting his partner on the head with a motorbike helmet). Alex had completed several programmes (enhanced thinking skills course, anger-control therapy, etc.) within the prison before release on licence. It could be argued that individual therapy is necessary in certain cases with other programmes as an adjunctive form of intervention to permit an idiosyncratic, personalised reformulation of the link between the offender's personality and the crime.

References

Cartwright, D. (2001). The role of psychopathology and personality in rage-type homicide: A review. *South African Journal of Psychology, 31*, 12–19.

Cartwright, D. (2002). *Psychoanalysis, violence and rage-type murder: Murdering minds*. London: Brunner-Routledge.

Eigen, M. (2002). *Rage*. Middletown, CT: Wesleyan University Press.

Fraser, K. A. (1988). Bereavement in those who have killed. *Medicine, Science and the Law, 28*, 127–130.

Hyatt-Williams, A. (1998). *Cruelty, violence and murder: Understanding the criminal mind*. London: Jason Aronson Press.

Kohut, H. (1972). Thoughts on narcissism and narcissistic rage. In P. Ornstein (Ed.), *The search of the self*. London: International University Press.

Megargee, E. I. (1966). The undercontrolled and overcontrolled personality types in extreme antisocial aggression. *Psychological Monographs, 80, Whole Issue No. 611*.

Meloy, J. R. (1992). *Violent attachments*. Northvale, NJ: Jason Aronson Press.

Pollock, P. H. (1999). When the killer suffers: Post-traumatic stress reactions following homicide. *Legal and Criminological Psychology, 4*, 185–202.

Pollock, P. H. (2001). Eye movement desensitization and reprocessing (EMDR) for post-traumatic stress disorder (PTSD) following homicide. *Journal of Forensic Psychiatry, 11*, 176–184.

Pollock, P. H., Broadbent, M., Clarke, S., Dorrian, A. & Ryle, A. (2001). The Personality Structure Questionnaire (PSQ): A measure of the multiple self-states model of identity disturbance in cognitive analytic therapy. *Clinical Psychology and Psychotherapy, 8*, 59–72.

Shapiro, F. (1989). *Eye movement desensitization and reprocessing: Basic principles, protocols and procedures*. London: Guilford.

Wertham, F. (1937). The catathymic crisis. *Archives of Neurology and Psychiatry, 37*, 974–978.

Wientrobe, S. (1985). Violence and mental space. *Bulletin of the Anna Freud Centre, 18*, 149–164.

Chapter 13

Adam and Eve in the forensic Eden

Boundary violations in forensic practice

Philip H. Pollock & Mark Stowell-Smith

Abuse in forensic mental health involves both the blurring of boundaries between the personal and professional life of the clinician and the failure to respect the power dynamics of the professional relationship. Anonymous surveys of clinicians indicate the severity of the problem, noting that the exploitation of the patient by the professional is more frequent than thought and sparking concerns about professional ethical standards and the dynamics of these 'fatal attractions' (Carr & Robinson, 1990).

The maintenance of boundaries is a central feature of all forms of psychotherapy and plays an essential role in the practice of forensic psychotherapy. Norris *et al.* (2003) define boundaries in psychotherapy as 'the edge of appropriate professional behaviour, a structure influenced by therapeutic ideology, contract, consent, and, most of all, context'. The same authors distinguish how boundary *violations* differ from boundary *crossings*. They describe the latter as 'harmless deviations from traditional clinical practice, behaviour, or demeanour' and cite as an example of this, helping up a patient who has fallen over. By contrast, they define boundary violations as harmful and exploitative, often involving sexual, affiliative or financial forms of inappropriate dependency. They cite as examples of this 'having sex or sexualized relations with patients, exploiting patients to perform menial services for the treater, exploiting patients for money or for financial demands beyond the fee, and generally using patients to feed the treater's narcissistic, dependent, pathologic, or sexual needs'.

The diversity of psychotherapeutic models allied to the diverse number of professional codes of ethics makes it difficult to provide a precise, universal definition of abusive practice in psychotherapy. Despite this, however, the literature seems be in some agreement that psychotherapists of all persuasions begin to abuse their clients when they use the therapeutic relationship to meet their own needs over and above those of the client. This form of abusive, exploitative relationship can have disastrous consequences for the patient.

The 'slippery slope' to professional abuse

The pathway to professional abuse is often described in terms of a progressive, insidious failure to maintain appropriate boundaries. This is an argument developed by, among others, Kroll (2001), who defines a 'slippery slope' in which seemingly innocuous boundary crossings may lead inexorably to more serious professional misconduct. Gutheil & Simon (1995) have defined the segment of the therapy session that occurs 'between the chair and the door' as the point where boundary violations might be initiated. This might be the start of the slippery slope, which, according to Simon (1998), follows an often predictable pattern. Simon says this path may be marked by several milestones, such as erosion of the clinician's neutrality, therapy becoming a social event looked forward to by both patient and therapist. The patient is treated as special, the clinician starts to self-disclose, physical contact occurs and extratherapeutic contact with greater intimacy follows.

This argument echoes the idea that the erosion of professional boundaries over a period of time leads to the gradual dismantling of the professional framework that regulates professional practice.

Why does the therapist abuse?

Kardener et al. (1976) argued that practitioners who engage in sexual relationships with patients hold idiosyncratic beliefs about the appropriateness and legitimacy of such actions. They surveyed 460 physicians by questionnaire regarding sexual contact with patients, identifying two groups, erotic practitioners and non-erotic practitioners, the former being a group that, at both attitudinal and behavioural levels, were freer with non-erotic contact with patients and, according to the authors, statistically more likely to engage in erotic contact.

Garfinkel et al. (1997a & b) have also speculated about the potential and actual characteristics of the abusive therapist. In one study (Garfinkel et al., 1997b), the authors used a series of troubling case vignettes which were discussed with a group of psychiatrists in terms of the doctor–patient relationship, sexual boundary violations and various forms of non-sexual exploitation. The authors concluded that psychiatrists with poor impulse control, exaggerated views of their own specialness, excessive need for affirmation or unacknowledged longings for care and nurturance are vulnerable to committing boundary violations. Subsequently, the authors conducted a small-scale, retrospective study (Garfinkel et al., 1997a), in which they identified psychiatrists' potential to abuse patients sexually by the therapists' psychopathic and narcissistic personality styles. They concluded that for some abusing therapists the sexual abuse of patients represents the continuation of a pattern of exploitative relationships. Averill et al. (1989) describe a loosely defined group of younger practitioners who are open to the possibility of exploiting the patients in their care. Pope (1991) argues that psychologists who have had sexual contact with a trainer are more inclined to cross sexual boundaries with patients as qualified practitioners. Thomas-Peter & Garrett (2000) cite both empirical and anecdotal evidence to suggest that female professionals can be equally culpable.

Situational variables, such as the therapist's circumstances and the nature of the clinical environment, have also been advanced as possible factors underpinning abuse in psychotherapy. A number of authors suggest that the therapist may be more inclined to abusive practice at times of personal pressure, a situation that may incline the therapist to use the relationship with the client for personal advantage. In this respect, Butler & Zelen (1977) report how therapists who engage in sexual or social relationships with clients are often lonely, and may be recently separated, divorced, or bereaved, and/or experiencing other personal difficulties. This theme is also taken up by Averill *et al.* (1989), who describe an additional subgroup of predominantly middle-aged men, disaffected by life events and seeking to find nurturance with patients as a way of repairing feelings of despair.

The professional–patient (offender) dyad is fertile ground for distorted relating given the nature and potency of the RRPs that can become apparent. Although the power differential between therapist and patient is typically perceived as biased toward the therapist's control and status, certain vicissitudes accompany the professional's interactions with the offender also.

The relational chemistry of offenders: Professionals' vicissitudes

The relational repertoire of many offenders does not augur well when predicting their capacity to forge a therapeutic alliance and to benefit from the process itself (Campling, 1996). An obvious example of this lack of connectedness is the psychopathic offender who lacks the capacity to attach, who tends to interact with the world through destructive patterns of relating, who harbours an impenetrable narcissistic self and who exhibits an ego-syntonic propensity for aggressive conduct. The depths of psychological deviance, primitive relations and perversity evident in the relating of many criminals and their actions to others may prompt the clinician to question whether any meaningful gains can be made. Such hopelessness and pessimism are often warranted (Meloy, 1992). Psychotherapy with offenders reveals that their relational repertoire can impinge upon the formation of the therapeutic alliance and every task of therapy itself. The professional encounters, and to some extent is exposed to, a variety of specific RRPs and procedures (in CAT terminology) which must be identified, understood and contained without collusion. The risk of harm to oneself or others is a facet of these procedures and can obscure the decision making, judgements, choices and actions of therapists, if they become sufficiently embroiled in the turbulence of these procedures. The dangers of forensic psychotherapy for the therapist include entrance into a dyad in which particularly potent, primitive and disordered relating materialises, most often implicitly.

Transference and counter-transference in forensic practice

Psychotherapy as a process is fertile ground for distorted, harmful and perverse relating. Chessick (1989) discussed the fact that therapists often use therapy and the patient to 'treat' themselves, and proposed that treatment rather than condemnation should be offered to the offending therapist, acknowledging the contributions of both parties. Apfel & Bennett (1985) refer to the fact that therapy is imbued with rescue fantasies and provokes such strong and intense recapitulation of early relationships and emotional neediness that it causes vulnerability for therapist and patient alike. Ciardello (1996) offers that the dyad within psychotherapy are essentially free to create their own reality and are open to the 'perverse temptation' and distortion of the relationship. Exploitation of one party is more frequent than thought within anonymous surveys of clinicians, sparking our concern about professional ethical standards and the dynamics of these 'fatal attractions' (Carr & Robinson, 1990).

Transference and counter-transference relationships when working with offenders can be potent, provocative and challenging. Strasburger (2001) cites counter-transference reactions, such as a fear of assault and harm (the 'menacing stranger'; Grant, 1978); helplessness and guilt, such as 'impotence in his [the therapist's] quest for change' (p. 198); a loss of professional identity in response to devaluation and narcissistic contempt; denial of danger and risk; rejection of the patient and experiences of hatred (which represent a type of attachment to be expected; Prodgers, 1991); and a rageful wish to destroy, a curious mixture of aversion and malice. Whether a concordant (*identifying*) or complementary (*elicited*) response is experienced within the transference (Racker, 1962), the therapist's task is to understand, formulate and manage the vicissitudes of these interactions to avoid collusion with these powerful transactions that are indicative of the offender's repertoire of relating (e.g. experiencing problems in trust, showing hostile dependency and envy, lying and deception, oscillation between extremes of devaluation and idealisation, and difficulty in ending therapy; Campling, 1996).

Referring to the original work of Racker (1962) on types of transference and counter-transference, Meloy (1988) described four types of relationship which can be observed when a person enters into an attachment with a psychopathic offender: sadistic, masochistic, hysterical and psychopathic. The sadistic and masochistic attachments are labelled as *concordant* transferences, representing relationships whereby the partner, typically a female, engages in ways that reflect parts of the offender's personality. The hysterical and psychopathic transferences are termed *complementary*, indicating an extension of the offender's personality. For the psychotherapist in forensic practice, a range of transference and counter-transference reciprocations and identifications can occur, yet often the 'pull' of the 'transitional game' is more intense, potent, provocative and deviant (Kiesler, 1988) than in treatment of other types of personality. Boundary violations within the therapeutic relationship require careful monitoring as the transference develops. Counter-transference responses must be checked and any deviations from the typical framework of therapy analysed to protect both parties.

The CAT model of transference and counter-transference was described by Ryle (1997) (see Chapter 1). Two types of transference (T) are noted. Firstly, an *identifying transference* is characterised by the patient or therapist mirroring an aspect of one or other's personality, causing a loss of separation and individuation through imitation. Secondly, a *reciprocating transference* is observed when one party responds by an enactment of the induced role of the RRP in a form of explicit or implicit collusion. Counter-transferences (CT) are of a similar nature. A personal CT is a response which is indicative of the therapist's reactions because of the elicitation of RRPs within his/her own history. Other elicited CTs include the identifying and reciprocating CTs, the latter being evidence that the therapist is being drawn into or stimulated to reciprocate the provoking pole of the RRP.

Case illustrations of CAT

An exploration of the CAT model applied to boundary violations with offenders is here described with two case illustrations to exemplify the transferences which can occur. The first case reports the development of an intimate relationship between a psychologist and a psychopathic killer within a prison setting and considers the response of the organisation and how CAT was employed to make sense of the matrix of responses to the events. The second case describes a psychiatric trainee's experience of an emerging intimate relationship with a psychopathic sex offender within a secure hospital and how CAT supervision was used to delineate the transference issues and their source, to promote appropriate management of the offender's case.

Case vignette I

The boundary violations in this case occurred between a prison psychologist and the sexual murderer of a female child. The offender's crime was the predatory enticement of the child to an isolated location, where he sexually assaulted vaginally and strangled her, and deposited her body in a sewer hole covered with a sheet of metal. The offender never admitted to killing the child over a 20-year period, claiming that she was murdered by a fellow member of a paramilitary gang when she stumbled upon them during gun-running activities. The offender had provided professionals with changing versions and accounts of the crime over many years. Diagnosed as having a psychopathic personality disorder, he had failed to make any progress through sex offender programmes in the prison or any other assistance. He constantly complained about his mistreatment and the prison regime and was considered negativistic and aloof.

The management of the case over many years had featured interesting developments. Successive professionals who dealt with the offender's case had engaged in a polarised struggle, certain professional groups claiming that this offender offered an acceptable risk of release, and other groups articulating a vociferous, conflicting opinion. The split in attitudes between all professional bodies involved was clear. During the 20-year period of imprisonment, the offender had availed himself of eight episodes of escorted paroles, the majority of these programmes collapsing because of his sexual innuendos or alleged sexual misconduct toward young female family members or other adolescent girls (e.g. shop assistants). On each occasion, he denied that any indiscretion had occurred, accusing the alleged victims of lying and fabricating allegations to continue his imprisonment.

The clinical psychologist was middle-aged, divorced and living with a teenage daughter. She had no prior experience of working with offenders but had considerable mental health training and skills. She was made aware of the offender's notoriety before assessing him because of the tensions which existed between professionals about his release.

Difficulties were first revealed when prison staff remarked about the length and frequency of sessions between psychologist and offender. The consulting room door was usually locked and a curtain drawn across the window. The telephone was switched off. The assessment report produced by the clinical psychologist about the offender, very much at odds with recent thinking about his case, recommended initiation of escorted paroles and an accelerated programme involving transfer to lesser security. The psychologist offered to assume the role of supervisor during paroles, arguing that this would provide opportunity to observe the offender. These paroles were granted and, during the third parole, while being supervised by the psychologist, the offender sexually assaulted a female niece in a garden shed. When asked to provide her account of his behaviours, the psychologist denied that any such incident had occurred and alleged that the victim had been flirting with the offender and enticed him to the shed. After the offender's parole programme was suspended, the psychologist disclosed to her supervisor that she had become involved in a sexual relationship with this offender, enacted regularly within the consulting room in the prison. The psychologist resigned, stating that she had obtained a position in another location. An internal inquiry was initiated by the prison authorities.

An independent clinician was asked to consult in the case by the authorities with the agenda of formulating an analysis of both accountability and responsibility for events, advising as to what action should be taken against the psychologist and making recommendations about the future management of the offender's case. An initial meeting with prison authorities indicated quite clearly that their stance was one of wishing to punish the psychologist. The psychologist had remained indignant and rigid in her attitudes, unrelenting in her advocacy of the offender and convinced of his victimisation by the authorities. The case was complicated further by the interventions of the head psychologist, who maintained that her employee was the victim of the offender's manipulation and deviant choreography of the situation, arguing that she was emotionally vulnerable and that the offender had taken advantage of her personal weaknesses.

A number of investigatory interviews were undertaken with the psychologist, the offender and the supervising psychologist. The interviews with the psychologist revealed that the relationship had developed as she had become convinced that the offender was wrongfully convicted and a victim of a conspiracy by the state and police. She had sight of all documentation, including crime scene and autopsy reports, and photographs, and she remarked, 'I know he didn't do it, so the crime doesn't bother me.' These beliefs had emerged during clinical sessions, the psychologist claiming that she had become indignant and angry about the offender's mistreatment and had decided, of her own volition, to become an advocate of his innocence and pursue his rightful release. She embarked on a crusading mission to 'clear his name and get him out'. As she assumed this role, the therapist–offender relationship became emotionally close, and sexual intimacy began within the prison establishment. The psychologist was asked to reflect upon the possible influences upon the developing professional–client relationship and the source of her intense, rigid and unfaltering perceptions of the offender. The psychologist did not perceive herself to be the object of any deviant RRPs or collusive inducement, declaring that the offender was 'the real victim in all of this'. The projective identification between professional and offender was not acknowledged by the psychologist (her inducement into a protective role toward the victimised offender). She argued that she was protecting the offender, and she denied that her professional ethics or conduct had become contaminated or compromised. She portrayed the offender as a 'patsy victim' and subject of a conspiracy by the state.

A review of all case material and interviews with the offender was undertaken. The offender presented as bemused by events, refusing to discuss the relationship with the psychologist and maintaining his secrecy about the matter. He denied any form of manipulation and focused upon the fact that he had been wrongfully accused of sexual misconduct on parole, arguing, 'I've been set up – I'm the vulnerable one here.' The psychologist and offender continued their relationship through prison visits and stated that they intended to live together on his release from prison. He allegedly told prison officers that he enjoyed the additional notoriety that he gained from the circumstances and liked the fact that 'there's a woman in there fighting for me, fighting my cause'.

A CAT reformulation was devised to decipher the RRPs within the case. The SDR is shown in Fig. 13.1. The matrix of professionals' perspectives is readily observed, portraying the differing collusions between parties. The 'crusading lover' position assumed by the psychologist in relation to the offender obscured objectivity and professional conduct. Her transference responses were indicative of a particular type of intense and fervent transference. She perceived the offender as a 'patsy victim' who was innocent and conspired against (victim state 2). The offender argued that he was the innocent victim of the girls who had enticed him into a vulnerable position while on parole (an enactment of the *manipulating/abusing-to-manipulated/exploited* RRP of victim state 1). The head psychologist viewed the psychologist as the 'duped victim' of the offender, given his history of relationships and ability to divide opinion between professional groups. The authorities wished to punish the psychologist for her misdemeanours, the head psychologist in contrast acting protectively (*protecting-to-wronged/rescued* RRP).

Walsh (1995) described the use of CAT within organisational contexts as a method of extrapolating the RRPs of different groups or parties and notating their interactions. The SDR permits the identification of intrapsychic, interpersonal and organisational responses and positions and articulation of each viewpoint. The varied and contrasting perceptions of the protagonists in these organisational scenarios can be defined through the diagrammatic reformulation. The location (at differing positions) of the '*victimised*' RP is interesting, as are the reciprocal roles enacted in response, particularly the offender being identified as a victim by the psychologist and the psychologist being assigned as a victim by her supervisor. The position of

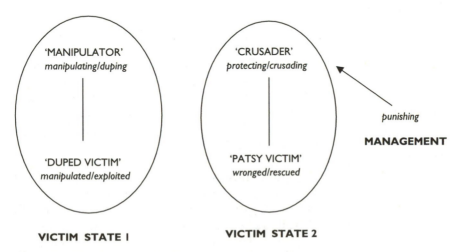

Figure 13.1 Case 1 – sequential diagrammatic reformulation.

the child victim of the original crime itself is omitted within the entangled relationships.

The offender had psychologically manoeuvred his position from perpetrator to victim, convincing the psychologist that he was innocent and maligned and that he was the target of enticing, entrapping females when on parole. The prison authorities were adamant about their desire to punish both offender and psychologist. The head psychologist's stance was disregarded and could not be sustained because of the psychologist's vociferous campaign on the offender's behalf, the supervisor being unable to argue simply that the psychologist was 'in denial' or 'smitten' by the offender's influence. She did state in defence of her employee, 'It would be unfair to punish her because you can't punish a victim, whether she's in love or not.' The psychologist's persistent crusading was viewed as 'admirable' by a prison-visiting fellowship, reinforcing the psychologist's endeavours.

Finally, a conference to decide upon a course of action with the authorities (the psychologist and the offender were excluded) used the SDR as a tool to reflect upon and understand the positions and roles of each party in the scenario. Responses varied on the management side, some articulating that they could perceive the psychologist to have become entrapped by the offender, and others claiming that her aggressive crusading was proof of poor reality testing. In view of the offender's past history of dividing the opinion of professionals, no further action was taken against the psychologist, given that she had resigned from her employment. The designation as a 'victim' in this case was difficult for management to decipher, and the decision was made not to punish the psychologist as the head psychologist prompted other professionals to perceive the psychologist as self-deceiving and manipulated.

Case vignette 2

A psychiatric trainee was offered supervision while working individually with a 23-year-old psychopathic sexual offender held in a secure hospital for the attempted rape of a 4-year-old girl in a park. He was a masculine, attractive, confident and somewhat arrogant person, who expressed his view that other mentally ill patients on the hospital ward were unworthy of his attention or friendship. He was visited by several women, and it was particularly noted that his female social worker from a previous hospital attended regularly and that they exchanged sexual intimacies during visits, despite close supervision. The trainee had commenced supportive counselling with the offender without any proper training in psychotherapy apart from 'reading books'. She had sought supervision because of difficulties which the consultant psychiatrist felt had become apparent in terms of the trainee's ability to cope with the therapeutic contact. The trainee entered supervision sessions displaying a timid, reticent and almost shameful demeanour. A psychological formulation had not been developed for the case, and the trainee expressed her feeling that she was unable to cope with the intense emotional reactions she experienced as a consequence of the sessions. A number of supervision sessions were devoted to deciphering the transference and counter-transference reactions and RRPs which had emerged between professional and offender.

The trainee's account of the developing therapeutic relationship was concerning, and she presented this information with tones of guilt, shame and anxiety. Her initial response to being asked to undertake work with this offender combined excitement, anxiety and being pleased that her supervising consultant felt she was competent enough to manage this type of case. From the first session, the trainee recalled that the offender 'was an Adonis, really attractive. He had piercing blue eyes, like he could see right through me. I remember feeling flustered and shy, a bit coy.' The offender complimented her on her 'looks', telling her she was the most attractive trainee he had ever met. A positive, eroticised transference developed in these early stages with mutual physical attraction apparent. The fact that the trainee's remit was unstructured and without psychological conceptualisation encouraged the development of transference RRPs without any understanding of their potential emergence.

The trainee reported that she looked forward to sessions with the offender and thought of him as her 'most prized patient' compared with the mentally ill offenders on her caseload (an early instance of identifying counter-transference in terms of her devaluing of the other patients). The sessions usually lasted for over 2 hours, and the trainee did not establish any therapeutic boundaries or frame, or impose any parameters on the sessions. She began to wear more revealing clothing to work on the days when sessions were to occur and acknowledged that the offender excited her and provoked fantasies of 'forbidden encounters'. The discussions between the parties quickly became sexualised.

The topic of the offender's sexual interests became part of the content of their discussions within three sessions, and the trainee felt this was appropriate given that the offender had committed sexual crimes. She offered that they discussed his past sexual history and she was amazed to discover that he was 'a virgin. He'd been caught when he was eighteen. I'd never thought of that, he was so sexually confident.' The offender appeared to have capitalised on this opportunity to talk about sexual matters and did so freely, wanting to discuss his fantasies with the trainee. She entered these discussions without rationale or consideration of the possible reasons for this request, the offender commenting that she might be able to help him modify his fantasies to more 'romantic and normal fantasies'. At the fourth session, the trainee claimed that the interactions in therapy had become blatantly sexualised with regard to their interactions and topics of discussion, the trainee providing personal details of her own sexual interests at the request of the offender. The transference had gathered momentum rapidly during these sessions and the trainee had sought discussion about the case with her consultant after the offender suggested that it would help him if he could masturbate in her presence in the consulting room as a method of modifying his repertoire of fantasies. The trainee agreed to participate in this type of incident and agreed to wear sexually enticing clothes for the scheduled session. The offender had masturbated until climax on four separate occasions until the trainee divulged these incidents to her supervising consultant. Therapy was terminated by the consultant prior to supervision being initiated.

In supervision, the trainee expressed her anxiety about failing her internship placement and spoke about the consultant's anger toward her – he called her 'a stupid little girl'. She felt humiliated and disgusted by her actions. The supervisor wondered about the transference and counter-transference RRPs which had transpired between the trainee and offender and requested that exploration of these issues be undertaken through a lens of curiosity and learning rather than a damning inquiry. It was felt necessary to acknowledge that the trainee had become embroiled in a pattern of reciprocal interaction that should best be used as a learning experience to encourage and nurture her professional development. The trainee's 'zone of proximal development' (ZPD) represents the area of learning in supervision (similarly for our patients) where self-development can be achieved. As stated by Thomas-Peter & Garrett (2000; p. 147), 'clinical supervision is a prerequisite for individual therapy. Supervisors should be unafraid of specifically raising matters of sexual feelings in order to alert those they are supervising to this danger.' It was felt that the CAT model of transference and counter-transference might be helpful to make sense of these interactions.

The trainee was encouraged to trace the transference and counter-transference she experienced when working with this offender. She acknowledged that her initial responses included feeling mesmerised, in awe and wonderment at the offender's physical attractiveness and his dangerousness. She had read his case file and knew about his crimes, expecting him to be 'a slimy, creepy, inadequate sex offender'. Her devaluation as anticipated was not borne out by the offender's presentation and she felt she began to idealise him immediately. The fact that offender and trainee were of a similar age appeared to improve their attachment. She recalled feeling that his interest in her was complimentary and beguiling to her.

The trainee reflected that her life at that time was lonely, as she was isolated from friends and living away from her family in a different part of the country. She had not been part of an adult relationship for some time, and her contact with the offender was the only source of positive reward. She was encouraged to think about the unexpected idealisation of the offender, given her anticipated reactions when reading the case file. She was helped to reflect upon how her perceptions of the offender had become idealised and the excitement she felt was part of the forbidden attraction of the scenario. The offender's obvious interest in her and his compliments appeared to fill a much-needed emptiness in her life. She recalled, 'I felt tingles, excitement – we seemed to click together.' The RRPs were identified through exploration of her own responses, the offender's behaviours toward her and within sessions, and the dyadic exchanges that materialised. The trainee felt the underlying RRPs could best be summarised as, on the explicit level, *appeasing/idealising (accepted)-to-approved of/wanted*, but, on the implicit level, as *exploited/used-to-exploiting/controlling*. The supervisor explored how the offender had manoeuvred the discussions onto sexual matters, how she had colluded with his wish to talk about these matters, and the reasons for wearing certain clothes and the fantasies behind these actions on her part.

The trainee disclosed during supervision that she felt that she was provoked to comply with the offender's requests because of her own history and repertoire of relating. Further exploration about these *personal* counter-transference insights revealed that the trainee had been brought up in a stoic, religious family in which sexual topics were forbidden and never discussed openly. Her father was a strict, disciplined man who wished his daughters to be 'ladies', and he would berate them if they acted inappropriately. The trainee declared that the supervising consultant's expressions of anger toward her had re-enacted this RRP from her past, causing her to feel humiliated and 'downtrodden, like a dumb child who was being ticked off'. Her past relationships with boyfriends had proven difficult to sustain because, 'me being a prude, I couldn't let them touch me or I felt dirty, as if sex was wrong, not allowed. I wouldn't be a lady then.' Her behaviours within relationships tended to be placating, subjugated and devoted, willing to please and 'like a lapdog, following, but always saying no to sex'. She felt that the interactions with the offender had become complicated by the fact that he was a sexual offender and she felt 'sex was in the room'. The decision to wear certain clothing was prompted by her desire to please the offender and to sustain his interest in her, in the hope that they might become romantically involved, yet also in anticipation of a forbidden encounter in the therapy room. The perversion of the therapeutic relationship and the contributions of the trainee's RRPs had resulted in the offender's manipulating the interactions into an exploiting, abusive and denigratory experience for the trainee, who felt that her position was one of compliance in an attempt to help the offender, a need to be approved of and accepted, and, on reflection, the enactment of a distorted transference which permitted the offender to achieve gratification at the trainee's expense. The collusive elements of the interacting RRPs were identified, and the trainee was asked to consider the reciprocal 'fit' between her own and the offender's RRPs and how the reciprocal 'pull' of their interactions compromised both the trainee and the therapy.

Discussion took place in a three-way meeting with the supervising consultant to decide the future of therapeutic work and to explain the potent RRPs which had subsumed the problems which had arisen. The trainee was withdrawn from the therapy process on this occasion, although it could be argued that her re-entrance into the relationship might have benefited both trainee and offender if CAT reformulation had been used to modify the offender's repertoire of relating and sexual deviance.

Commentary

The two illustrative cases do not encompass the full range of procedural exchanges and repertoires which are typically seen in forensic practice. Hatred of the offender is a common response felt by the therapist (Prodgers, 1991). Who is exploited and who is vulnerable in forensic work is very much dependent upon the contribution of each participant in the dyad and the relational chemistry that develops. Similarly, within therapy generally, the role of the offender can be distorted and misplaced. CAT's relational focus allows the therapist who feels drawn into compromising exchanges with patients to ponder and deliberate the unfolding RRPs and to act without collusion. Conceptualising the offender-to-therapist's unique combination of RRPs facilitates decision making and measured, advised choice about managing the dyadic relationship in the patient's best interests.

References

Apfel, R. J. & Bennett, S. (1985). Patient–therapist sexual contact. II. Problems of subsequent psychotherapy. *Psychotherapy and Psychosomatics, 43*, 63–68.

Averill, S., Beale, D., Benfer, B. & Collins, D. T. (1989). Preventing staff–patient sexual relationships. *Bulletin of the Menninger Clinic, 53*, 384–393.

Butler, S. & Zelen, S. L. (1977). Sexual intimacies between therapists and patients. *Psychotherapy: Theory, Research and Practice, 14*, 139–145.

Campling, P. (1996). Maintaining the therapeutic alliance with personality-disordered patients. *Journal of Forensic Psychiatry, 7*, 535–550.

Carr, M. & Robinson, G. E. (1990). Fatal attraction: The ethical and clinical dilemma of patient–therapist sex. *Canadian Journal of Psychiatry, 35*, 122–127.

Chessick, R. D. (1989). In the clutches of the devil. *Psychoanalysis and Psychotherapy, 7*, 142–151.

Ciardello, J. A. (1996). Therapist–patient sexual contact. *Psychoanalytic Review, 83*, 761–775.

Garfinkel, P. E., Dorian, B. & Sadavoy, J. (1997a). Boundary violations and departments of psychiatry. *Canadian Journal of Psychiatry, 42*, 764–770.

Garfinkel, P. E., Bagby, M. & Waring, E. M. (1997b) Boundary violations and personality traits among psychiatrists. *Canadian Journal of Psychiatry, 42*, 758–763.

Grant, V. W. (1978). *The menacing stranger: A primer on the psychopath.* Oxford: Open University Press.

Gutheil, T. G. & Simon, R. I. (1995). Between the chair and the door: Boundary issues in the therapeutic 'transition zone'. *Harvard Review of Psychiatry, 2*, 336–340.

Kardener, S. H., Fuller, F. & Mensh, I. N. (1976). Characteristics of 'erotic' practitioners. *American Journal of Psychiatry, 133*, 1324–1325.

Kiesler, D. G. (1988). *Therapeutic metacommunication: Therapist impact disclosure feedback in psychotherapy*. Palo Alto, CA: Consulting Psychologists Press.

Kroll, J. (2001). Boundary violations: a culture-bound syndrome. *Journal of American Academic Psychiatry Law, 29*, 274–283.

Meloy, J. R. (1988). The psychopath as love object. In J. R. Meloy, *The psychopathic mind: Origins, dynamics and treatment*. Northvale, NJ: Jason Aronson.

Norris, D., Gutheil, T. G. & Strasburger, L. H. (2003). This couldn't happen to me: Boundary problems and sexual misconduct in the psychotherapy relationship. *Psychiatric Services, 54*, 517–522.

Pope, K. S. (1991). Dual relationships in psychotherapy. *Ethics and Behavior, 1*, 21–34.

Prodgers, A. (1991). On hating the patient. *British Journal of Psychotherapy, 8*, 144–154.

Racker, H. (1962). Transference and countertransference. New York: International Universities Press.

Ryle, A. (1997). Transferences and countertransferences: A CAT perspective. *British Journal of Psychotherapy, 14*, 303–309.

Simon, R. I. (1998). Boundary violations in psychotherapy: From gray areas to malpractice. In L. E. Lifson & R. I. Simon (Eds), *The mental health practitioner and the law: A comprehensive handbook*. Cambridge, MA: Harvard University Press.

Strasburger, L. H. (2001). The treatment of antisocial syndromes: The therapist's feelings. In R. J. Meloy (Ed.) *The mark of Cain: Psychoanalytic insights and the psychopath*. Hillside, NJ: Analytic Press.

Thomas-Peter, B. & Garrett, J. (2000). Preventing sexual contact between professionals and patients in forensic environments. *Journal of Forensic Psychiatry, 11*, 135–150.

Walsh, S. (1996). Adapting cognitive analytic therapy to make sense of psychologically harmful work environments. *British Journal of Medical Psychology, 69*, 3–20.

Wegman, R. J. & Lane, R. C. (2001). Therapist–patient sexual contact: Some dynamic considerations regarding etiology and prevention. *Journal of Psychotherapy in Independent Practice, 2*, 73–90.

Chapter 14

Cognitive Analytic Therapy analysis of the errant self and serial sexual homicide

An encounter with the extremes of human conduct

Philip H. Pollock

Those who commit serial homicides can attain iconic status in societies, capturing the imagination of the public and media, almost reifying the stealthy, predatory and rapacious archetype. Watching the cinematic portrayal of the human predator is fascinating and titillating, knowing such a criminal is loose in one's community is frightening and direct contact with the serial sexual homicide perpetrator is disarming. The closer we get, the more that grotesque realism substitutes for theatrical licence. The predatory, repetitive killing of other human beings for psychological reasons implies a psychopathological state of mind or abnormal personality (Gacono & Meloy, 1994; Meloy, Gacono & Kenney, 1994; Pollock, 1995). The 'apparent craziness' of these types of crimes (Geberth & Turco, 1999; p. 51) is an immediate perception, given the 'senseless' way that the offender acts toward others (Shrapec, 2001; p. 47). Excluding psychotic illnesses as explanation, we are stretched to project our understanding into the mind of the serial killer (Fox & Levin, 2000). To gain insight into the serial killer's actions, we must enter a perverse and distorted personal universe, a journey which can be warping and traumatising.

For most of us, dedicating time and energy to carrying out a macabre and dehumanising fantasy which entails the killing of an innocent victim is an incredulous deed. The serial killer's predation reflects a motivated and formulated plan of action. In anyone's conception, serial killing is an extraordinary behaviour that distends the observer's imagination to comprehend the driven part of the offender's personality that spawns these actions against humanity. Shrapec (2001; p. 50) cogently remarked, 'serial murder tends to be analysed as an objective event, not as a subjective experience' and 'to understand serial murder we must go beyond mere description of the offender, the crimes and their victims' (p. 48). Dietz (1986; p. 487) asserted, 'even mental health professionals have great difficulty accepting the possibility that certain individuals enjoy killing people'. The facets of these behaviours, such as premeditated fantasy, conscious design, investment of energy, organisation and the requirements of 'careful execution' (Dietz, 1986), are indicative of a determined enterprise on the part of the offender. Society's desire to ensnare and capture these offenders is glamorised and depicted in dramatic terms such as 'hunting down' these predators (Ressler, Burgess & Douglas, 1990; Godwin, 2000); such language testifies to the collective anxieties they inflame. Many myths and much folklore have developed around the subject of serial homicide, and our heightened awareness has caused some theorists to speculate on whether or not this crime is increasing within society (Schlesinger, 2001).

The killing act and criminal investigations

Understanding the phenomenological world of serial killers requires us to make inferences about their internal, subjective dynamics, derived from behaviour during the crimes. Investigative psychology (Canter, 1994; Salfati & Canter, 1999; Salfati, 2000a & b), as a specialist strand of forensic work, has advanced our knowledge of the actions of these killers, and a variety of classification systems and models have been developed to aid law enforcement and mental health professionals. Ressler *et al.*'s (1990) study of 36 sexual killers and the emergence of criminal profiling initiated a flurry of interest in investigating and devising systems to facilitate the apprehension of these offenders. Several typologies, classification systems and models have been developed for the sexual and serial killer. Keppel & Walter (1999) applied the power-assertive, power-retaliation, anger-retaliation and anger-excitation model of rape to sexual killings, suggesting that differing attributes and characteristics are associated with each type of killing. Arrigo & Purcell (2001) provided an integrative model of 'lust murder', defining sexual killings. Kocsis, Cooksey & Irwin (2002) report the use of multidimensional scaling techniques applied to 84 cases in Australia, defining four themes and patterns termed, respectively, fury, predatory, perversion and rape. Beauregard & Proulx (2002) report an analysis of 36 sexual killers, deciphering distinctive 'pathways', called the anger and sadistic pathways. Salfati & Canter (1999) used the instrumental/expressive violence distinction to examine stranger murders. Geographical profiling (Rossmo, 2000) has been developed to permit a different type of analysis of the killer's behaviours. These models aim to facilitate an understanding of serial homicide and assist the investigative process for law enforcement services tasked to apprehend the serial killer, and are, essentially, focused at the level of the actions and behaviours of the offender (Turvey, 1999).

Motivations and internal dynamics

Other theories and models have been proposed which concentrate on the offender's alleged motivations (e.g. Holmes & DeBurger's (1988) typology of visionary, missionary, hedonistic and power-control types) and psychiatric diagnoses. Ressler *et al.* (1990) validated the original motivational model of Burgess, Hartman, Ressler, Douglas & MacCormack (1986), which attempted to explain the functioning of the offender and the crimes through the organised/disorganised distinction, a model which has proved controversial (Godwin, 2000). Hickey (1991) described the trauma-control model of multiple killers and a classification system based on the extent of the serial killer's mobility (place-specific, local and travelling). Castle & Hensley (2002) and Wright & Hensley (2003) proposed a social learning theory model of serial murder. Giannangelo (1996) provided a comprehensive model of serial homicide that accounts for the internal and external processes observable. It is important that the neurobiological evidence is not ignored when speculating about the reasons for extreme, repetitive violence (Lang & DeWitt, 1990; Raine, Buchsbaum, Stanley & Lottenberg, 1994). As asserted by Mitchell (1997), no single explanation can account for this type of violent action.

These models are created for the specific purpose of the criminal investigation of serial homicide and assisting law enforcement. When faced with the serial killer, either within the criminal justice system or during imprisonment and detention, the clinician must look to differing sources and theories for insights into the psychological functioning of the offender.

The psychopathology of sexual homicide

Our knowledge of the link between the functioning of the personality and homicide, sexual homicide and serial homicide has improved greatly over the past years. Liebert (1985) speculated that borderline and narcissistic disorder lies at the centre of the personalities of serial killers. Pollock (1995) and Geberth & Turco (1999) offer that Kernberg's (1995) concept of malignant narcissism, a form of antisocial personality disorder, is present in some serial killers with evidence of pathological grandiosity, overt antisocial behaviours, derivation of pleasure from sadistic or ego-syntonic aggression, and paranoid tendencies. Pathological narcissism is fused with a lack of attachment or concern for others, an absence of conscience, and a failure of object integration and associated stimulus hunger. Holt, Strack & Meloy (1999) argue that sexual sadism and psychopathy are entwined in the pathology of these offenders.

Gacono & Meloy (1994) report the Rorschach study of 20 sexual killers, identifying a range of pathological indicators and offering a tentative theory that these types of crimes are driven by an abnormal personality structure featuring a narcissistic, pathological entitlement and grandiosity, interpersonal detachment, a 'hungry' mode of relating, borderline or psychotic reality testing, formal thought disorder, chronic anger and deviant sexual arousal patterns associated with sadistic fantasies and preferences. Projective identification of this pathology is evident in terms of the offender's targeting and choice of victim, his perceptions about what the victim represents to him symbolically, and how the offender relates to the victim during and after the killing. Idiosyncratic acts of violence and relating to victims during premeditated homicides have been interpreted to reflect the internal world of the offender (dismemberment, rearrangement of body parts, destruction to the body, manner in which it is disposed, etc.). For example, Weinshel & Calet (1972) speculated that acts such as mutilation suggest a desire to re-enter and explore the mother in psychodynamic terms. The way that a killing is conducted may be considered to hold significant implicit meaning and symbolic value for the offender, and it is only on a unique case basis that the crime can be understood from a subjective perspective.

Gacono (1990) found the sexual psychopath's violence to 'serve as an intrapsychic regulatory function helping to restore narcissistic equilibrium and stabilise affect' (p. 217), in agreement with Liebert's suggestion that sexually violent impulses restore the offender for a period of time (similar to the relief encountered during catathymic crisis; Wertham, 1937), only to be repeated when dysphoria and dissatisfaction re-emerge, requiring solution through additional killings.

The crucial function of fantasy in the mental lives of homicide perpetrators and other criminals has been described within many psychological models (MacCullough, Snowden, Wood & Mills, 1983; Prentky, Burgess, Rokous, Lee, Hartman, Ressler & Douglas, 1989). Fantasy serves a compensatory, survival function for sexual offenders and permits the rehearsal and conditioning of the deviant actions, often through compulsive masturbation. As Gacono & Meloy (1994) succinctly described, the offender's isolative fantasies surrounding imagined objects are translated into 'violent forays' against external objects in the real world. Chronic detachment, and feelings of being alone and empty are typical fantasies generated as the gratuitous, introspective vehicles and catalysts for sexual violence.

The offender's idiosyncratic method of committing the crime is often a reflection of elaborate, much nourished fantasies creating a 'death tableau' (Biven, 1997). The elements of the death tableau expressed in the crime must be 'decoded', Biven arguing that serial killers develop fantasy-driven, action-oriented disorders, the offence representing the acting out of the core fantasy that has evolved. The uniqueness of the crime reflects the 'aggregate of meaningful things and themes, a collage, an amalgam, grotesque parody in the offence, the desire to freeze their perverse murderous creation' (p. 47). As proposed by Segal (1985), our conscious and more implicitly omnipotent fantasies influence many aspects of our everyday lives, yet incubation of aggressive fantasies and their execution signals a qualitative difference in human capacities.

The psychiatric diagnoses observed within homicide as a crime vary considerably, and no homogeneous disorder has been noted (Yarvis, 1990). The role of psychopathic personality disorder and its association with sexual sadism or 'characterological sadism' (Kernberg, 1995) are obvious deductions, and the analyses of serial sexual homicides does testify to the strength

of this connection (Lowenstein, 1992). The majority of serial homicide perpetrators are not found to be suffering from psychosis or severe mental illness, and the link between the personality and the homicides should be considered when attempting to understand the subjective world of the serial
killer and the acts of homicide and their meaning.

The errant self in serial homicide

It is well documented that serial homicide offenders, despite the gravity and
perversity of their actions, are observed to present without distinctive peculi-
arities. Carlisle (1993) claimed that many serial killers operate in a dual existence, compelled to live a dissociated psychological existence with separate
selves, one self compulsively homicidal. Carlisle cites the process of dissociation in response to trauma to generate this split, Jungian shadow-like, dual
mentality, the offender killing episodically, yet returning to equilibrium and
'normality' until sexually aggressive or homicidal impulses resurface. Carlisle
referred to the killer's experiences of 'oppositional motivational forces'
(p. 28) while living a dual psychological existence. The process of dissociation
is used to explain the apparent divided experience of the self and its contradictory features. This is similar to Hickey's trauma-control model in that a
dissociated, violent part of the self develops, hidden by the façade of normality within other aspects of the offender's lifestyle. This apparent 'healthy' side
of the personality veils the concealed, secretive, errant violent conduct which
emerges episodically.

Few people who know the serial offender note any markers that would
indicate that this individual has extremely violent tendencies. Canter (1994)
eloquently remarked of serial killers that 'they have much more about them
that is normal, everyday, than is not' (p. 220). These ideas are reminiscent of
the distinction between the development of the true and false selves which
function to maintain a sense of self (Shrapec, 2001). Whether this is an
accurate formulation of the secrecy, stealth and shadow self of the serial
killer is debatable. Goldberg (2000) offers cases which describe what he
termed the 'errant self', a compulsive, often destructive and driving part of
the personality that overwhelms the individual's inhibitions and is expressed
through wayward and unruly actions, often with damaging effects for both
the person and others. The compulsive nature of the serial killer's repetitive
and maverick behaviours has been noted to be suggestive of an addictive
process or obsessive compulsive disorder (Lowenstein, 1992).

In her case analyses of a number of serial killers, McKenzie (1995) noted,
within the constellation of factors, that 'although many serial murderers
have had relationships of long duration, they appear to have a hidden or
compartmentalized self that thwarts all attempts to find satisfaction. The
distinction between reality and daydreaming is blurred in an intoxicated state
and the individual finally puts into action what he believes will make him

"happy" only to discover it is short-lived' (p. 8). And so the killings continue, the first killing an experiment in the enactment of fantasy, the second encouraging the offender to refine his predatory projects, the following homicides fuelling his taste in an addictive process, or becoming a ego-syntonic, compulsive, unwanted necessity, escalating to recklessness.

A case is presented of a serial sexual homicide perpetrator who requested psychotherapy after 11 years of detention in a maximum-security hospital for mentally disordered offenders. Case studies of serial killers proliferate in the literature, yet there is an absence of descriptions of the psychotherapy for such an offender. This case is tendered as a rare and unusual therapy in which Cognitive Analytic Therapy (CAT) was chosen to reformulate the offender's disorder and as the method of treatment. In the UK, serial sexual killers are provided with psychotherapy like other offenders, and the following case illustrates the reality of engaging such a killer in individual forensic psychotherapy.

Robert's clinical presentation

Robert requested to be assessed after 11 years of detention. He was a well-dressed, composed and articulate man who had been found to be of superior intellectual abilities. He was well read in literature and enjoyed discussing philosophy and abstract topics with anyone he could engage in conversation. There was no objective evidence of anxiety or agitation, Robert showing arousal only when talking about subjects that interested him or his offences. His behaviour was appropriate on the hospital ward, and he was selective about his companions, preferring to spend time with nursing staff rather than other patients. Nursing staff declared that they found Robert to be polite, courteous and compliant, showing no indications of aggression or questionable conduct. Robert had been assessed to be personality disordered rather than mentally ill at his criminal trial. Formal psychological testing had revealed no abnormality of particular note. Despite these observations, Robert's crimes were considered to be perverse and deviant in the extreme. It was felt by all professionals involved that Robert's veneer of normality belied a sinister personality capable of hidden destructiveness.

On occasion, Robert was noted to be irritable and intolerant of other patients, and he lived a disengaged existence studying for a doctorate in social sciences. Robert was permitted escorted paroles from the hospital into the local community and had not posed any management problems.

Initial sessions with Robert found him to be a plausible, genteel patient and very interested in what therapy might provide for him. He expressed his curiosity about the therapy process and wanted to know more about the 'experience' of therapy. Robert had never entered therapy for any problems in the past and expressed his wish to engage in therapy 'to see what comes up. We might be able to sort this stuff out.' He was perceived to be emotionally controlled and modulated in his presentation.

Robert knew that he was entitled to therapeutic intervention and strongly stated his wish to avail himself of such programmes. He was offered 24 sessions of individual CAT as part of his rehabilitation plan. Robert was cognisant of the fact that the risk element of his sentence was problematic for him, given the seriousness of the crimes, the public notoriety of the case and the responsibility of the reviewing body who would appraise his progress. Robert argued that he was entitled to therapy and that he should be judged on his participation. The gravity of the offences in terms of the depth and perversity of the pathology involved, the nature of the killings and the likelihood that Robert would never be released into the community were relevant factors when initiating therapeutic work with him. When the referral was made for psychotherapy, the potential risks of engaging in such a therapy process and its benefits for Robert were debated, given the fact that his risk potential would be evaluated by a commission when the deterrent component of his sentence was expired. However, Robert was entitled to receive therapy, and the review body which would oversee his case and assess the risk potential he presented expected psychological therapy and prison programmes to be offered to address Robert's risk, as for any other prisoner.

Robert's history

Robert's personal history was self-reported as follows. He was the first-born child of working-class parents; he had a younger brother. His grandparents lived close by and there was no family history of social or psychiatric problems. Robert's mother and father had marital problems because of his father's 'womanising', which appears from records to have occurred repeatedly. At the age of 8, Robert found his mother hanging in the family home when he returned from school one morning because he had forgotten school textbooks. It was thought that the discovery of another of his father's extramarital affairs had prompted her suicide. Robert recalled being 'mesmerized. I stood and looked and looked and looked at her, she was sort of grotesque. My mother was a glamorous woman, always looking her best and keeping up with the Jones. I sat for a long time, cross-legged on the floor, just staring. Then I eventually went to my grandpa's house and told him.' This formative event changed Robert's life dramatically in a negative direction. He was placed into care because of his father's 'nervous breakdown' and the family unit fragmented. Robert's father did not maintain regular contact and the relationship disintegrated. His brother was placed in a different children's home and contact with him was lost also.

Life in the children's home was difficult and abrasive for Robert. Social Services records show that Robert was well known as a bullying, aggressive ringleader in the children's home, one report describing him as 'a bright child, probably much more intelligent than his peers who he sees as below him in every direction. Rob can be charming, deceptive, beguiling and every-one's friend, yet below this is another side to his personality that we know has come out to terrorise his peers. I refer to claims by frightened children who say that Rob has intimidated, threatened and harmed them in all man-ner of ways. . . . Rob is worrying in the way he adeptly operates and manipu-lates his environment to get his own way . . . he was confronted by the staff to no effect. He is seen as either a precociously talented child or a bully. We wonder about when he will enter politics or the paramilitaries.' Concerns were documented about Robert's early, perhaps unhealthy, age-inappropriate interest in sexual matters, the staff querying whether he had been sexually abused.

Three incidents from the ages of 10 to 15 are worthy of note. At 10, Robert was involved in a riot within the children's home, instigating the gang rape of a male resident, who was taken hostage for several hours. Robert denied any direct action during this alleged offence. Secondly, Robert was accused of the attempted abduction of a 12-year-old girl with a group of youths, the inten-tion being to rape the victim. Once again, his involvement could not be proven. Thirdly, he was accused of the abduction at knifepoint of an 8-year-old boy, the victim being threatened, gagged, tied to a fence in a field, sexually assaulted, and left naked and restrained. Robert was not convicted for any of these alleged crimes. At interview, Robert refused to discuss his experiences within the family home and would disengage if this subject was discussed. A reference and subsequent referral for therapy were documented in Robert's Social Services case file whereby he did disclose that he had been sexually abused when aged 7 by a male adolescent neighbour in a local wood. This referral was not initiated, and no further mention is made of this event in the file.

Robert's later years of schooling saw a dramatic change in his behaviours. He exhibited strong academic abilities throughout his schooling and was capable of concentrated study. He showed talent for drama and sports and was voted by fellow students into positions of authority and leadership. Des-pite a record of sporadic instances of worrying violence and intimidation, Robert was considered an 'achiever of some promise'. He was perceived as intellectually able, resourceful and self-directed with ambition and goals for his future. On testing when arrested, Robert showed superior intellectual abilities.

On leaving school and statutory care, Robert's first job was installing 'gaming machines', an entrepreneurial enterprise of his own initiative. He claims that he always considered this occupation as a 'sideline', and he gained management and business qualifications that permitted entry into a leading management consultancy. After a few years, he had forged alliances with many in the upper echelons of the organisation and was perceived as a 'rising star' in the company. No criminal activities were recorded from the age of 16 until his arrest for multiple homicides. Robert appeared to have lived a productive life for many years, marrying and having children, and holding down a lucrative and responsible position as his career blossomed.

At the age of 25, Robert married Donna, who worshipped him. Family life was described by Donna as 'just normal. Rob went to work, came home, did his own things most of the time, but everything was great.' Certain problems did arise after 2 years of marriage when Donna found gay pornographic magazines in Robert's briefcase. This was resolved through Robert's explanation to Donna that he was 'minding' these magazines for a work colleague. On another occasion, Donna had questioned him about his periodic absences for days on end without explanation, but Robert was able to assuage her concern and suspicion by stating that his work required secrecy and she would have to tolerate these absences without being informed or 'kept in the loop'. When his wife announced her first pregnancy, he recalled, 'I was angry, panicked, but I also thought that this was a chance for me to prove to myself that I could fix a lot from my own past.' Robert stated that the birth of his daughter was 'an amazing, life-changing moment'. He involved himself with every aspect of parenting care and was considered to be a devoted father, continuing this dedication to his second child, a son. Between the times of his children's births, Robert had begun targeting victims through homosexual chatlines in magazines and preparing for the first killing. When aged 29, Robert had formulated his plan with organised precision and killed his first victim. Interview with Donna revealed that she was shocked by the accusations against her husband and did not believe that she was aware of or had ignored any indications of concerns. Robert was idealised in Donna's eyes, although she admitted that she knew little about his background, that they rarely had sexual relations after their son's birth, and that Robert, as the children grew up, had become distant with them and did not involve himself in their care. Donna noticed how strained and challenging Robert found fatherhood, and shielded him from extended contact with the children or caring responsibilities. The apparent normality of Robert's lifestyle was remarkable.

Interestingly, medical records showed a distinctive pattern of physical complaints. Robert presented with a variety of unspecified ailments on eight occasions from the age of 26 until his arrest. He reported varied physical and psychological symptoms such as lethargy, fibromyalgia-like pain, low mood, poor motivation, disturbed sleep and loss of pleasure and interest. He was diagnosed as having viral fatigue, and Robert spent 2–3 months off work until he recovered. A mental health referral was never made. At no time did Robert report to his medical practitioner any history of substance misuse or dependency. He did not drink alcohol habitually. These episodes of malaise were the only notable signs of problems in Robert's functioning.

Psychological analysis of the offences: Robert's serial killings

Robert was convicted of three killings over a period of 10 years. His fourth attempted homicide was incomplete and resulted in his capture. His first victim was a 10-year-old boy, who was abducted in a local street, gagged, tied, raped anally, strangled and mutilated post-mortem. The second victim was an 11-year-old boy, who was enticed by Robert to follow him to a glade in a wood (under the pretence that Robert knew his father), bludgeoned with a stick, gagged, sexually assaulted, strangled and mutilated post-mortem. The third victim was a 10-year-old 'rent boy', who suffered a similar fate, Robert abducting him and taking him to a secluded car park, where he bound, tortured and strangled him before sexual intercourse and mutilation. The fourth victim was an 11-year-old boy, who managed to struggle free from Robert's binding after a blitz-type attack, having been knocked unconscious with a hammer. Investigators had attempted to convict Robert of three additional offences of a similar nature, but there was insufficient evidence. By general consensus of definition (Egger, 1984; Busch & Cavanaugh, 1986), Robert was considered a serial killer.

As in the pattern described by Norris (1988), that is, seven key phases, namely, aura, trolling, wooing, capture, murder, totem and depression, Robert would withdraw from others and reality before the hunt, entrapment and murder of the victim, and then reimmerse himself in his family life and job between each killing until 'something started to build up again, a dissatisfaction. I'd think about how I hated myself. Memories from the past, clear memories, they'd like tap me on the shoulder and drift in and bother me, even when I was on the computer at work. It would distract and occupy me. I'd get lower and lower, then angry and all worked up, irritable with everyone and everything, the kids at home, my wife.'

One of the most significant disclosures from Robert was that, after he had killed, he would spend perhaps 2 hours watching the victim. 'Like in a serene garden, I had transformed the world. I had someone with me who felt the same, in the same state, together.' This act was secondary to the killing itself, but an important facet of the offence for Robert. Discussion of this with Robert revealed that he felt that he shared a 'deadness' with the victim, and the killing permitted him to experience a communicative reverie with the dead victim. Robert also commented that strangulation of the victim and the alternation of strangling and then reviving him was 'maybe like what happens in cartoons. You know, the way cartoon characters are squashed, like Wily Coyote, then he springs back to life – Tom and Jerry, like that. Nobody dies or gets killed.' Robert's reality testing was questioned on the basis of these comments, and psychological testing was administered to formulate his personality functioning and its relationship to the crimes.

After 11 years of detention, psychological testing indicated high scores on factor 1 (aggressive narcissism) on the PCL–R (Hare, 1991), with relatively low scores for factor 2 (antisocial lifestyle). The profiles observed suggested that Robert was an affectionless, detached and interpersonally manipulative personality. The MCMI–3 (Millon, Millon & Davis, 1994) produced a schizoid, narcissistic, sadistic and compulsive profile with no depression or anxiety. The Thematic Apperception Test (TAT) stories obtained were superficial in terms of the narratives gleaned. The content analysis of Robert's Rorschach protocol was rife with imagery suggestive of omnipotent creatures, gods and sinister characters who were engaged in sexual or violent degradation of weak, vulnerable, yet masochistically gratified others. His reality testing was somewhat compromised. Robert scored 24 on the Personality Structure Questionnaire (Pollock, Broadbent, Clarke, Dorrian & Ryle, 2001), indicating some identity disturbances. Robert declared that he felt that there were 'many sides' to his personality and that many people would know him differently. His scores on the Dissociation Questionnaire revealed identity fragmentation with no evidence of amnesia or loss of behavioural controls (Vanderlinden, Van Dyck, Vandereycken, Vertommen & van Verkes, 1993). The reported dissociation and identity disturbances alerted the clinician to the relevance of these experiences, yet little evidence of such phenomena was directly apparent in his history or presentation.

Robert's offences were analysed from two perspectives. Firstly, the therapist relied strongly upon the forensic evidence in the case and the retrospective construction of the crimes (the death tableau; Biven, 1997). Secondly, Robert's own subjective accounts of the offences were interwoven to flesh out the internal facets of his criminal acts. The forensic evidence indicated that Robert had selected four known victims, all male, between the ages of 10 and 11. He had commenced these crimes when aged 29, the crimes occurring approximately 7 months apart. Medical records suggested that Robert had attended for help during this intervening period for queried chronic fatigue symptoms of profound tiredness, excessive sleeping and lack of energy.

The offences were meticulously planned, and Robert acknowledged that he had spent many hours preparing the offence scenarios in fantasy before their implementation. The most consistent features of the offences included luring the child to a solitary location through different ruses, the administration of an overwhelming blitz of aggression to subdue the victim, and the enactment of sexually intrusive assaults before and after death. Each child was tortured in a variety of sexually aberrant ways before strangulation. Robert tended to dispose of the bodies in locations far removed from the site of the killings, driving over 100 miles to bury the victims in shallow graves in peat bogs. Photographs were taken of each victim naked with comments written on the back of the photographs (a reflection of what Norris (1988) refers to as the totem phase of serial murder as a means of sustaining the psychological rewards of the acts). Robert was known to have reimmersed himself in his typical, organised lifestyle after each killing with no recognisable signs of disturbance in his demeanour or behaviours.

When asked about his behaviours throughout the time of the killings, Robert volunteered that he experienced episodes of stress which affected him greatly. A pattern was noted whereby Robert would devote his time and interest to his work and family, describing these episodes as 'trying to be normal, but bored, empty, feeling dull, flat, depressed, unfulfilled'. He would then entertain fantasies about committing an offence and become pre-occupied with the planning of a crime, a state in which he felt some exhilaration and improved mood. As this fantasy gripped his attention and interests, Robert felt that he struggled to cope with his mounting compulsion to translate fantasy into action, and it was at these times he felt that his psychological and physical energies were sapped and depleted as he struggled with this dilemma about offending. He would seek help from his doctor, yet, he ultimately succumbed to his desires. Robert claimed that he would feel 'like a vampire that needs the blood of someone to stay alive. I hated myself for being dependent on these kids to feel alive. I suppose I thought that it was like I was on the top of the food chain and these kids were there to service me. I needed them to exist, or for that part of me to exist.' After each killing, Robert reported, 'I would go as low as I went high when I did them', using the photographs as a method of sustaining the feelings he obtained from the killings. Robert was patient, deliberate, organised and strategic in his planning of the crimes with an awareness of forensic evidence. He did refer to returning to the crime scenes on two occasions, but in order to ensure that he had not left any evidence rather than to savour his crimes.

It became apparent that the offences served multiple functions for Robert. He divulged that he perceived himself as punishing the victims, expressing his rage and anger through the initial violent attack. He perceived the victims as 'full of innocence, ready for the taking, ripe for the picking'. The sexual acts were varied and tended to be sadistic and indicative of prolonged torture (strangulation–revival cycle), Robert admitting, 'I took my time with them, did what I felt I needed to. The only constraint was my imagination.' The victims served as props within his sexually violent fantasies: 'I was god-like, they were sacrifices to me.' He was 'feeling alive, like an explosion of excitement, buzzing'. Robert claimed that the sexual acts of the offences were particularly revitalising because the visceral sensation of contact between the victim and him (either through violent or sexual actions) brought on sensations of 'being electrified'. After the sexual acts, Robert claimed that he strangled the victims and spent time savouring the situation. When asked why he spent so much time with the dead victims, Robert replied, 'The fact that he [a victim] was dead was like being with someone I knew, who knew me, what I felt like inside, together, dead.' Robert's killing of the victim permitted him to communicate through projective identification his own internal deadness and lack of vitality. A sense of 'aliveness' was achieved through each of the crimes, but vanished just as quickly. Robert was encouraged to reflect upon his connection to the 'dead boy' inside himself and the victim he created. Therefore, there were two specific phases to the killings, and Robert's violence appeared to bring him alive internally, his sexual behaviours expressing hate and rage and, latterly, the killing of the victim serving to communicate his inner 'deadness'. He denied any empathy for the victims or that they were relevant to his thinking after an offence. The psychological rewards of killing were numerous for Robert and the therapist questioned whether the depth of disorder in his personality could be addressed through therapy.

Robert's ability to compartmentalise his sinister and destructive tendencies while living a socially acceptable, undisturbed existence was remarkable. In many respects, the subjective tension felt as each killing episode was incubated was reminiscent of the errant, rampant, wayward parts of personality described by Goldberg (2000). Exploration of this capacity suggested that Robert was entirely aware of the duality of his psychological functioning, and he voiced his belief that 'there are two of us inside here, one that's deep and dark, the other's a really nice guy'. He could identify the strain and stresses that emerged from the tension between these dual aspects of his personality. There was no amnesic barrier for the differing states, and Robert's experiences did not feature any particular dissociative phenomena or symptoms. He was not considered to exhibit a dissociative disorder. He did speculate that he had become addicted to the act of killing and wondered how long he would have been able to maintain this behaviour because of his desire to accelerate the frequency of the murders. The psychological formulation was based on the hypothesis that early traumatic and adverse childhood experiences had caused a structural dissociation of his personality, which became configured into a duality consisting of a pseudo-normality that helped him cope with the world (chameleon-like) and a veiled, errant, dissociated, violent and traumatised state detached from human connection and seeking expression through sexual violence and homicide. Robert was not amnesic for these facets of his personality and could reflect upon, discuss and describe them.

The 'deadness' described by Robert appeared to be indicative of the traumatic experiences he had endured, and he reported that the accumulation of 'disappointments' (his term) and losses had caused a detachment, a shutting down emotionally and a retreat and removal from the living world. His single method of attachment was manifested through sexual violence that was rewarding in terms of its excitement and stimulation and, later, the resonance with a dead victim. This successive process of dissociative recoil from human contact was an ingrained feature of Robert's emotional existence and directly related to his crimes, and their functions and derived rewards. His repertoire of relating to others was a deceptive façade to conceal narrow, limited choices within relationships, Robert realising that it was imperative to hide the sinister rumblings of his sexually violent desires and fantasies.

CAT with Robert

The provisional Reformulation Letter was derived after session 6. The target problems and underlying target problem procedures were agreed, and 24 sessions of CAT were offered to Robert, although he stated that he disliked the time-limited nature of CAT. This was not considered to indicate any dependency but more likely to reflect Robert's appreciation that his difficulties required longer-term work to deal with the potency of his risk potential and to convince decision-making authorities that this risk was addressed sufficiently.

The draft SDR was presented to Robert (Fig. 14.1). Robert's initial engagement changed after the reformulation tools were introduced, and almost immediately certain transference and counter-transference developments surfaced that threatened the integrity of the therapy relationship. The therapist had begun to experience the therapy as overwhelming in certain respects and wondered whether there was any merit in continuing to work with Robert. His disorder was so profound that the therapist questioned the capacity of any form of therapy to address Robert's underlying sexual perversity and pathological relating. His more authentic or 'true self' was considered to reflect the sinister, exalted, pathological self-state rather than the

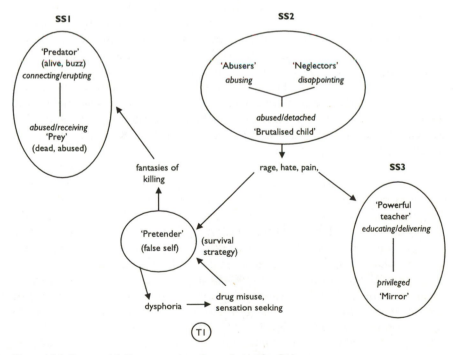

Figure 14.1 Sequential diagrammatic reformulation for Robert.

'false self' displayed through his socially appropriate actions. Healthy capacities were notable in Robert's personality, and his struggle to suppress the sexual aggression he harboured was acknowledged within the reformulation.

The reformulation elicited a paranoid withdrawal by Robert, who voiced his dislike of the explicit nature of the process. His demeanour changed toward the therapy and the therapist, an emerging narcissistic transference being noted. Robert vacillated between statements and attitudes, suggesting that he was teaching the therapist about 'people like me who are rare, get books written about them', and expressing the view that his secrets were no longer his own and that the therapist had 'something on me now, this could be used against me'. His sense of vulnerability was acknowledged, and Robert was encouraged to discuss his distrust of the therapist's motives. The narcissistic grandiosity that was lacking previously became a prominent feature of the sessions, Robert stating that he would provide the therapist with insights into serial killers which had never been written about or known before. During session 10, he brought along a copy of the 'Moors Murderer' Ian Brady's book *The Gates of Janus*, sniggering at and denigrating Brady for his 'vanity publishing, the rantings of a madman', and Brady's self-appointed position as a deliverer of insights into murder. His envy was tangible and intense. At session 11, Robert appeared to lack interest in discussing anything and deflected all conversation and focus away from the reformulation. He belittled the therapist's competence and stated that he believed that his case was too complex ('maybe we need a special type of therapy for special types of criminals') for the therapist, who was simply not intelligent enough or brave enough to deal with his psychological intricacies. The therapist felt inadequate, incompetent and dismissed (because of his own countertransference responses and the patient's accusations). The transference RRPs shown by Robert were reminiscent of the malignant narcissism fused with aggression and paranoid influences described by Kernberg (1995) and often evident in the personalities of serial killers (Myers, Reccopa, Burton & McElroy, 1993; Pollock, 1995).

It was felt that Robert's engagement with the therapy was distorted through the narcissistic transference, the therapy being used as a process of self-absorbed aggrandisement whereby the therapist was required to mirror his grandiosity and resonate Robert's omnipotence. This pattern within the transference was noted within supervision, and the impact of the interaction required sensitive management to prevent collusion and perversion of the therapy relationship. Within the Reformulation Letter, the possible influences of these RRPs (*mirroring-to-aggrandised*, as a deliverer of knowledge) were explicitly stated. Robert's response was one of annoyance and dismissal of the therapist's comments: 'You're trying to prevent me from getting the help I need.' A rupture in the relationship occurred in reaction to this observation, and Robert failed to attend his next three sessions, claiming that he was busy completing his degree. The therapist pondered that the reformulation process had failed to mirror narcissistically Robert's desire to bind the therapist into narcissistic introspection for self-serving purposes.

Robert requested the next session and attended in a more cooperative mood. He remarked that he had been contemplating the Reformulation Letter and SDR and wished to discuss a variety of issues. He commented that he had always known that his dual internal and outer life had been constructed to cope with many of the experiences he had suffered at the hands of others throughout his upbringing. Robert acknowledged and spoke at length about the 'brutalised child' (a label used by the therapist) who had endured abuse, abandonment, traumatic and tragic loss, neglect and sexual exploitation. Robert could talk of his decision to detach from others as a protective mechanism and the 'deadness' he felt inside. Using the SDR, Robert could decipher that this 'deadness' was composed of a deep-seated rage and hatred against others, and feeling alone, unwanted, and disregarded or abused. Robert explained, 'I have a child in the back of my head looking out at the world, but it's kept well out of the way.' He was asked to reflect upon the adversity he had experienced, how he had configured his personality to cope with this psychological pain and the 'survival strategies' he had adopted. Robert and the therapist conceptualised the 'deadness' as a description of his traumatised, recoiled, disconnected states, most probably a vestige of his exposure to his mother's tragic suicide.

In contrast, his sexual violence was viewed as his action-oriented way of relating to others to re-enact traumatic abuse that pressed for expression and release, achieving a sense of 'alive-ness'. This need to express his rage and hatred through annihilation was construed as a perverted method of communicating the 'psychic deadness' he felt inside and externalising these experiences in an extreme, fatal way. Robert explained that he found these topics difficult to discuss, and a number of sessions were unproductive because of his open request not to talk about these matters, he preferring to enter into philosophical discussion with the therapist. It was decided to collude with Robert's pattern of engagement because this appeared to allow him to 'dose' himself episodically to tolerate discussing these subjects.

Robert did state that he recognised that he had developed a coping mode which he labelled 'pretending', representing the false self which helped him deal with the world through chameleon-like acting. Robert's duality of existence included trying to convince himself that he could be a sociable, accepted father and employee to cover up these pathological and perverse states. He accepted that this presentation was difficult to sustain, caused tension and required energy to manage without the emergence of sexually violent fantasies that affected his thinking. Dysphoria would set in, and Robert could manage his distress only through drug misuse or sexual misdemeanours (e.g. homosexual contact with rent boys in risqué public places, and gambling with large amounts of money in late-night drinking dens).

The predatory, organised nature of Robert's crimes was obvious. When this aspect of his offending was discussed, Robert spoke about his states of mind when preparing to commit the crime and when fantasising. Part of the CAT reformulation process entailed the identification of the dialogical sequence of RRPs and the positions within self-states that culminated in the offence itself and developing an appreciation of the offender-to-victim relations. Robert was asked to reflect upon the internal states of mind (thoughts, feelings and perceptions of himself and others) which formed the preoffence and offence interactions. The location of his 'peak' risk potential was determined to be lodged in SS1, labelled 'predator' (a mixture of underlying RRPs describing the offender-to-victim relations named as *connected-to-understanding* – through 'deadness' – and *erupting/exploding-to-receiving* – the sense of 'alive-ness'). In this state, Robert was omnipotent, in control, powerful and animated.

The dialogical sequence of self-states and the offender-to-victim (*self-to-other*) RRPs were analysed with Robert. It was put to him that it appeared that his perceptions and choice of victim, his actions during the crimes and manner of relating to them, and the functions his offences served could be best interpreted within the SDR positions and RRPs. The offences indicated a process of projective identification with several elements apparent. Firstly, Robert perceived the victims as being 'privileged. I felt hatred towards them, as if I hadn't had a chance. They did. Innocent, I was told I was a deviant all my life.' The victim role created during the offences incorporated the projection of Robert's states of mind in that he used the offences to recapitulate his own history and its effects. Robert was asked to think about the position, feelings and role he forced the victim to assume (reflective of the 'brutalised child' state). The relevance of being alone, abused, desecrated and spoiled through sex during the offence was considered. It was suggested that Robert used sexual torture to master his own abuses and to achieve a sense of being 'alive' and stimulated, releasing his rage, hurt and hatred by creating an irrevocably damaged child. The killing of the child and Robert's communicative resonance with the victim's deadness were linked to the traumatic re-enactment of his own feelings in response to his mother's suicide. The fusion of sexual aggression and communication of deadness as an identification was discussed at length with Robert to encourage further reformulation of his offending. In many respects, the brutalised child could be said to have been identified with the stranger self-object (Meloy, 1992) and to have become an internalised aggressor role that Robert re-enacted through the offences. His predatory crimes and their elements could be explained via the SDR, allowing Robert to contemplate the mixture of motivations. Robert's peak risk potential was located in the RRPs within SS1, fantasies fuelling the enactment of these procedures through crimes.

Outcome and risk prediction

Forensic psychotherapy with an offender who has committed serial homicide must acknowledge the realities of what can possibly be achieved. For Robert, changes were noted within therapy.

Robert did report improved recognition of the target problems and insight into the nature of and motivations for the offences. An offer of several options to address the underlying feelings associated with the brutalised child was refused by Robert, fearing that he could not cope with the likely sense of vulnerability because of the abuse he had endured. Robert developed insight and understanding about the origins and functions of his sexual violence and the killing of the victim (the hatred and rage of the brutalised child emerging from the actions of abusing and neglecting others), yet resolution of these complex feelings could not be claimed. He felt that these events and experiences were too difficult to think about. Robert's capacity to empathise with the victim was too entwined with his own adversity and abuse, and he did fail to translate insight into his own abuse into the development of any awareness of the likely experiences of the victims of his crimes.

On several occasions, Robert's self-aggrandisement re-emerged through boastful, arrogant and contemptuous behaviours. Furthermore, the function of the 'pretender' was monitored, and Robert did acknowledge that he understood the therapist's concerns about whether he was simulating engagement in CAT. Robert made progress in dealing with his tendencies to seek sensation to cope with the internal deadness he reported and also worked toward genuine interaction and attachment with other people as a means of learning to engage in authentic relationships. The false 'pretender' was designated importance as an idealised state which Robert had perceived as a hoped-for state he might aspire to achieve.

Robert's case was reviewed at 13 years after sentence, and the gravity of his offences was considered an obstacle to further rehabilitation (parole or liberty) by the state. Despite this agenda, Robert had made progress in CAT, acknowledged when the clinician gave formal evidence to the commission. Somewhat sarcastically, a commissioner remarked at the hearing, 'Therapy has made a difference. We now have an insightful multiple murderer who has the vocabulary, but can't talk his way out of this one.'

Commentary

This CAT was unusual in terms of its application and the offender's willingness to engage. It is perhaps simplistic to devise psychological formulations of extremely violent, sadistic killers which rely upon the influences of childhood traumas, harsh caregiving environments, faulty learning and mechanisms such as dissociative disorder to explain the actions of these offenders (Meloy, 1992; Pollock, 1999). Nevertheless, it is clear that the repetitive killings and the pathological relating to the victim underlying these actions (as vehicle or object; Canter, 1994; Godwin, 2000) can be analysed by the CAT model. Forensic psychotherapy, CAT or otherwise, can aim to achieve only a modicum of positive changes within the rehabilitation process for these types of offenders.

CAT, as a method of reformulation and analysis, helps to link the killer's early experiences, development of the self and its configuration, the ways in which the offender develops RRPs and the self-states implicated directly in the commission of the crimes. Not every serial killer exhibits a linear recapitulation of past abuses which are discernible in a projective identification system or are so clearly manifest in the offender-to-victim RRPs. CAT does provide a method of formulating intrapersonal and interpersonal processes that are evident in the action-oriented harmful procedures within the crimes. The natural obstacles to rehabilitation in these types of cases may disqualify the merits of delivering therapy to serial homicide perpetrators, yet, in certain circumstances, CAT may illuminate the offender's personality-to-offence link, facilitating a measured, astute decision-making process with more perceptive comprehension of the risk potential in these cases.

References

Arrigo, B. A. & Purcell, C. E. (2001). Explaining paraphilias and lust murder: Toward an integrated model. *International Journal of Offender Therapy and Comparative Criminology*, *45*, 6–31.

Beauregard, E. & Proulx, J. (2002). Profiles in the offending process of nonserial sexual murderers. *International Journal of Offender Therapy and Comparative Criminology*, *46*, 386–399.

Biven, B. (1997). Dehumanization as an enactment of serial killers: A sadomasochistic case study. *Journal of Analytic Social Work*, *4*, 23–49.

Burgess, A. W., Hartman, C., Ressler, R., Douglas, J. & MacCormack, A. (1986). Sexual homicide: A motivational model. *Journal of Interpersonal Violence*, *7*, 593–600.

Busch, K. A. & Cavanaugh, J. L. (1986). The study of multiple murder: Preliminary examination of the interface between epistemology and methodology. *Journal of Interpersonal Violence*, *1*, 5–23.

Canter, D. (1994). *Criminal shadows: Inside the mind of the serial killer*. London: HarperCollins.

Carlisle, A. L. (1993). The divided self: Towards an understanding of the dark side of the serial killer. *American Journal of Criminal Justice*, *2*, 23–36.

Castle, T. & Hensley, C. (2002). Serial killers with military experience: Applying learning theory to serial murder. *International Journal of Offender Therapy and Comparative Criminology*, *46*, 453–465.

Dietz, P. E. (1986). Mass, serial and sensational homicide. *Bulletin of the New York Academy of Medicine*, *62*, 477–491.

Egger, S. A. (1984). A working definition of serial murder and the reduction of linkage blindness. *Journal of Policy, Science and Administration*, *12*, 348–356

Fox, J. A. & Levin, J. (2000). Serial murder: Psychological myths and everyday realities. In M. D. Smith (Ed.), *Homicide: A sourcebook of social research*. Thousand Oaks, CA: Sage.

Gacono, C. B. (1990). An empirical study of object relations and defensive operations in antisocial personality. *Journal of Personality Assessment*, *54*, 589–600.

Gacono, C. B. & Meloy, J. R. (1994). *The Rorschach assessment of aggressive and psychopathic personalities*. Hillside, NJ: Lawrence Erlbaum Associates.

Geberth, V. J. & Turco, R. N. (1999). Antisocial personality disorder, sexual sadism, malignant narcissism and serial murder. *Journal of Forensic Science*, *42*, 49–60.

Giannangelo, S. J. (1996). *The psychopathology of serial murder: A theory of violence*. Westport, CT: Praeger.

Godwin, G. M. (2000). *Hunting serial predators: A multivariate classification approach to profiling violent behaviour*. Boca Raton, FL: CRC Press.

Goldberg, A. (2000). *Errant selves: A casebook of misbehaviour*. Hillside, NJ: Analytic Press.

Hare, R. D. (1991). *Manual for the revised psychopathy checklist*. Toronto: Multi-Health Systems.

Hickey, E. (1991). *Serial murderers and their victims*. Pacific Grove, CA: Brooks/Cole.

Holmes, R. & DeBurger, J. E. (1988) *Serial murder*. Newbury Park, CA: Sage.

Holt, S. E., Strack, S. & Meloy, R.J. (1999). Sadism and psychopathy. *Journal of the American Academy of Psychiatry and Law*, *27*, 23–32.

Keppel, R. D. & Walter, R. (1999). Profiling killers: A revised classification model for understanding sexual murder. *International Journal of Offender Therapy and Comparative Criminology*, *43*, 417–437.

Kernberg, O. F. (1995). *Aggression in personality disorders and perversion*. New Haven, CT: Yale University Press.

Kocsis, R. N., Cooksey, R. W. & Irwin, H. J. (2002). Psychological profiling of sexual murders: An empirical model. *International Journal of Offender Therapy and Comparative Criminology*, *46*, 532–554.

Lang, J. E. T. & DeWitt, K. (1990). The Ripper syndrome: A perspective on serial murder. Unpublished.

Liebert, J. A. (1985). Contributions of psychiatric consultation in the investigation of serial murder. *International Journal of Offender Therapy and Comparative Criminology*, *29*, 187–200.

Lowenstein, L. F. (1992). The psychology of the obsessed compulsive killer. *Criminologist*, *16*, 26–38.

MacCullough, M., Snowden, P., Wood, P. & Mills, H. (1983). Sadistic fantasy, sadistic behaviour and offending. *British Journal of Psychiatry*, *143*, 20–29.

Meloy, J. R. (1992). *The psychopathic mind: Origins, dynamics and treatment*. Northvale, NJ: Aronson.

Meloy, J. R., Gacono, C. & Kenney, L. (1994). A Rorschach investigation of sexual homicide. *Journal of Personality Assessment*, *62*, 58–67.

Millon, T., Millon, C. & Davis, R. (1994). *The Millon Clinical Multiaxial Inventory* 3rd edn (MCMI–III). Minneapolis, MN: National Computer Systems.

Mitchell, E. W. (1997). The aetiology of serial murder: Towards an integrated model. Unpublished. University of Cambridge.

Myers, W. C., Reccopa, L., Burton, K. & McElroy, R. (1993). Malignant sex and aggression: An overview of serial sexual homicide. *Bulletin of the American Academy of Psychiatry and Law*, *21*, 435–451.

Norris, J. (1988). *Serial killers: The growing menace*. New York: Doubleday.

Pollock, P. H. (1995). A case of spree serial murder with suggested diagnostic opinions. *International Journal of Offender Therapy and Comparative Criminology*, *39*, 258–268.

Pollock, P. H. (1999). When the killer suffers: Post-traumatic stress reactions following homicide. *Legal and Criminological Psychology*, *4*, 185–202.

Pollock, P. H., Broadbent, M., Clarke, S., Dorrian, A. & Ryle, A. (2001). The Personality Structure Questionnaire (PSQ): A measure of the multiple self states model of identity disturbance in cognitive analytic therapy. *Clinical Psychology and Psychotherapy*, 8, 59–72.

Prentky, R., Burgess, A. W., Rokous, F., Lee, A., Hartman, C., Ressler, R. & Douglas, J. (1989). The presumptive role of fantasy in serial sexual homicide. *American Journal of Psychiatry*, *146*, 887–891.

Raine, A., Buchsbaum, M. S., Stanley, J. & Lottenberg, S. (1994). Selective reductions in prefrontal glucose metabolism in murderers. *Biological Psychiatry*, *36*, 365–373.

Ressler, R. K., Burgess, A. W. & Douglas, J. E. (1990). Sexual homicide: Patterns and motives. Lexington, MA: Lexington Books.

Rossmo, K. D. (2000). *Geographical profiling*. Boca Raton, FL: CRC Press.

Salfati, C. G. (2000a). The nature of expressiveness and instrumentality in homicide. *Homicide Studies*, *3*, 265–293.

Salfati, C. G. (2000b). Profiling homicide: A multidimensional approach. *Homicide Studies*, *4*, 265–293.

Salfati, C. G. & Canter, D. V. (1999). Differentiating stranger murder: Profiling offender characteristics from behavioural styles. *Behavioural Sciences and the Law*, *17*, 391–406.

Schlesinger, L. B. (2001). Is serial murder really increasing? *Journal of the American Academy of Psychiatry and the Law*, *29*, 294–297.

Segal, H. (1985). *Phantasy in everyday life: A psychoanalytic approach to understanding ourselves*. Northvale, NJ: Aronson Press.

Shrapec, C. A. (2001). Phenomenology and serial murder: Asking different questions. *Homicide Studies*, *5*, 46–63.

Turvey, B. (1999). *Criminal profiling: An introduction to behavioural evidence analysis*. San Diego, CA: Academic Press.

Vanderlinden, J., Van Dyck, R., Vandereycken, W., Vertommen, H. & van Verkes, R. (1993). The Dissociation Questionnaire (DIS-Q): Development and characteristics of a new self-report scale. *Clinical Psychology and Psychotherapy*, *1*, 21–27.

Weinshel, E. & Calet, V. (1972). On neurotic equivalents of necrophilia. *International Journal of Psychoanalysis*, *53*, 67–75.

Wertham, F. (1937). The catathymic crisis: A clinical entity. *Archives of Neurology and Psychiatry*, *37*, 974–977.

Wright, J. & Hensley, C. (2003). From animal cruelty to serial murder: Applying the graduation hypothesis. *International Journal of Offender Therapy and Comparative Criminology*, *47*, 71–88.

Yarvis, R. M. (1990). Axis I and Axis II diagnostic parameters of homicide. *Bulletin of the American Academy of Psychiatry and Law*, *18*, 249–269.

Chapter 15

A case of dissociative murder

Mark Westacott

Murder is a complex and intensely interpersonal offence. The act of obliterating someone can be viewed as an extreme form of projective identification whereby murderous rage finally achieves its aim and the victim is forced violently into the reciprocal position.

The murderous act

What lies behind the murderous act will clearly vary from patient to patient. Occasionally, the act will be set firmly within the context of an elaborate delusional system, and such patients are often considered too unwell at the time of their offence to have been responsible for their crime. The victim may well be a stranger or might be someone known to the patient. Treatment usually takes the form of medication, interventions to improve treatment compliance, and sometimes cognitive-behavioural therapy to reduce the tenacity of delusional beliefs. In other cases, the act may result from a more circumscribed set of irrational beliefs, as in erotomania, or may arise from a cold and calculated act of instrumental violence, typical of psychopathy.

The type of murder to be discussed here, though, differs from these. In this case, the victim is rarely a stranger but is usually someone with whom the individual has some close contact. There may be a deep emotional link, or the attachment may be more symbolic, perhaps representing a figure from the patient's past. Usually, there is sufficient contact between the two for the victim to be the recipient of the patient's projections.

The murderous act itself is usually sudden and explosive, often without apparent motive, and leaves the murderer deeply shaken and relieved that the entire episode is over. There is often a feeling of unreality, disconnection and maybe some amnesia of the event itself. Extreme levels of violence may be used, such as multiple stabbings or the breaking of bones, leading writers such as Cartwright (2002) to refer to them as 'rage-type murders' (see Chapter 12). Meloy (1992) has also written extensively in this area and refers to this form of murder as 'catathymic homicide'. Here, catathymia is used to mean 'in accordance with emotions', to indicate that this is an intensely emotional, interpersonal, and yet often wholly or partially dissociated act of murder.

Given this description of the crime, it is not surprising that these patients often fail to give a very good account of their motives. Recollection may be poor, they may report simply not knowing or they may describe seemingly bizarre experiences such as experiencing the victim as someone else at the time of the assault. As a result, their risk of reoffending is usually judged as high, they may be seen as deliberately obfuscating the truth, and hospital staff may become polarised in their attitudes and responses to them.

Cognitive Analytic Therapy (CAT) and dissociative murder

From what has been said above, there are at least three areas in which CAT theory can contribute to the treatment and management of these patients. The first is that of formulating the act of murder itself and, on the basis of this, informing a course of treatment that might be undertaken by patient and CAT therapist. Patients can be deeply traumatised by what they have done and will invariably be struggling for an explanation. They may never have fully disclosed this and may find reawakening these memories deeply disturbing. Affect might be managed through self-harm, aggression or withdrawal, and brief periods of psychotic decompensation can follow periods of stress. In these cases, a great deal of 'pretherapy' work on establishing a relationship, gaining a sufficient level of trust and discussing background factors, such as the limits of confidentially, involvement in tribunals and relationships with solicitors, will need to be done before formal therapy begins.

The particular contribution of CAT to understanding these patients is the multiple self-states model (MSSM) (Ryle, 1997; see Chapter 2), which suggests that dissociation originates in a failure to integrate experience as a result of trauma or neglect. This results in the existence of self-states that are partially dissociated from one another and that are associated with intense, undermodulated emotions and poor self-reflection. In violent patients, the reciprocal role templates underlying these states are usually derived from earlier abusive relationships and are typically described in terms of persecutor or predator and victim roles. The victim role is invariably associated with intense feelings of shame or humiliation, a fact which can make this an acutely painful as well as dreaded and potentially dangerous place for the person to be (Horowitz, 1998). Patients may switch rapidly from one self-state to another, or may oscillate between persecutor and victim roles (i.e. a role reversal). A clear example of the latter was provided by Pollock & Belshaw (1998) in their description of a sexually violent male offender who forced his victims to injure him while he was committing the sexual assault.

The second area in which CAT can make a contribution to the management of seriously violent patients is with respect to risk assessment and management. Clearly, risk assessment needs to be based on an adequate formulation of the client's behaviours and a clear description of risk indicators. The identification of triggers into and out of particular states is central to the CAT process of developing a shared understanding of the patient's problems. This understanding, based on the self-states model, and its graphic description in the form of the self-states sequential diagram (SSSD), provides an exceptionally powerful tool for helping staff identify states – with their corresponding behaviours and emotions – that are associated with increased risk of harm to self or others. In terms of risk management, the procedural loops of the diagram indicate the pathways into and out of the various states and naturally lend themselves to various interventions for interrupting movement into states that might be associated with crude and poorly modulated emotions. However, in many ways, this mapping of problematic procedures is merely icing on the cake, for the most important contribution of the SSSD to risk management is the help it gives staff to avoid being pulled into particular reciprocal role relations that might exacerbate the patient's anger or distress and lead to heightened risk of injury to self or others.

The final area to be discussed here is related to risk management and is that of assisting the multidisciplinary team to understand and work with these individuals. As was mentioned earlier, patients who have murdered often elicit complex and intense emotional reactions in those charged with their care. I emphasise that these reactions are complex because they can and do vary from extremes of dislike and a desire to punish to, at the other extreme, erotic excitement and admiration. Because interpersonal relations are central to the CAT understanding of the client, and the reformulation diagram clearly predicts what reciprocal role pressures staff will face, unwitting recruitment into these positions can be avoided or worked with constructively when it occurs. This approach is not of course confined to work with offenders. The use of what has come to be called *contextual reformulation* has been used to help staff in a variety of contexts (e.g. Walsh, 1996; Kerr, 1999), and once again it is the diagram, and elaborations of this to include the various responses of staff to the patient's self-states and roles, that forms the main CAT tool for promoting understanding and change.

The following case study describes the use of CAT with an in-patient diagnosed with antisocial personality disorder. It emphasises the importance of working closely with the team and highlights the contribution of CAT to risk assessment and management.

Case example: Simon

Simon, aged 35, was born in central Liverpool. At the time of his birth, his mother was working as a waitress in a central nightclub and had been involved with various members of a notorious Liverpool gang. His father was well known locally for his brutality and gangland status. Simon had two older brothers and a younger sister, all by different fathers. His older brother had been killed in his 30s in a car accident caused by his driving while intoxicated. Simon grew up in this family until he was 8 years of age. He remembers his father coming home drunk and being physically violent to his mother, brothers and himself. He would often be hit violently across the head and locked in his room. Shortly after Simon's eighth birthday, his father left for another woman, and his mother soon took a new partner, who turned out to be considerably more violent and sadistic toward the children. He was a prize-winning bare-knuckle boxer and was also very much involved in the Liverpool criminal underworld. Simon remembered feeling the odd one out in the family, less aggressive than the rest and less interested in theft and street fighting than his new stepfather would have liked. He was taunted, periodically beaten for no apparent reason, and often left to stand outside the house in just his underwear.

From the age of about 14, life became so intolerable for Simon that he started leaving the house and sleeping rough. It was at this time that he was befriended by a man who, unbeknown to him, was a well-known paedophile. He initially enjoyed the attention and liked being given alcohol and cigarettes and treated like an adult. However, after about 6 months, this man took him to the house of a stranger where he was sexually assaulted by both men. He was told that his brother would receive similar treatment if he disclosed to anyone what had happened.

Simon then entered a different phase of his life. He did occasional jobs, mainly delivering drugs, for his stepfather but continued to be beaten and chastised for no apparent reason, and the atmosphere in the house became unbearable. He already had something of a drug habit, using amphetamines, alcohol and cannabis regularly. He also began to go into the centre of Liverpool to pick up men in lavatories, occasionally going home with some of them. Initially, he said that he had always been paid for going back to people's houses, but later denied this and said that he often wanted companionship. On one occasion, he remembered going home with a large Irishman he had met in a bar, who then sexually assaulted him violently.

At the same time this was happening, he began to visit a secluded gay cruising area just outside the city. He attacked gay men here, always in the same way. He would sit in the dark on a park bench holding a concealed iron bar. Eventually, he would be approached, and when physical advances were made, he would begin clubbing the victim until he was unconscious. This continued over a 2-year period, during which he attacked over 30 men.

The index offence occurred when Simon was 22 years old. A few months earlier, he and a mate had been doing some work for a local man who was known to be paedophile. On the evening of the offence, Simon was drinking heavily with two mates when they decided they would return to the house to burgle it. On their approach, they saw no lights on, and they entered through a window at the back. Simon remembered being in the lounge when he heard movement in the next room. He said that he turned around and saw his stepfather standing in the doorway. Suddenly overcome with rage, he ran at him and began to pound his head and chest. The man collapsed, and Simon continued to punch him until his skull was fractured and he was unconscious. He died on the way to hospital. When the rage subsided, Simon saw that this was not his stepfather but the owner of the house, and fled in panic.

Simon was later convicted of murder and detained in a number of prisons until the age of 33. He proved extremely difficult to manage, and his experiences there compounded his difficulties. While he witnessed assaults on other patients and sexual abuse, he also used violence and intimidation to protect himself. He took drugs regularly, harmed himself, and on a number of occasions assaulted prison officers. Shortly before being transferred to a medium-secure unit in the North of England, he began to describe psychotic symptoms of persecutory voices, and his behaviour become increasingly paranoid and disordered. He had also made death threats against a number of prison officers and the prison governor.

CAT for Simon

Psychotherapeutic work occurred in a number of phases. The first phase involved making an initial assessment of suitability for psychological treatment and the development of a sufficient level of rapport and engagement for therapy to begin. The emphasis was on hearing Simon's story while also clarifying anxieties, such as anxiety about confidentiality, what would be written in the notes and who would have access to them. At the same time, an assessment was made of his motivation for change, his capacity for engagement in the work and his self-reflective abilities. This phase of treatment with weekly sessions lasted about 12 weeks.

Alongside this, work was begun with other key staff involved in his care. Forensic patients often have a very powerful transference to the hospital and to the clinical team as a whole. It is crucially important that the staff group is as cohesive as possible, with clear lines of communication, and that the therapist should be seen as having a good relationship with the rest of the team (Welldon & Van Velsen, 1997). Plans for the use of CAT with this patient were discussed soon after admission, and the training requirements for new staff were identified. Regular meetings were held between therapist and key worker so that information from the initial therapy sessions could be used in developing the care plan and the initial risk assessment. This was important, as details of the patient's history not contained in previous notes were being disclosed in these initial sessions, and much of this was relevant to the assessment of risk and the construction of an initial risk management plan. An example of this was his tendency to be easily angered by young female staff who he thought were trying to humiliate him. Because he had had little contact with young women in prison, this trigger had not previously been identified.

After 3 months of weekly contact, it was agreed that sessions would continue for a further 30 sessions. These could then be followed up by less frequent sessions to monitor progress as needed. By this stage, Simon was much more relaxed in sessions and had been able to give an account of his earlier life and traumas. On measures of personality functioning such as the Millon Clinical Multiaxial Inventory–2 (MCMI–2) (Millon, 1987) and the Personality Assessment Inventory (PAI) (Morey, 1991), he scored high on borderline, narcissistic and antisocial features. He also scored highly on posttraumatic disorder symptoms and measures of traumatisation. He completed the Psychotherapy File, wrote a brief life history, and brought his journal to the sessions. The journal, which he had kept for a number of years, contained reflections on moods and thoughts about his family, friends and those he came into contact with each day.

On the basis of this information, the SSSD (Fig. 15.1) was constructed over a number of sessions. The diagram identified three main states that seemed to underpin his difficulties. The admiring state (*admired rescuer-grateful admirer*) existed in fantasy only and was a place he would retreat to when the world seemed overwhelming. A typical fantasy here would be that of rescuing children from lions in the Colosseum and consequently being hailed as a hero. The second self-state (SS2) was associated with feelings of abandonment and humiliation (*neglecting, dismissive-hurt, sad, humiliated, angry*). It was usually from this state that staff were perceived as insufficiently responsive or as favouring other patients. On these occasions, Simon would

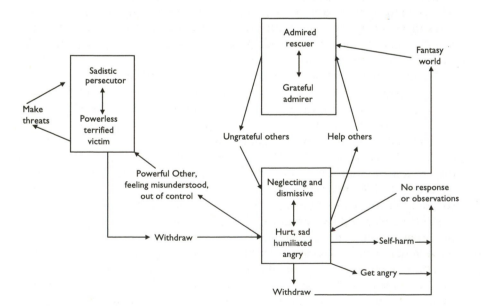

Figure 15.1 Simon's self-states sequential diagram.

withdraw, superficially harm himself or become verbally aggressive toward staff. The final self-state was one of extreme and violent emotions, and, to use a phrase coined by Horowitz (1991; 1998), it was called the 'dreaded place'. This state was rarely entered into but remained a place that terrified him. The commonest trigger for a shift to this place was when a staff member responded in such a way as to leave him feeling persistently humiliated and powerless. Once in this self-state, he would oscillate between powerless terror and intense hatred for the individual. It became a question of who would survive. Staff on the receiving end of this would feel terrorised and refuse to come on the ward. Meloy (1992) has clearly described this *self–object* relationship in catathymic murder, where self and object representations are either good or bad across time and are not held constant despite the vicissitudes of reality. For Simon, it became a question of who would be destroyed, himself or the member of staff. Once he was in this state, risk management and work with staff became imperative, as the persecuting state, once activated, could be re-entered much more easily. The risk of suicide at these times was simultaneously heightened.

Fortunately, in this case, Simon was able to form sufficiently positive relationships with a number of staff, so that he never disengaged totally from therapy. There were a number of areas that were identified for intervention. Some of these were centred on sustaining contact with staff when he was feeling dismissed and humiliated, thus breaking the cycles of withdrawal and anger. Staff provided regular times to review progress with him and worked hard to engage with him when he was angry rather than simply encouraging him to let off steam in a 'time-out' room. During the construction of the SSSD, different coloured pens were used for each self-state and the procedures that arose from it. Diary entries were made in the same colour to help Simon map the shifting of states. In the initial stages of treatment, emphasis was placed on self-state identification rather than on monitoring of individual procedures, which came later. State-shift mapping became particularly helpful in ward meetings, which were initially experienced as dismissing and irrelevant. Simon would occasionally walk out of these meetings in anger. Later on, he was able to take the SSSD into the meeting and trace his movement into the abandoning and humiliating state as this was happening. His immediate response when he did this for the first time was to laugh. From then on, he was able to communicate more openly what it was about the meetings he disliked, leading to a subsequent change in the structure of the meetings and an end to his walking out in anger.

As mentioned earlier, discussions about using CAT with Simon started soon after admission and arose from the availability of a therapist trained in CAT and also a sense that his management on the ward might be helped by this model. A number of training sessions were held with staff, focusing specifically on CAT concepts such as states, reciprocal roles and countertransference, although these terms were not necessarily used. The next very important step came from Simon, who asked whether he could do a training session for staff on his own diagram. This proved very powerful in strengthening the bond between himself and members of the clinical team, and it later enabled a joint risk-management plan to be drawn up, largely written by Simon himself. The final part of work with the team consisted of work on their responses to the patient and linking this with his SSSD. It might have been useful to draw up a complete contextual reformulation of the case. However, this work was done individually with staff who had close involvement with Simon and who therefore tended to be pulled into particular roles. The responses most typically reported by staff were of admiration, intimidation, wanting to care for him, irritation, finding him sexually provocative or of being afraid. These different reactions were discussed at team meetings, and staff were free to discuss their reactions and how they managed them. The SSSD was produced at all of these discussions and seemed to be a tool that people could engage with and use quite readily after some initial training.

The value of doing all of this contextual work was immense and confirms what others have already said about the usefulness of CAT with care teams (see Ryle & Kerr, 2002). Although Simon initially failed to get along with his key worker and had finally refused contact with him, he was able with his second key worker to use the reformulation to gain some distance from his initial fears and continue the relationship into a period where these anxieties were largely overcome. Interestingly, this shift coincided with a reduction in judgement-laden evaluations of the patient and is similar to Walsh's (1996) observation that contextual reformulation locates individual reactions in a non-judgemental system of causality. In the present case, this allowed staff to talk more openly about their feelings and reactions to the patient, reducing anxiety and guilt, and providing rich information that deepened understanding of the patient and assisted risk assessment and management. It also helped staff cope when they were the recipients of very intense reciprocal pressures, as when Simon was feeling persecuted. Frank discussion using the diagram and relating this to Simon's history of abuse increased empathy with his more fearful and humiliated aspects and decreased the impulse to reciprocate his persecuting state by complete withdrawal.

Commentary

The outcome of this case was the successful management and eventual release of a patient who might otherwise have spent a considerable time in medium security. One of the values of reformulation is that behaviours that can often seem random and impulsive become more understandable and predictable. In the case of this patient, the result was that a pass to leave the unit was granted relatively early, and he was able to take part in rehabilitative activities outside the hospital that eventually promoted his move to a less secure environment.

The collaborative nature of the treatment helped Simon overcome some of his initial feelings of mistrust. Although this required preliminary work, the joint construction of the diagram in particular helped to anticipate and work with difficulties as they arose. Of course, the diagram became the main tool used by the team in thinking about and planning his care. A particular benefit of therapist and team using the same, clearly presented, formulation was that the psychotherapy, and the therapist–patient relationship, became more transparent.

A particular contribution to risk assessment and management was the systematic use of the SSSD. This very powerful tool can show clearly the internal and external setting conditions for various risks and the triggers for shifts into particular states. In the case of Simon, it was clear that his *persecutor-to-terrorised* victim state was entered mainly from feeling hurt and misunderstood in the setting of a relationship perceived as unbalanced. If his feelings were not acknowledged and he continued to feel misunderstood, he would eventually switch into this more dangerous state. In a team used to working with CAT, the diagram can be placed at the front of the risk assessment document, although I would recommend that this be supplemented with a written description of the relevant target problem procedures.

A further point regarding risk management is the way in which CAT can contribute to improved staff–patient relations and so reduce risk behaviours. The CAT reformulation also provides a historical context for problematic behaviours and reduces the likelihood they will be viewed as 'intentional' (usually with the implication that they are aimed at provoking staff) or irrational and arising from disorder. Keeping the patient's history alive in the collective mind of the care team is vitally important and is accomplished very successfully through the reciprocal role procedures of the diagram (the letter remains a more personal document between therapist and patient).

The CAT reformulation can help staff identify the relationship between particular collusive reciprocations and heightened risk. In the case of Simon, feeling irritated and attempting to set firm boundaries with him when he was feeling humiliated and angry simply led to withdrawal, self-harm or increased aggression. CAT calls for risk management in these contexts to become a shared responsibility, not something implemented by staff simply in order to contain him. If, as happened in the present case, the plan can be developed as a collaborative tool, there is even greater chance of establishing joint understanding and risk reduction. Given all these benefits of using the CAT model in secure contexts, there are clearly very strong arguments for the further application and extension of the CAT model in various forensic settings.

References

Cartwright, D. (2002). *Psychoanalysis, violence and rage-type murder*. Hove: Brunner-Routledge.

Horowitz, M. J. (1991). *Person schemas and maladaptive interpersonal patterns*. Chicago: University of Chicago Press.

Horowitz, M. J. (1998). *Cognitive psychodynamics: From conflict to character*. New York: Wiley.

Kerr, I. B. (1999). Cognitive-analytic therapy for borderline personality disorder in the context of a community mental health team: Individual and organizational psychodynamic implications. *British Journal of Psychotherapy, 15*, 425–438.

Meloy, J. R. (1992). *Violent attachments*. Northvale, NJ: Aronson.

Millon, T. (1987). *The Millon Clinical Multiaxial Inventory-2*. Minneapolis, MN: National Computer Systems.

Morey, L. C. (1991). *Personality Assessment Inventory Professional Manual*. Odessa, FL: Psychological Assessment Resources.

Pollock, P. H. & Belshaw, T. D. (1998). Cognitive analytic therapy for offenders. *Journal of Forensic Psychiatry, 9*, 629–642.

Ryle, A. (1997). The structure and development of borderline personality disorder: A proposed model. *British Journal of Psychiatry, 170*, 82–87.

Ryle, A. & Kerr, I. B. (2002). *Introducing Cognitive Analytic Therapy*. Chichester: Wiley.

Walsh, S. (1996). Adapting Cognitive Analytic Therapy to make sense of psychologically harmful work environments. *British Journal of Medical Psychology, 69*, 3–20.

Welldon, E. V. & Van Velsen, C. (1997). *A practical guide to forensic psychotherapy*. London: Jessica Kingsley.

Chapter 16

The contribution of Cognitive Analytic Therapy to court proceedings

Philip H. Pollock

The role of the expert in court

Clinicians who venture among the dramas of courts and decision-making boards enter forums that are akin to theatres of mental chess and often involve outright psychological warfare between parties. Taking part in the unfolding dramas in these situations is not for the faint-hearted or self-doubting. The dramaturgical metaphor (Goffman, 1959) can be applied to the role of the clinician as expert witness in that the 'theatre' of the courtroom has well-defined roles for each protagonist or actor. In this chapter, the relevance of Cognitive Analytic Therapy (CAT) is illustrated for specific functions and features of the court process and decision-making boards or commissions in different contexts.

Most clinicians entering the court arena are relatively naive about the intricacies of the strategies and tactics that are likely to be used in dealing with the evidence we supply. The dynamics of the court process and courtroom are littered with pitfalls, traps and tricks (Brodsky, 1991). An understanding of the machinations of the court process and one's roles and responsibilities within it are essential for the provision of proper and professional evidence. A lack of knowledge and a dose of naivety render the clinician potentially vulnerable to harmful, esteem-sapping experiences.

Firstly, a CAT analysis of the dynamics of the courtroom drama is offered, and consideration is given to the expert's professional roles and how the court process can influence the clinician's thinking and behaviours and affect the evidence provided. The use of CAT reformulations for training and supervision of the clinician to improve the evidence proffered and sustain one's own psychological health is reported also.

Secondly, the application of CAT to 'inform' the jury and judge in certain cases is reported, providing an illustrative case study in which CAT helped explain the nature of a criminal's motivations and actions.

Thirdly, the relevance of CAT to decision-making and risk-assessment boards or commissions is described where assessment, prediction and forecasting of risk are required pending release into the community for certain offenders. CAT is presented here as one of many theoretical frameworks to address these matters.

Contributing, informing and the dynamics of court adversity: Roles in the drama

The roles assigned to each party in court proceedings are well defined. Certain positions (RRPs) can be assigned to protagonists in relation to each other. The prosecuting and defending agents (the state, prosecutors, advocates, defenders, etc.) tend to assume relatively adversarial, polarised sides and attitudes and construct a narrative story with the objective of convincing the adjudicating party of matters such as innocence and guilt. The victim is, in criminal cases, afforded a position of moral righteousness toward the offending party. Into this melée of arguing positions and clamouring voices enters the expert witness in some form. The roles played by the expert or professional witness and the tasks undertaken in this split, dichotomised drama are less defined and more amenable to the 'pull and push' of the court dynamics (Brodsky, 1999).

Brodsky (1999) clarifies the varied tactics and strategies of legal advocates used in relation to expert witnesses. For example, he warns clinicians about harbouring any naive assumption that their impartiality, independence and neutrality will not be challenged, or that their opinions and the process of how they were arrived at will not be undermined and distorted. He also warns that their expert status is ripe for insult, demeaning, criticism and attack. The tactics and approaches to be anticipated from legal advocates aim to damage and undermine the expert's evidence (i.e. to make the clinician appear to demonstrate poor integrity, professionalism and practice in order to induce a sense of inadequacy, guilt and even stupidity). The intention is to damage the worth of the testimony, its foundations, the processes culminating in its derivation and the expert's integrity. These traps are obvious, yet the 'green' clinician entering court is liable to face these tactics immediately. The expert's personal and professional vulnerabilities must be acknowledged before undertaking any form of court work or provision of evidence or opinion.

Brodsky (1999) set out the four, hierarchical levels of witness obligations that must be kept in mind. The roles of the professional and expert witness are clearly set out in guidelines which state that clinicians should adopt a stance of autonomy and internal integrity toward the task of informing the court and facilitating its decision making, avoid the conflicts which emerge from the demands of the court drama and its protagonists, and adhere to ethical standards of conduct. Klawans (1991) suggested that the expert should assume the posture or position of 'teacher' to the adjudicating authority (e.g. the jury, judge or panel) and employ dynamic communication styles of relating in the witness box that involve the audience, and clear communication of the evidence, the opinions and the authenticity of the clinician in the role of scientist and professional. Of course, the integrity of the evidence offered should be matched by the integrity of the clinician who, as an imperfect human being and professional, proffers his/her evidence to the court, appreciating its origins, conception and robustness and acknowledges his/her own limitations.

The designated roles of the expert witness can become distorted as the drama unfolds through influential social processes. The expert is expected to conform to certain 'codified' obligations and rules within the process (Childress, 1989). The description of these roles has included the 'whore in the court' (Hagen, 1997), the 'bought courtesan' and 'hired gun' (Brodsky, 1999). The inducement to collude with the instructing party is well documented and the first 'pull' affecting the expert. Collusion based on a desire to affiliate and avoid rejection by the instructing side is an immediate force upon the expert and must be resisted emphatically (Brodsky, 1991; Ziskin, 1995; Blau, 1998). Other difficulties arise when, for example, the perhaps naive and narcissistic clinician is cajoled into believing that his/her expertise and experience have encouraged the legal representative to choose and select him/her for the specified case. The mere status implied by the term 'expert' can activate grandiose aspirations for some clinicians and weaken the neutrality of the clinician's stance toward the case.

Deviations from the expert role: A CAT perspective

The dyadic exchanges within the court process are often characterised by differing 'push and pull' interactions that induce the expert to deviate from the stance of advising and informing the court. A range of tactics and strategies can be identified which lead the professional away from the intended stance to deviate into more compromised or weaker positions in relation to the legal representatives' advantages. The expert can feel provoked and induced in subtle or major ways and forced to assume unwanted, compromised positions when offering evidence. In CAT terms, the intended stance of the expert can be described as an *advising/teaching/informing* RRP or position to the court with the objective of supplying a competent opinion to facilitate and enhance decision making. Guidelines for experts incorporate the adoption of such a stance and way of relating to the court and professional behaviour. The clinician's ability to maintain this stance of impartiality and independence of either party with responsibility to the court is imperative to the proper and effective task of advising the court or teaching the jury or decision-making body. A number of patterns of deviation from this stance can be identified, and they highlight the process of manipulation and inducement experienced by the expert in response to a variety of tactics and strategies. The paramount importance of the expert's own self-monitoring and self-regulation is clarified by an understanding of the types of processes affecting his/her stance and also the need for internal supervision as these influences are applied. Figure 16.1 provides a schematic depiction of the typical RRPs and positions involved in the expert's performance in court and suggests a series of deviations which can compromise the expert's ability to inform impartially the court or decision-making party.

The aspired RRP and position is located in the centre of the diagram ('stance'; Fig. 16.1). The first deviation (deviation 1) occurs when the expert is provoked or induced to depart from this intended position through tactics by legal representatives which attack, criticise, undermine, condemn or humiliate the expert, in terms of the evidence offered itself, the expert's professional identity and personal identity. The RRP assumed by the legal representative who harbours intentions to corrupt the expert's testimony is first noted and can be 'felt' as attempts to wound narcissistically the expert both profession- ally and personally. These strategies, if not noted and managed, tend to induce the expert to assume defensive or self-protective stances, deviating from the task of informing and advising. Defensive reactions by the expert can consist of 'digging in', 'fighting one's corner', becoming resistant to debating other evidence offered, intransigence, inflexibility and obduracy. This represents the RRP in response to the provoking tactics of the legal representative designed to undermine and damage the expert at many levels. Typical reactions of the expert include anger, loss of perspective, loss of confidence, confusion and a sense of being victimised. The naive expert's psychological vulnerabilities and sensitivities can be triggered and tapped to sinister advantage. Such attacks on professional and personal identity can elicit seeking of allies (e.g. identifying with the 'side' who has instructed the expert) or adamant and rigid adherence to evidence without open consider- ation of the alternative arguments proffered. In the worst, dreaded scenarios,

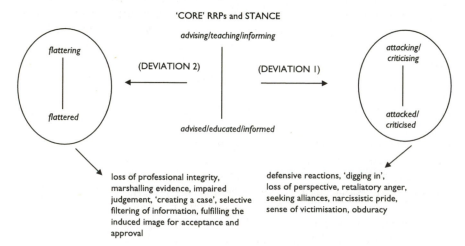

Figure 16.1 RRPs, 'stances' and their deviations in experts' performances in courts.

the professional's integrity, competence and abilities are so undermined and disintegrated that narcissistic wounding is prolonged to the point whereby the expert can feel trapped in relentless attacks, defeated and unable to combat the assaults. The expert may feel that the only survival strategy available is to submit and to await reprieve, a similar psychological position in evolutionary terms within dominant–subordinate contests (Birtchnell, 1993).

An additional type of deviation (deviation 2, Fig. 16.1) can materialise when an expert is approached to provide an opinion on a case with a specific agenda either implicitly or explicitly stated. Legal representatives may appeal to the expert's narcissistic self through flattery (telling the expert that s/he was chosen for the case because of expertise, eminence in the clinical area, reputation for constructing pleas in mitigation, etc.). If the expert is cajoled into this position, a different type of deviation from the *advising/teaching/informing* stance occurs and the expert forms an alliance, with an immediate loss of perspective. The expert, when conducting the evaluation, may be prone to filtering or selectively focusing on the evidence with a lack of objectivity, articulating a view designed to please and gratify the instructing representative's image of the expert. Such behaviour compromises the expert and indicates a collusive, conspiratorial relationship preserving the narcissistic self of the expert. Approval seeking, a desire to be accepted and to live up to the image the expert feels must be presented, can create deviant allegiances which go beyond the true role and evidence.

The importance of 'internal' supervision

The necessity to seek and benefit from professional supervision is critical for the expert, no matter how experienced. Internal supervision (Casement, 1991) at the time of offering evidence requires permitting oneself the psychological space to analyse the unfolding process and readjusting one's stance through repeated reference and feedback about the expert's own performance. When in the witness box, the clinician is alone. The expert who has not developed self-awareness or cannot reflect on his/her reactions is vulnerable to the traps and foibles of the court process and its vicissitudes. For example, the expert clinician who believes that he has intellectual prowess that should not and dare not be challenged because of a sense of narcissistic entitlement is susceptible to criticism and attack, often on other aspects of his evidence and argument. Sensitivity to criticism renders the expert vulnerable to deviation from an objective stance and to react in an inappropriate manner with a loss of perspective. All clinicians as experts are fallible, and acknowledgement of our shortcomings (even while in the witness box) is necessary to ensure professional conduct and performance of our role as required in these circumstances.

CAT reformulation in a case of homicide: Explaining the crime

CAT reformulation can provide a method of explanation of many of the internal and interpersonal facets of criminal behaviours. The power of psychological formulation in comparison with psychiatric diagnosis has been debated at length (Newnes, 2000; Pilgrim, 2000), and it is argued that presenting a coherent, lucid and explanatory description of the offender's personality functioning and its relation to the crime can enhance decision makers' grasp of complicated concepts. As stated by Newnes (2000) in this debate in the British forum, if psychologists cannot speak in a language understandable by the general public, they should 'keep quiet'. The link between psychopathology and crime can be explained through diagnosis (e.g. paranoid schizophrenia and arson explained through reference to delusional thinking), yet such a level of analysis lacks the thread of psychological understanding that animates the offender's intentions, motivations and their relationship to the idiosyncratic expression of the crime. Psychiatric diagnosis is not explanation, and, for example, expressions of anger and rage can be so contextually bound that violence by a narcissistic personality in response to criticism is very different from the abandonment rage of the borderline personality (Benjamin, 1996). Although experts make inferences about criminals' intentions and motivations from many sources of data, the construction of a psychological formulation translates the personal expression of the offence act and aims to explicate the ways in which the offender's internalised procedures are manifest in unique action-oriented procedures.

The case presented here is that of a 33-year-old Caucasian man, David, who was tried for the murder of a young woman. The clinician was asked to provide an evaluation for the court after prior expert opinion had failed to identify a definite psychiatric diagnosis–offence link that was considered helpful to the court. The application of CAT is described and its use in advising the jury of the personality–offence relationship and the offender's intentions and motivations.

David had killed a young woman in his home after luring her there through promises of drugs. He had met her in a local takeaway shop after a night of heavy drinking. David vaguely knew the victim, who, he recalled, was willing to travel to his nearby home for drugs, having been released from an addictions clinic 2 days previously. The construction of the crime scene based on all of the evidence indicated that, on entering the house, David had offered the victim alcohol and they drank for an hour. David made sexual advances to the victim, who spurned him. David then passed out on the settee and slept for a short time while the victim searched his home for the promised drugs. The victim became impatient and made repeated demands for drugs from David, becoming irritated and argumentative, and eventually waking him. David attempted to engage the victim in sexual contact upon awakening, only to be rebuffed once more. The victim launched into a tirade of abuse of him and attempted to leave the house. However, she could not open the front door. In response, David grabbed the victim by the hair, punching her on the face repeatedly, kicking her indiscriminately as she lay in the hallway and spitting on her. The victim lay bleeding with a crushed nose and severe injuries to her head and body. When prompted during interview in prison, David recalled, 'I thought, "no woman walks away from me." ' He was unable to identify any sense of rejection or reactive anger prior to the assault on the victim or think about how he perceived himself. David's later actions were fatal and decisive. He returned to sleep on the settee and awoke to the victim's moaning, calling David names and threatening revenge. He kicked the victim several more times, and then found and applied high-strength glue to the victim's lips, securing them together. The victim died of asphyxia, as she was unable to breathe through either her damaged nasal passage or her glued lips. A weapon was not used. David went to sleep and awoke to realise that he had killed the victim.

David stored the body in his garage for 2 days before disposing of it in a shallow grave in a local country park which he knew from his childhood. During the 2 days after the killing, and despite his reported shock and sense of numbness and denial, David had reunited with his wife, taken her to a luxury hotel and engaged in sexual relations, enjoying the newly established relationship with her. He claimed that he was 'wracked with remorse. I couldn't stop thinking about what I'd done. It was like a dream. Then I went back to the house and the reality of it all hit me when I looked in the garage and she [the victim] was still there.' His actions in disposing of the body were selfish and callous, showing a self-interest and strong need to preserve both himself and the renewed relationship with his wife.

David had a significant antisocial history dating back to his adolescence. He was an overindulged child who was poorly disciplined by both parents and known for criminal activities with his two brothers in the local community. This criminal, unruly and wayward identity was idealised by the family, David lacking any accountability for his actions or response to punishment. His education was stifled by his placement in Borstal and other institutions, his offending escalating to armed robbery, burglary and numerous lesser offences. David's alcohol misuse began at age 13 and persisted to the time of his index offence. He was recognised as a dangerous individual by the police and thought of as a 'street fighter' who would seek brawls and confrontations in public bars, intimidating others. David became involved in paramilitary racketeering and drug dealing but never used substances. He considered imprisonment to be an occupational hazard.

David's finicky relationships with woman were turbulent and of minimal importance to him: 'If women gave me shit, I just walked away. They're two a penny, you just get another one. They're only good for one thing, sex.' He admitted that he was a 'player' who exploited women, and was interested only in sexual conquests. His relationship with his partner at the time of the index offence appeared different in quality. Initially, the relationship had followed the typical pattern, David selfishly disregarding his partner's feelings and showing minimal consideration or investment. The triggering events that altered David's behaviours within the relationship were the pregnancy of his wife and the birth of the couple's first child. David reflected that he began to feel that he was dependent upon his partner, tending to her every need and anticipating the birth of what he believed would be his 'heir' and 'another me'. When born, his child was physically handicapped with a severe heart disorder. Despite these difficulties, David proved to be a devoted father who invested in his son's development and cared for him. The birth of his son also coincided with a change in the relationship with his partner, who began to attempt to curtail his criminal activities, threatening that if he did not comply with her demands, she would leave him and take his son with her. Six months after his son's birth, David was imprisoned for 1 year for drug dealing, placing additional strain on the partnership.

On release, David's partner insisted that he refrain from crime, and the escalating conflict between them resulted in several instances of domestic violence, triggered by her demands. She had separated from him repeatedly in the 3 months prior to the index offence, taking their son and not permitting contact, arguing that the child was witness to the violence and that David needed to seek professional help for his temper. He coped through alcohol bingeing and fighting in local public bars, being arrested for assaulting police officers. His wife had left the family home 3 weeks prior to the offence after numerous incidents of serious domestic violence against her by David. During the corroborating interview, David's wife reported that, on one occasion, he had beaten her severely in front of the child and his parents-in-law, as she attempted to leave the family home. David claimed that he felt depressed, regretful and suicidal on the day of the crime, making several 'begging' telephone calls to his partner, who rejected any suggestion of returning to the family home. David had withdrawn from company, had been prescribed antidepressant medication and was drinking heavily day and night.

At his trial, David pleaded guilty to manslaughter and denied intent to murder, claiming that he did not know that applying the glue to the victim's lips would result in her death (his argument was that at the time he did not know that she could not breathe through her broken nose). A psychological report was requested by the prosecuting counsel to examine the defendant's personality and its relationship to his formed intent at the time of the crime.

Clinical interview of David was compromised by his initial reluctance to discuss the offence or his history because of his religious conversion while imprisoned. Several sessions were required to encourage him to talk freely about events. He completed the psychological testing, which indicated an undercontrolled, primary psychopathic personality with narcissistic, antisocial and sadistic features. The PCL–R assessed David as above the cut-off

score for psychopathic personality disorder (Hare, 1991). Additional diagnoses of alcohol dependency and antisocial personality disorder were made.

CAT reformulation was applied in this case to tease out the RRPs and self-
states involved in his offence and to trace the sequence of internal and
external events which culminated in his actions. Importantly, the focus was
placed on the RRPs underlying the offender-to-victim relations and explaining the intentions and motivations driving his specific, idiosyncratic actions.
The SDR derived is shown in Fig. 16.2. It was apparent that David was a
narcissistic, psychopathic offender who had habitually resorted to alcohol
misuse as a coping strategy when distressed, and had shown extreme violence
against others throughout his life, particularly toward his wife after the birth
of their son and in response to the changes within the marital relationship.
The SDR permitted an analysis of the RRPs underlying David's narcissistic
and antisocial personality and its relationship to violent conduct toward his
partner on repeated occasions (e.g. the changes from David's *exploiting/using*
procedures toward women to an enmeshed, *controlled, rejected, dependent
and spurned* RRP which evoked his anger and depression). It was argued that
there was evidence that the transaction between victim and offender had
begun as an enactment of the *exploiting/using-to-exploited/used* RRP, as
David lured the victim to his home for sexual reasons, her behaviours causing
David to perceive her as demanding (insisting he give her the drugs he promised), rejecting of his sexual advances (making him feel spurned; name calling)
and threatening.

A partial SDR was presented to the jury and court at the trial and explanation given at length about the origins and sources of the RRPs and self-
states. The sequences of procedures which culminated in the climax of the
offence were discussed and the offender-to-victim RRPs and positions were

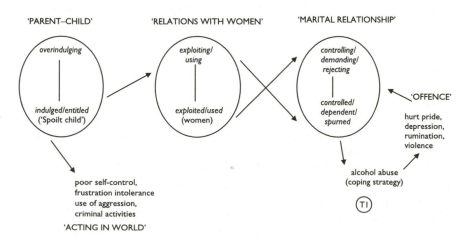

Figure 16.2 Sequential diagrammatic reformulation: Homicide case.

described (from an indulged and entitled criminal who exploited women for his own gratification to a controlled, dependent, spurned killer; the victim was initially exploited and then attacked for her rejections and 'walking away' from David). It was explained to the jury that David's behaviours toward the victim were a recapitulation and re-enactment of his wife's leaving, David expressing violence against the victim in a form of mastery and narcissistic repair for perceived wrongdoing by his wife in a displaced offence. The killing was callous because David's angry arousal was reignited by the victim's moaning and threats, causing him to silence her in a fatal act which echoed his statement that 'no woman walks away from me'. It was accepted by the jury that his gluing the victim's lips was not indicative of premeditated intent, yet he had acted callously and deliberately at a time when other choices could have saved the victim's life. The jury were informed that RRPs represented 'ways of relating' and consisted of a self and other perspective, the offence being formed through an interaction between offender and victim, in this case a displaced recapitulation of the RRPs within his marriage. Traps were discussed as 'cycles of acting' and survival strategies as 'ways of coping with distress'. The critical components of the SDR were the offender-to-victim positions. From the analysis of the RRPs which were manifested during David's offence actions, inferences could be made regarding his motivations, intentions and reasons for behaving in this unique manner toward the victim during the crime.

CAT and risk assessment and prediction

Assessing and predicting an offender's risk potential is the most challenging task for the forensic clinician or worker. The plethora of actuarial methods and theoretically derived tools to assess and forecast risk is testament to the magnitude of this duty. The identification of static and dynamic factors and their combination for differing types of offence category has greatly improved over recent years, and valuable guidelines and methods for estimating risk potential have been established (Quinsey, Harris, Rice & Cormier, 1998). The contribution of CAT reformulation to risk assessment and prediction is debated here. It is hoped to present CAT as a way of thinking about the offender's personality and the offence that permits construction of an 'aerial map' and explicit schema that facilitate prediction of reoffending in the future through identification of RRPs, positions, self-states and crime-related procedures.

CAT assumes that the offence has occurred at a point of climax or location within the offender's personality, an expression of an underlying series of RRPs and positions emanating from a number of self-states. The *offender-to-victim* self-states form the pivotal point of analysis of the offence and the interpretation of intent and motivation. This position represents the location of the offender's most potent risk and the *dominant offence position* underlying the criminal act. This is located through conducting a *dialogical sequence analysis* of the states and positions, exploring the offender's perceptions of him/herself in relation to others, particularly the victim. Perceptions of the victim can change significantly as the offender 'moves' through different states of mind and self-states. *Risk potential* is located within the offender's personality and viewed as a part that requires scrutiny and analysis to develop an appreciation of its sources and origins, operation and manifestation in action. Relapse-prevention plans can be better designed when the offender is made explicitly aware, within this mental model of him/herself, of the internal and external combination of 'ingredients' that indicate inflation of the risk potential. These RRPs and positions are the dominant points of climax and the sequence of psychological passage whereby thresholds that have been surpassed must be identified. Examining the unfolding patterns of procedures helps to identify the sequence of escalating actions leading to the offence. In other cases, an offence RRP can be considered to indicate the expression of a position within a self-state that is deliberately galvanised to alter the offender's internal state or mind, when fantasy is translated into action.

The traced procedures and recognised critical junctures that are evident before an offence occurs are explored, agreed and inserted in the Reformulation Letter and SDR or SSSD. The *dialogical sequence analysis* permits tracking and self-monitoring of crucial RRPs and positions (e.g. paying attention to states such as the emergence of jealousy and envy, hatred and rage, depressed states of mind) to derail the advancing movement toward commission of an offence. The RRPs of the offender-to-victim positions should also be explored and defined. Within the SSSD or SDR, marking or highlighting the particular sequence of shifts, switches and transitions (e.g. using a coloured line, an asterix, and other methods) distinguishes the offence RRPs and the sequence which culminates in the climax of the criminal act. When the RRPs and position are noted, the self-state of the offender-to-victim state is articulated, and then the offender can be prompted to contemplate the 'voice' and emotional states associated with this RRP.

For example, a rage-type killer recognised that his offence emerged from an RRP of *controlled/enmeshed* with a *controlling/crushing* partner. He typically coped by obliterating his thinking in alcohol and drug binges, but never felt able to alter effectively his situation or relationship. After the offence had occurred, the offender could recall emotions of unexpressed, incubated anger, perceiving himself as humiliated, emasculated and weak in relation to a threatening, bullying partner. At the material time of the index offence, he reported shouting 'leave me alone!' repeatedly during his stabbing of the victim with feelings of emancipation and relief after the killing. In such a contextually bound offence, the location of his risk potential can be traced to his induced state of helplessness and RRP of inadequacy and defeat. The 'voice' (the shout he emitted during the killing act) and associated emotions of rage were readily identified. The task for this type of offender is to develop insight, the capacity to self-reflect, and to monitor, control and regulate those aspects of his personality which are linked to the risk potential for offending in the future. Identifying the dynamic flow of internal psychological processes promotes acknowledgement and ownership of risk potential and its management by the offender. Promoting self-awareness, an ability to self-monitor and plans that empower the offender to take corrective or decisive action and apply self-control and regulation can be accomplished through the CAT reformulation and therapy. Unfortunately, in contrast, despite their value, actuarial methods and tools do not equip the offender with any portable tools to think, understand and act in a manner that helps in real-time situations.

References

Benjamin, L. (1996). *Interpersonal diagnosis and treatment of personality disorders* (2nd edn). New York: Guilford.

Birtchnell, J. (1993). *How humans relate: A new interpersonal theory*. Westport, CT: Praeger.

Blau, T. H. (1998). *The psychologist as expert witness* (2nd edn). Chichester: Wiley.

Brodsky, S. L. (1991). *Testifying in court: Guidelines and maxims for the expert witness*. Washington, DC: American Psychological Association.

Brodsky, S. L. (1999). *The expert's expert witness: More maxims and guidelines for testifying in court*. Washington, DC: American Psychological Association.

Casement, P. (1991). *Learning from the patient*. New York: Guilford.

Childress, J. F. (1989). The normative principle of medical ethics. In R. M. Vaetel, (Ed.), *Medical ethics*. Boston, MA: Jones & Bartlett.

Goffman, E. (1959). *The presentation of self in everyday life*. Malden, MA: Blackwell.

Hagen, M. A. (1997). *Whores of the court: The fraud of psychiatric testimony and the rape of American justice*. New York: Regan.

Hare, R. D. (1991). *The Hare Psychopathy Checklist–Revised*. Toronto: Multi-Health Systems.

Klawans, H. L. (1991). *Trials of an expert witness: Tales of clinical neurology and the law*. Boston, MA: Little, Brown.

Newnes, C. (2000). Psychiatric diagnosis: More questions than answers: Comment. *Psychologist, 13*, 390–391.

Pilgrim, D. (2000). Psychiatric diagnosis: More questions than answers. *Psychologist, 13*, 302–305.

Quinsey, V. L., Harris, G. T., Rice, M. E. & Cormier, C. A. (1998). *Violent offenders: Appraising and managing risk*. Washington, DC: American Psychological Association.

Ziskin, J. (1995). *Coping with psychiatric and psychological testimony* (5th edn) (vols 1–3). Los Angeles, CA: Law and Psychology Press.

Chapter 17

Fragile states and fixed identities

Using Cognitive Analytic Therapy to understand aggressive men in relational and societal terms

Karen Shannon, Abigail Willis & Steve Potter

> *Humpty Dumpty sat on a wall:*
> *Humpty Dumpty had a great fall.*
> *All the King's horses and all the King's men*
> *Couldn't put Humpty together again.*

A relational approach to treating male aggression

Mental health professionals in forensic settings are increasingly aware of the complexity of formulating a therapeutic response to aggression. The range of social issues of which aggression is a component include: sexual offending, domestic violence toward partners and children and violent offences within the public arena, including psychiatric and penal institutions.

Physical aggression against individuals has been considered predominantly a phenomenon of men. Reports indicate that the incidence of men cautioned or convicted for violence against person offences was 70 per 10 000 persons in the 16–24 age group and 47 per 10 000 in the overall population (Home Office, 2001). Men are also most frequently the victims. According to the British Crime Survey, one in five males aged 16–24 in England and Wales were the victims of violence in 1999 (Home Office, 2001) (notably, women are more often the victims in domestic violence; Home Office, Patterns of Crime Group, 2002). While women's convictions for more serious offences have increased in recent years (Chesney-Lind, 1977; Campbell, 1984; Poe-Yamagata & Butts, 1996), there remains a significant difference in the frequency of violent offences recorded (10 women per 10 000 cautioned or convicted for violent offences in the 16–24 years age group and 7.8 women per 10 000 in the overall population; see previous statistics provided for men (Home Office, 2001)). The causes for, and motivation behind, women's offending may be different, but, while important, they are not the focus of this chapter.

In this paper we use Cognitive Analytic Therapy's (CAT) integrative and relational framework to help with the formulation of the interaction between the states of mind, social identities and status positions which shape some men's experience of, and predisposition to, aggression. Among other influences, CAT draws upon the basic shift in psychoanalytic thinking from a predominantly drive theory to a more relational perspective (Mitchell, 2000; Nathanson, 1994; Fonagy *et al.*, 2004). The shift to a relational perspective is one which combines developments in object-relations theory, self-psychology and interpersonal therapy. However, CAT has further enriched both the therapeutic practice and theoretical foundations of this relational perspective through its ideas of reciprocal role procedures (RRPs), dialogical sequences and an integrative framework for understanding self–other restrictive and damaging interaction in the past and present. We feel CAT's integrative relational approach offers a way of working with aggressive men because it is capable of holding in view at the same time the intrapersonal, interpersonal and social dynamics that are constructing their behaviour.

Distinguishing anger from aggression

Williams & Barlow (1998) distinguish definitions of aggression and anger. Aggression is defined as 'any form of behaviour directed toward the goal of harming or injuring another living being or object'. This harm could be inflicted physically, verbally or by behavioural threat/intimidation. In contrast, anger is 'an emotional state experienced as the impulse to behave in order to protect, defend or attack in response to a threat or a challenge' (p. 54). Anger could thus be seen as a normal and healthy emotion experienced as part of a continuum of feeling and only sometimes precipitating aggression.

Anger has been considered from a variety of perspectives. Classically, it is seen as the 'moral' emotion inasmuch as it is perceived as a felt reaction to a sense of infringement or injustice (Power & Dalgleish, 1997). In cognitive-behavioural terms, anger is seen as a response to threat or the transgression of expectations; for example, in antisocial personality disorder, Beck, Freeman and associates consider anger as arising from the feeling of injustice that others seem to have what they deserve (Beck & Freeman, 1990). Anger has been seen as a stress response from the evolutionary perspective (Gilbert 1992; 2000; Dixon, 1998). Lazarus (1991) offers a view of anger and other key emotions as dependent upon an overall system of appraisal that he theorises in cognitive-relational terms. Within psychoanalytic literature, the focus has been more on the social requirements for the inhibition of emotion and their unconscious influence on character as repressed desires, which are defended against to maintain ego identity (Mitchell, 2000). With the more relational perspectives of object-relations theory, ego psychology and self-psychology, the focus has been on character disorder arising from restrictive or damaging experience of self-expression and regulation (Nathanson, 1994).

In this vein, our perspective is to move away from approaches that reductively see aggression merely as a behavioural element of anger and toward the more integrative psychosocial and relational framework that CAT offers. This suggests shifting the treatment focus on aggression from a narrow focus on anger as an emotion and towards the relational context in which aggression is enacted. Moreover, the focus on the causative role of anger in relation to aggression ignores the other contributing factors such as social exclusion, status positioning and use of aggression to achieve instrumental aims. A narrow focus may be adequate for more simple case formulations but is not enough to help the more complex and treatment-resistant cases with which we are working. We propose to explore aggression at the more general level of self-functioning and maintenance as a particular set of relational coping procedures. Our emphasis, as per CAT, is on high-level, accurate, shared description and understanding. CAT takes the RRP sequence (Ryle & Kerr, 2002) as its basic unit of study with a view to avoiding an atomistic reduction to bits of thinking, feeling or behaviour, thus losing sight of the larger and more socially situated relational pattern. We believe this more holistic perspective of CAT allows the multiple aspects of aggression to be worked with therapeutically and avoids reducing psychotherapeutic responses to aggression as only involving anger management.

Existing frameworks for working with this client group

Numerous authors cite a lack of robust studies evaluating psychological interventions for anger and fewer studies evaluating interventions directly targeting aggression (e.g. Novaco, 1997; Renwick, Black, Ramm & Novaco, 1997). A variety of approaches are to be found in the literature (Tafrate, 1995). Novaco, Ramm & Black (2001) highlight the fact that different approaches have varying levels of sophistication and individual tailoring. Reflecting this, Novaco's (1975; 1977) popular, cognitive-behavioural treatment package has been extended to include traumatic life experiences, addressing more widely distressing emotions, and utilising transference and counter-transference methods. This extension might reflect the need to frequently address the individual's victimisation, and, in a more relational way, widen the context for and function of, our view of aggressive behaviour. This approach is strengthened by the observation that anger is used to heighten self-esteem for individuals in secure environments. The clients in these environments see themselves as having low status and low personal control and consider talking about emotions to be at odds with a manly masculine identity, and to be a sign of being 'soft'. This seems to us to be a prompt to include status positions and identities associated with aggression in the formulation of the therapy. These ideas are echoed by Polaschek & Reynolds (2004) in describing the work of Guerra, Tolan & Hammond (1994): 'An exclusive anger control focus ignores other common motivational biases for violence . . . such as its normative and status restorative functions' (p. 211). Within restrictive reciprocal interactions, such as gang leader to gang member, abusive husband to abused wife, abusive parent to abused child, it is 'usually the most dominant who is more free to express anger and aggression and use it as a means to assert their rank, authority and control' (Allan & Gilbert, 2002; p. 553).

In the literature on the treatment of male anger, compliance rates with current therapy frameworks remain low even in recent studies (Siddle, Jones & Awenat, 2003). It may be that a narrow and restricted conceptualisation of these complex clients can explain some of these engagement difficulties. From the observations, it seems that historically, 'there has been an absence of an adequate conceptual framework to guide theoretically coherent programme development' (Serin & Brown, 1996; p. 79; Howells *et al.*, 1997). We propose a framework using CAT that takes this social and relational construction further. While few psychological studies have explored the role of the victim of aggression between men as opposed to the role of the offender (Price, 1988; 1991), we believe a relational approach would also be relevant in this context.

The role of aggression in establishing, maintaining or restoring status positions is culturally and socially determined. A sociological description of the complexity of these culture and identity processes is beyond the limits of this study. However, the social dynamics of men's aggression does need to be included in the therapeutic formulation. In this respect, we intend to use CAT as a broad-enough framework to offer a combined description of intrapersonal, interpersonal and social dynamics. Aggressive activity in CAT terms is understood as a procedural sequence of intentions, feelings and interactions which relate to assumptions arising out of a dialogue between personal history, states of mind, sense of self and social identity. Previous thinking has tended to locate aggression as a problem within the individual and in so doing problematised him. What seems to be lacking is a more fine-grained relational analysis of how some men exhibit aggression in response to seemingly unmanageable status and identity requirements, such as being dominant without any legitimate social authority, or to unmanageable emotional role requirements, such as maintaining composure while inhibiting emotional reactions to experiences of humiliation and abandonment. Our concern is to see how an individual's aggression is nested within harmful or restrictive masculine social identities and relational roles.

Future ways of conceptualising and providing intervention for this client group

We hope this chapter is also a contribution towards a more respectful approach to this client population by virtue of striving to be less reductive. It seeks to offer a more versatile relational framework based on narcissistic personality difficulties and their solutions, which are gender specific. The idea of narcissistic solutions is outlined in the section below.

Our starting point is to make use of the cognitive-analytic formulations of narcissistic personality disorder (NPD) (Ryle, 1995a) and borderline personality disorder (BPD) (Ryle, 1997). Ryle (1990) views individuals with both borderline and narcissistic presentations as having poorly integrated personalities with two or more distinct sets of reciprocal roles. NPD is conceptualised as a set of reciprocal roles coupled with a predominating grandiose self-concept and an inordinate need for recognition from others in order to avoid, or dissociate from, intolerable feelings of contempt. On the other hand, BPD is characterised by reciprocal roles reflecting the tension between longing for ideal care and fearing abandonment, while coping with the feared recurrence of abuse through the use of various dissociative states. Both personality disorder presentations have elements of dissociation that contribute to a lack of integration and reduced capacity for self-reflection. It is important to note that both types of personality disorder produce entangled expectations of self and others. For instance, in the case of individuals with NPD presentation, the other must be admiring in order for the self to experience being valued. In BPD, rescue from an abusive, inconsistent or absent other can be secured only through the provision of ideal care. What constitutes the other in these patterns of relating must not be seen as simply another person but as the role expected of, or played by, another, perhaps within a group or societal context. Admiration or ideal care might then be linked to a particular social identity or status position.

In working with the aggressive, male-offender population, it seems to make sense (for both us as clinicians, and the client group) to make use of aspects of both the NPD and BPD formulations. Aggressive men seem to alternate between warding off threats to self-esteem and safety by seeking a dominant grandiose position (as in NPD) and by seeking ideal care (as in BPD). Commonly, these men may covertly seek care in a way that to them seems legitimate and unthreatening to their self-esteem; for example, by declaring to a social worker their fear of harming someone. In our experience, the aggressive, male forensic client group has, like other NPD and BPD clients, typically experienced trauma and traumatic relationships, profound loss, deprivation and abuse. As with NPD and BPD, the internalisation of this traumatic relationship is understood in CAT terms as a polarised and restricted reciprocal role repertoire forming separated or dissociated self-states. These result in a fragmented sense of self, unmanageable feelings and untried feeling skills with the consequent inhibition of new learning, self-reflection or integration. We propose that for this particular client group NPD and BPD are closely linked, as detailed in our diagrams in Figs 17.1 and 17.2.

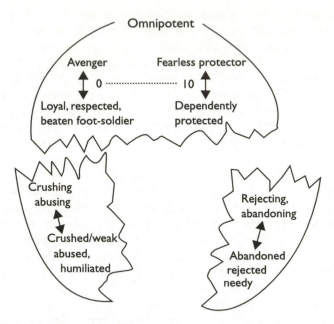

Figure 17.1 The broken-egg formulation.

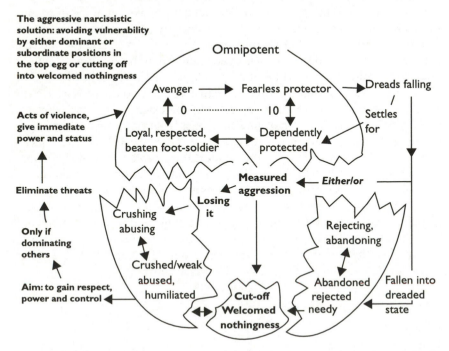

Figure 17.2 Sequential diagrammatic reformulation of client's attempts to maintain the dominant position.

Narcissistic solutions: An introduction to the framework

Having conducted a series of case reviews, we suggest that the damaged or unmet needs for care and attention are partially, and destructively, resolved by male, forensic clients in a narcissistically disturbed search for safety and control through aggressive domination. This is partly expressed through abuse and humiliation of the other and partly through co-opting or being co-opted as a respected and included subordinate to a powerful other. This is often enacted through a very restrictive male group dynamic. A stereotypical example in our culture would be the main doorman of a nightclub; he represents a larger-than-life male figure, able to control the response of the other by whatever means necessary in a powerful, dominating and avenging fashion. A novice doorman looking on might be in awe and admire his power and ability to control others. He may value the apprenticeship role and welcome his subordinated status to this more powerful individual, including accepting a loyal and respected foot-soldier position when undertaking menial tasks for him. Both the dominant and subordinated men are working in collusion to avoid the abused position familiar to them in childhood and a more profoundly dissociated position of abandonment and neglect to which we now turn.

In addition to the narcissistic and more easily recognisable socio-cultural element of this client group of top dog and subordinate loyal foot soldier, there also appear to be elements of BPD. We have incorporated these in the framework; in particular, the pattern of seeking ideal care or protection in a way that avoids any experience of dreaded vulnerability and abandonment. This can be seen in the narcissistic need to impose care on others and elicit care in quite restrictive and rigid ways such as through the controlling but protective social identity offered by group/gang membership. In this vein, we conceptualise the adoption of a reciprocal role relationship of fearless protector to dependently (submissively or compliantly) protected. If we take our example further, the doorman may coexist as a 'bruiser', superdad figure who can protect 'weaker' individuals in the face of any adversity, leaving the junior doorman in a protected but dependent position.

Rather than viewing these sets of reciprocal roles as separate, we view them as coexisting on a sliding scale (see the top half of Fig. 17.1). The scale goes from *avenger-to-fearless protector*, with an overarching theme of omnipotence (powerfully controlling) for both positions that can be used either for protection or to subordinate others. For example, the teenage son of the main doorman could experience his father as an omnipotent avenger. He is required to follow the behavioural code of his father and is subordinated to do this, with 'fear of' and 'control by' responses enmeshed with admiration and inevitable dominance (foot-soldier to avenger). Or, in the same example, the son could experience his father as an omnipotent protector (fearless protector to dependently protected), if there were threats of attack from others outside the family. The position of omnipotent, powerful avenger to foot-soldier on the one hand, and fearless protector to protected dependent on the other may be interchangeable expressions of early experiences of family modelling. The states may indeed co-act. An individual is unlikely to go into a fearless protector position without the avenger state/status in the wings ready to 'kick off' if their protective manoeuvres are felt to render them too vulnerable. These reciprocal roles may have developed in response to early relationships with parents, the experience of gangs and peer relationships and in combination with responses to subcultural styles and status pressures. They shape interpersonal and intrapersonal functioning and the choice of social identity as they serve to regulate otherwise unmanageable states. The idea of a sliding scale helps the therapist and the client see how violent behaviour may be justified in terms of a protector or avenger position. It also offers a self-monitoring framework for the recognition in therapy showing how less damaging (less extreme) enactment of these self–other states and patterns may be achieved.

An important element to note is that both of these reciprocal roles tend to be subjectively experienced as inevitable or destined for both the doorman and the son. They seem destined because societal influences emphasise both these roles but with a preference for the protector role as opposed to the dependently protected role.

Diagrammatically, we have incorporated the sliding scale between two linked reciprocal roles within what was dubbed in CAT a 'split-egg' diagram to emphasise the fragmentation of these individuals into two core states (Ryle, 1995b). In our review of a series of cases and from continuing supervisory and clinical experience, the bottom of the two states seems best understood as broken off into two further parts, with the abandoning to abandoned state as the painful and disallowed core from which subsequent positions and experiences are restrictively built. We have dubbed this the 'broken' egg rather than the 'split' egg. Use of the broken-egg diagram resonates with clients' sense of an acute and powerful division within their masculine identity of either being on top and dominant or falling to a weak, vulnerable and humiliating position. Working with these aggressive men has shown that it makes sense for them to prefer putting themselves in the top half of the egg and to favour the dominant reciprocal role (*omnipotent avenger-omnipotent protector*). However, the less dominant position of foot-soldier or dependently protected is favoured over the reciprocal roles in the bottom half of the egg. The two bottom states contain reciprocal roles derived from earlier abuse and trauma, characterised by humiliation and abuse on the one hand and abandonment and neglect on the other. We believe that the experience of aggressive male offenders is often understandable as a linked series of dreaded, desired or endured mental states embedded in a particular group or social status position.

These reciprocal roles represent the internalisation and reactivation of the abuse and neglect experienced by these men in their life histories. There is likely to be constant vigilance as part of an effort to avoid the intolerable positions in the bottom parts of the 'broken-egg' diagram. These men recognise that despite this striving to remain at the top, it is an unstable and fragile place, and they fear falling into the dreaded and unyielding positions depicted in the bottom broken parts of the egg. The time spent in each self-state can vary to a greater or lesser extent depending on the relative stability of the narcissistic and borderline elements. We have made use of the split-egg diagram, which has been superseded in CAT theory and practice by the multiple self-states model (MSSM) diagram (to capture more fragmented patterns of personality organisation; Ryle & Kerr, 2002), because we believe there is a hierarchical, sequential and social coherence to the changing states experienced by these men that adds up to a particular type of aggressive masculine identity. Much of it is socially orchestrated in tandem with the internal processes of dissociation. It is probable that only the earliest and most painful part depicted by the broken egg – that associated with being abandoned and neglected and experiencing vulnerability – is partially dissociated. Hence the diagrammatic depiction of this reciprocal role as slightly more broken off.

Top egg: maintaining the 'hard man' image

In maintaining the top-egg self-state, there are limits to acceptable social behaviour defined by the subcultural rules of a gang, which tend to emphasise rigid leadership and conformist membership. Intimacy and vulnerability are ritualistically controlled by a tight code of conduct. In this context, prison mirrors the dynamics of gang life and can be experienced as *the* omnipotent power, with individuals adopting respectful subordination, in response to a more powerful entity. This allows the individual to maintain a sense of agency in a restrictive environment in the foot-soldier position. Society also sanctions some of the means of adopting the omnipotent avenger and foot-soldier positions and, in doing so, endorses some forms of violent behaviour. It is common for clients to believe that society affirms their self-identity, and that aggression is acceptable if it is carefully measured and justified, as in acts of retribution. In this view, although an individual may feel responsible for violence, this is as much likely to be associated with pride and self-righteousness as guilt or remorse. Indeed, this type of aggressive retribution is glamorised or condoned at times in the media; for example, when the newspapers supported a campaign of vigilante attacks on sex offenders by printing their personal details and residence. Within the idealised position, there are alternative positions to aggression that can be adopted; thus, whether aggressive avenging is chosen, or acts of protection or subordination, will depend on a variety of factors both external and internal to the individual.

Such procedures fit with masculine social identities and the power of a group of men to see these positions as self-evident. Society's endorsement can offer a temporary sense of self-coherence. However, such coherence can mean analysis of an aggressive incident, or empathy for the other party, is prevented by not being able to get beyond the barrier of the self-evident identity procedure: 'this is our way of life' and 'this is what a man has got to do'. Empathy and any sense of personal choice or autonomy are lost by the justification that one is only applying prescribed rules of thought and behaviour. Society tends to put socially disadvantaged men (without sanctioned ways of being dominant) into the acute psychological dilemma of either being powerful only through being dominant and aggressive or being a weak, inadequate failure.

Where the dominant position is hard to sustain (through lack of social power, status or opportunity) and the humiliated position is barely tolerable, pressure is placed on others to play the reciprocal and more tolerable position, the loyal foot-soldier. In this way, they may participate in the idealised position of powerful avenger/protector vicariously, as a bystander or assistant (the example of the inexperienced bouncer). This mirrors some male-dominated recreations, such as football fans feeling the reflected glory of their team winning. This is also reflected in society's view that men should be able to cope, adopting the position of the coping foot-soldier who is able to continue despite pressures to follow the leadership or authority, and not cry or show weakness (fall into the inadequate and vulnerable position). However, being positioned in the intolerable bottom half of the egg may occur in response to external triggers such as experiencing others as abusive or abandoning and being pushed to the weak, humiliated reciprocal position. For example, an individual experiencing physical aggression may feel crushed and humiliated though later adopting the position of a beaten opponent. Other internal triggers for falling to the lower parts of the broken egg are those of trauma and the unpredictability of intrusive symptoms. Various methods of avoidance and the 'cut-off' state maintain these symptoms. Furthermore, as described before, adopting a cut-off state may be a means of moving from and gaining respite from this intolerable position.

In our experience, the idealised position at the top of the egg diagram also cannot be sustained when an individual recognises his own behaviour as 'extreme' and abusive rather than that of a just and powerful avenger, as for example, if he realises that an act of retribution has gone too far and the victim is perceived as one having been crushed and humiliated rather than a suitably beaten opponent. If the idealised position cannot be achieved or is not opted for, the alternatives to remaining crushed and abused are to become abusive oneself (as in performing acts of cruelty not within one's own rules of conduct, such as acts of domestic violence or cruelty), or to shift into dissociation by cutting off, being numb and unfeeling. The latter is frequently achieved through substance misuse, social withdrawal and blanking out of others. This state appears to exist across clients on a continuum from zombified blankness, numbness to conscious withdrawal. This has been described by clients as 'welcomed nothingness', a respite position from the constant striving to maintain the dominant, controlling, 'top of the egg' position, and away from the dreaded and intolerable vulnerable and crushed or abandoned state.

Case study

Nathan, aged 39, was referred by the probation service for an assessment of his risk of violence. He had a long history of violent offences, which had resulted in numerous prison sentences. With confidentiality limitations firmly in place, he proudly alluded to numerous other offences that had gone unreported due to the code of the macho subculture of which Nathan was a key member.

Nathan was one of four brothers. He exhibited behavioural problems at an early age, including bullying of peers, setting fires and general defiance. He described his father as a he-man figure employed on building sites. His father always used his strength to overcome adversity, and he belittled signs of weakness and vulnerability in others. Therefore, his father offered little in the way of emotional care or support. As a child, he often witnessed his father's violence toward his mother. He felt powerless to protect her from his father, and she had few emotional resources left to offer Nathan. In order to cope with his disallowed feelings of rejection, abandonment, powerlessness and neediness, Nathan developed means to cut off from emotion (Fig. 17.2, 'welcomed nothingness'). He achieved this by disappearing on his own for miles on bicycle rides, hiding alone in coal sheds, and later misusing alcohol and drugs. In mid-adolescence, he especially liked to ride his bicycle on stormy nights to pit his strength and courage against the elements, seeking to gain his own sense of power, control and omnipotence (Fig. 17.1, procedure to maintain the top-egg state). He also took to swimming out to sea to experience the feeling of being alive.

In his late teens, his grandfather and father reinforced his aggressive behaviour when they periodically had him adopt the vigilante role. Gradually, he gained a reputation within his locality as a 'just avenger' and a prestigious status within a gang subculture where people gave him their loyalty and respect (see Fig. 17.1, top half of the broken egg). Periodically, gang members attempted to climb the hierarchy past him, but, when beaten by Nathan, they resumed a position of admiring loyalty to him. Nathan found that not only did he achieve power and status in his role of avenger, but also he was, all powerfully, able to protect weaker gang members and girlfriends. Vicariously, he experienced being close to others in his protector role while not losing credibility or status. Positively for Nathan, they became dependent upon protection from him (Fig. 17.2). Each party needed the other to ensure their needs were met.

Although Nathan had achieved his position within the subculture over years, he always felt a lack of security. Nathan feared there was someone waiting in the wings to knock him down, and he was therefore tense and hypervigilant for signs that others were challenging him. He was also unsure how he would maintain his position as he grew older and his physical strength declined. Furthermore, when avenging, he was required to measure carefully just the right amount of violence or he risked losing the respect of the gang for being an 'out-of-control nutter' (Fig. 17.1, bottom half of the broken egg). All of these pressures meant that Nathan, although apparently dominant and intimidating, still experienced the underlying feelings of vulnerability and weakness he had sought to overcome.

Bottom parts of the broken egg: The 'sneaky' narcissistic solution

Early experiences contribute to the development of the reciprocal roles depicted in the lower parts of the broken-egg diagram. Feeling crushed and abused in response to experiences of humiliation is common, as is the feeling of being neglected and abandoned in response to withholding and absent care. In early experiences, the feelings of the bottom egg state, being crushed or abandoned, are either chronically endured or fearfully avoided (usually through attempts to adopt instead the abusive or abandoning role, or through the cut-off state). These reciprocal roles are listed in the bottom part of Fig. 17.3.

The need or aim to escape hurt and damage (i.e. feeling crushed and abandoned), referred to by one client as 'the pits of hell', may lead to assumptions about the need for control. It can feel more tolerable to be at the abusing and abandoning poles rather than their reciprocals. (Sometimes this is achieved to the degree that individuals may have almost no awareness of their opposing experience, e.g. *crushed* and *abandoned*.) However, neither of these positions is rewarding or stable. States of dominance or control that may feel like escape from dreaded states of humiliation may also feel unstable. More widely, they constantly invite retaliatory response, or escalation, which in return requires constant vigilance and the shoring up of the control position. This instability results in the individual's falling back into feared hurt and damage, and feeling constantly unsafe, producing hyperarousal similar to post-traumatic states (Horowitz, 1998). Thus, one can see the cycling or 'shimmering' (as described by Horowitz) between omnipotent control and vulnerability evident in these clients.

Unlike the situation represented in Fig. 17.2, where an individual's aggression and dominance are overt, other clients with a history of aggression

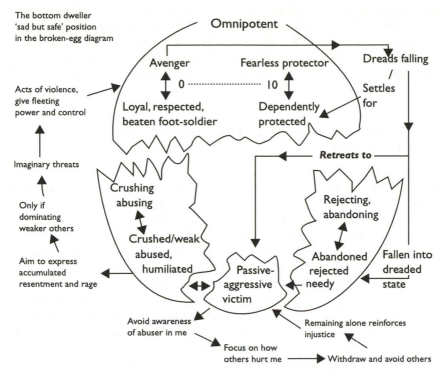

Figure 17.3 Sequential diagrammatic reformulation of the 'sneaky' narcissistic solution.

conceal their rage and their sense of omnipotence. All too aware of their painful 'bottom-egg' state, they often adopt a victimised stance as opposed to that of aggressor, and although they yearn for the top-egg state, they position themselves to be retraumatised and trapped in this humiliating and degraded bottom-egg position. These clients assume that any attempts at moving from this position would result in their inevitably being positioned back in the humiliated state. Therefore, they do not attempt to assert goals or strive to achieve the top-egg state, as returning to the 'gutter' again heightens and compounds intolerable psychological pain. But adopting a 'preferred' sad but safe position instead, with certainty and predictability, ensures that they can 'fall no further'. However, this pattern does not account for the self-loathing and rage these men experience. Often a rich internal fantasy life or projective social identification is utilised as a means of entering into the top-egg state and gaining fleeting omnipotence and dominance. Even in reality, they may somewhat 'sneakily' and fleetingly enter into the top egg in an abusive fashion, defending their core of weakness, humiliation and inadequacy. This may be done through concealed acts of avenging, such as attacks on those they see as 'lower than them' (e.g. racially motivated attacks, domestic violence and offences against children), yet they quickly return to the seemingly safe, victimised position in the lower half of the egg as this behaviour transgresses moral codes. This client group struggles to acknowledge the sneakily abusive, crushing and controlling aspects of their personality by adopting a self-protective stance as victim. This is illustrated in Fig. 17.3.

The societal context: States, social identities and status positions

In formulating our approach above, we are seeking to combine an understanding of the internalised patterns of states of mind associated with aggression and masculine group social identities and status positions. In considering the sociology of social identity, Giddens (1991) and Jenkins (1996) are examples of writers who take an integrative and dialogical view in ways that resonate with CAT. For Giddens in particular, the twentieth century saw the emergence of a new kind of self-identity with an associated life politics where a more exposed and reflective self has continuously to negotiate meaning and position in society. For Giddens, the speed and uncertainty of social change are key and historically unique features. In his perspective, one can note that men's social identities have undergone a continuing process of profound changes, which, for many men, are opportunities for a more rounded and balanced sense of self. However, we feel that this newly exposed and uncertain life politics compounds the isolation and deprivation of men with very limited social support and resources. Some men have lost their place in a variety of ways at work, at home and in the community. These men lack the internal coherence or basic security of self to respond to changes in previously fixed gender positions for handling intimacy, love and care that have been freed and replaced by a more enlightening but more diverse set of possibilities. Within feminist theory and practice (Flax, 1990; echoed by Giddens above), there has long been a focus on a politics of self and identity and new and rich relational discourses for how men and women should handle intimacy, conflict and difference. While these changes have brought many benefits in terms of gender equality and challenges to discriminatory and sexist assumptions, they demand greater emotional and psychological literacy and adaptability. These changes have been the subject of varied responses and discussions. However, for the purposes of this chapter, for some men who have lost traditional economic and social position or who have very limited social opportunities for esteem and status, or for whom traditional masculine identities remain an important defence against humiliation and vulnerability, there can feel far less room to move toward positive or enlightened change. They may have less access to privilege and fewer ways to hide more self-consciously exposed aspects of self. Such men may be less able to adapt to the more informal relational competencies required for these changes (Goleman, 1998) and the life politics described by Giddens. They may feel chronically exposed and unsure how to reconcile new and old conflicting masculine identities unless this social context is openly built into some form of psychoeducational programme alongside any therapeutic intervention. With the combination of their history of trauma and deprivation, their retreat into the narcissistic and sneaky means of coping described by us and these restrictive social opportunities, these men may further retreat into an outsider position in society. Such a retreat further compounds their reduced exposure to changes in men's identity and their less gender-defined, more relationally adaptive ways of coping. The development of the highly restrictive, internal self-management procedures which we describe, and their reinforcement by a narrow social identity, leave the population of men with whom we work with limited options for a more varied sense of self and reflection.

We feel our work requires us to link more closely society's role in moulding aggressive patterns of coping and to provide a means to understand the complex interaction between social control mechanisms, welfare institutions, social identities, and self-states. We need to assist aggressive men to see their social positioning within an emotionally unmanageable and restricted space. Often, through therapy, monitoring the most painful aspects of unmanageable procedures and feelings allows men with whom we work to avoid disabling forms of self-blame and shame. They can recognise deficits in the capacity for self-reflection and regulation of feelings and behaviour in relation to themselves and others. Better understanding and coping skills and increased access to their own warded-off feelings allows the development of empathy for others and, hence, the modulation and inhibition of aggressive behaviour and assumptions.

Mental states, social identity and status positions are all interwoven in complex and changing ways, but they offer useful analytic distinctions. For example, Nathan may say that he feels invincible and powerful (a state of mind) and sees himself as a gang leader (a social identity) who is above all others (status position). Nathan cannot say any of these things without drawing upon the society within and through which he is relationally woven and by whom he is categorised. Nathan can know only himself and have a sense of himself through his dialogue with others and for himself. His self is social. Some of the states he gets into and the social identities he occupies will be partly outside his awareness and are only activated in certain situations.

The two self-states described in our narcissistic solutions framework may thus be associated with differential status positions and identities, as illustrated in the diagram in Fig. 17.4. Each layer is associated with a network weaving between states, status, reciprocal roles and identities.

Individuals shimmer, slide and switch between top and bottom broken-egg

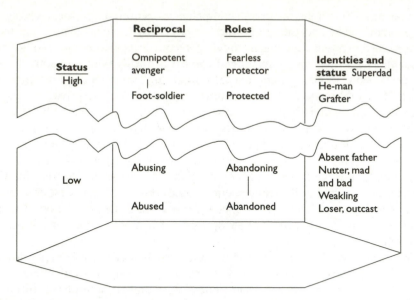

Figure 17.4 The layered relationship between states, identity and status.

states in a way related partly to functional masculine subcultural identities and partly to collusive processes of self-justification. Thus, an individual may move between identities such as he-man and superdad, mad and bad, and absent father, depending on the subjective experience of demands both internally and externally. Moves across bands will be associated with changing status as well as identity. Thus, the oscillations in these men's lives promote a culminating sense of chaos and insecurity. This insecurity may be compounded by the changing gender roles and identities offered to men, some of which conflict with the deeper emotional roles these men wish for or are driven to adopt.

In moving away from the dilemma of either romanticisation or demonisation of aggression, we begin to understand violence as a narrow narcissistic repertoire of desperate solutions. We see reciprocal role analysis as a means of creating dialogue, which extends beyond interpersonal relations to social action, identity and culture. CAT as a descriptive framework helps us explore how adult social identities link with early relational roles and emotional experience to produce problematic and dangerous states of mind and associated patterns of behaviour that thwart attempts at healthy self-regulation and development.

Formulating and using narcissistic solutions in therapy

Developing individual sequential diagrammatic reformulations allows therapist and client to work collaboratively within a shared framework of feeling and understanding. For this group of aggressive male offenders, seeking therapy is incredibly difficult, as they fear exposure to the crushed, humiliated, abandoned role. A common ambivalent dialogue regards emotional exploration and a preference at times for 'safety' in familiar positions and places, including incarceration in prison, instead. The framework provides an explanation for this, the strong subcultural influence and the high attrition rates associated with this client group. Therapists can gain a purchase on these men's social positions and their reality and, importantly, the realistic perception of, and degree of potential for, therapeutic change. Emotional exploration can be collaboratively graded within the client's zone of proximal development incorporating empathic listening to both dissociated parts. The utility of this framework requires further investigation to see whether these benefits can be achieved more widely.

The broken-egg framework can conceptualise identities including culture, class, gender, ethnicity and the complex means by which these reciprocally interface with social status, states of mind and the self-state. Clinically, without this framework, therapeutic change can be impeded. It seems the reality of these aggressive offending men's lives is not merely constrained by restricted internal reciprocal roles but also by the limited social/gender identity opportunities and the antagonistic position of attempting to gain a 'valued' status in a marginalised subculture.

Lack of recognition by the therapist of the impact of therapeutic change on masculine identity and status risks the aggressive offender's being 'laid bare' and exposed to or open to abuse and humiliation by his peer group (which pushes him to the bottom state on the left of the diagram), or exposed to the more often dissociated, intolerable state of feeling, and being, abandoned. The scaffolding provided by the broken-egg diagram, with the *abandoning-to-abandoned* reciprocal role somewhat split off, provides some security in tracking this potential. In this way, a poignant aspect of intervention is the utilisation of the CAT reformulation in a way that can help join with the client to open dialogue and empower the individual regarding the choice, timing, or degree of therapeutic change. Moreover, with the therapist's and client's full awareness of the implications of change for their masculine identity, status and their sense of self, the framework enables the therapist to empathise with this dilemma and assist. To some extent, using this CAT approach addresses the dilemma described by Smail (2001), who states 'one should not . . . underestimate the value psychotherapy might have as a means of clarifying their [the client's] situation . . . but nor should one overestimate its ability to change them' (p. 351).

Our approach suggests that aggressive men offenders shimmer between experiences of 'omnipotent avenger' and fearless protector/loyal foot-soldier, both of which are elements of masculine social identities and are equally (in a contradictory way) powerfully reinforced and punished by society. These men experience society as intrigued by and admiring of them sometimes, yet denigrating and dismissive at other times. In focusing upon the denigrating aspect, it could be argued that this group of individuals provides a societal function of blame for society's ills whereby blaming others helps reduce society's collective responsibility. The argument runs: only if their 'animalistic criminal behaviour' is eradicated, will society then be capable of being ideal. Hidden within the denigration of these men is a collusive reciprocation between social expectation and their life experience which encourages dissociation and denial. Perhaps we have our own idealism in the hope that therapy should promote in the individual the development of a more benign 'safe', supported and self-monitoring position in relation to a supportive, watchful but trusting society. The implication of this approach at the level of policy and politics suggests a need for change in society toward providing support, balanced monitoring of, and response to, aggression.

We have now begun to deliver this intervention in the form of four individual reformulation sessions followed by a small therapeutic and educational group experience, including from six to eight aggressive male offenders, and lasting for 16 sessions. We hope the group experience will provide these men with a shared perspective on the fears of vulnerability and the restrictive practices and powerful cultural pressures that frustrate change. Of particular interest will be the opportunity to address the reciprocal role of feeling abandoned and needy, which is hardest to acknowledge. We have begun to apply this approach with a case series, and it seems increasingly likely that therapeutic success depends upon accessing this early and recurring core pain in a constructive way.

We hope our approach has value for conducting therapy not just in measuring up to the complexity of working with this group of men in therapy, but also its valuable contribution to the assessment of risk of offending behaviour. For example, the broken-egg framework offers an individually-tailored risk assessment tool for potential offending/reoffending behaviour and the conditions that make it probable (such as procedures leading to either avenging or humiliating aggression). Moreover, because this is achieved collaboratively with the client, it encourages understanding of, and accountability for, behaviour. Ultimately, this approach reframes an understanding of the behaviour not only for the client, but also for other agencies around them, and, more generally, for society as a whole. Perhaps it is a case of all the king's men and all the king's horses could not put Humpty together again, but a carefully planned relational and integrative therapeutic intervention can.

References

Allan, S. & Gilbert, P. (2002). Anger and anger expression in relation to perceptions of social rank, entrapment and depressive symptoms. *Personality and Individual Differences, 32*, 553.

Beck, A. T. & Freeman, A. (1990). *Cognitive therapy of personality disorders*. New York: Guilford Press.

Campbell, A. (1984). *The girls in the gang*. London: Basil Blackwell.

Chesney-Lind, M. (1977). Judicial paternalism and the female status offender: Training women to know their place. *Crime and Delinquency, 23*, 121–128.

Dixon, C. (1998). Ethological strategies for defence in animals and humans: Their role in some psychiatric disorders. *British Journal of Medical Psychology, 71*, 417–446.

Flax, J. (1990). *Thinking fragments: Psychoanalysis, feminism and postmodernism in the contemporary West*. Berkeley, CA: University of California Press.

Fonagy, P., Gergely, G., Jurist, E. L. & Target, M. (2004). *Affect regulation, mentalisation and the development of the self*. London: Karnac.

Giddens, A. (1991) *Modernity and self-identity*. London: Polity.

Gilbert, P. (1992). *Depression: The evolution of powerlessness*. Hove: Lawrence Erlbaum.

Gilbert, P. (2000). Varieties of submissive behaviour: Evolution and role in depression. In L. Slogan & P. Gilbert (Eds), *Subordination and defeat. An evolutionary approach to mood disorders*. Hove: Lawrence Erlbaum.

Goleman, D. (1998). *Working with emotional intelligence*. London: Bantam.

Guerra, N. G., Tolan, P. H. & Hammond, W. R (1994). Prevention and treatment of adolescent violence. In L. D. Eron, J. H. Gentry & P. Schlegel (Eds), *Reason to hope: A psychosocial perspective on violence and youth* (pp. 383–403). Washington, DC: American Psychological Association.

Home Office (2001). Offenders found guilty of, or cautioned for, indictable offences by type of offence and age. *Social Trends, 33*. www.statistics.gov.uk/StatBase/ssdataset.asp

Home Office: Patterns of Crime Group (2002). *Crime in England and Wales 2001/2002*.

Horowitz, M. J. (1998). *Cognitive psychodynamics*. Chichester: Wiley.

Howells, K., Watt, B., Hall, G. & Baldwin, A. (1997). Developing programmes for violent offenders. *Legal and Criminological Psychology*. In C. Hollin (Ed.), *Handbook of Offender Assessment and Treatment* (pp. 2, 117–128). Chichester: Wiley.

Jenkins, R. (1996). *Social identity*. London: Routledge.

Lazarus, R. S. (1991). *Emotion and adaptation*. Oxford: Open University Press.

Maple, N. & Simpson, I. (1995). CAT in groups. In A. Ryle (Ed.), *Cognitive Analytic Therapy: Developments of theory and practice*. Chichester: Wiley.

Mitchell, S. A. (2000). *Relationality: From attachment to intersubjectivity*. New Jersey: The Analytic Press.

Nathanson, S. M. (1994). *Character styles*. London: Norton Press.

Novaco, R. W. (1975). *Anger control: The development and evaluation of an experimental treatment*. Lexington, MA: DC Heath.

Novaco, R. W. (1977). Stress inoculation: A cognitive therapy and its application to a case of depression. *Journal of Consulting and Clinical Psychology, 45*, 600–608.

Novaco, R. W. (1997). Remediating anger and aggression with violent offenders. *Journal of Criminological Psychology*, 2, 77–88.

Novaco, R. W., Ramm, M. & Black, L. (2001). Anger treatment with offenders. In C. Hollin (Ed.), *Handbook of Offender Assessment and Treatment*. Chichester: Wiley.

Poe-Yamagata, E. & Butts, J. A. (1996). *Female offenders in the juvenile justice system: Statistics summary*. National Centre for Juvenile Justice, USA.

Polaschek, D. L. L. & Reynolds, N. (2004). Assessment and violence in offenders. In C. Hollin (Ed.), *Handbook of Offender Assessment and Treatment*. Chichester: Wiley.

Power, M. & Dalgleish, T. (1997). *Cognition and emotion*. London: Psychology Press.

Price, J. S. (1988). Alternative channels for negotiating asymmetry in social relationships. In M. R. A. Chance (Ed.), *Social fabrics of the mind*. London: Lawrence Erlbaum.

Price, J. S. (1991). Homeostasis or change: A systems theory to depression. *Journal of Medical Psychology*, 64, 331–334.

Renwick, S. J., Black, L., Ramm, M. & Novaco, R. W. (1997). Anger treatment with forensic hospital patients. *Legal and Criminological Psychology*, 2, 103–116.

Ryle, A. (1995a). *Cognitive Analytic Therapy: Developments in theory and practice*. Chichester: Wiley.

Ryle, A. (1995b). Transference and counter-transference variations in the course of the Cognitive-Analytic Therapy of two borderline patients: The relation to the diagrammatic reformulation of self-states. *British Journal of Medical Psychology*, 68, 109–124.

Ryle, A. (Ed.) (1997). *Cognitive Analytic Therapy and borderline personality disorder*. Chichester: Wiley.

Ryle, A. & Kerr, I. B. (2002). *Introducing Cognitive Analytic Therapy*. Chichester: Wiley.

Serin, R. & Brown, S. (1997). Treatment programs for offenders with violent histories: A national survey. *Forum on Corrections Research*, 9 (2).

Siddle, R., Jones, F. & Awenat, F. (2003). Group cognitive behaviour therapy for anger: A pilot study. *Behavioural and Cognitive Psychotherapy*, 31, 69–83.

Smail, D. (2001). *Why therapy doesn't work and what we should do about it*. London: Robinson.

Tafrate, R. C. (1995). Evaluation of treatment strategies for adult anger disorders. In H. Kassinove (Ed.), *Anger disorders: Definition, diagnosis and treatment*. Washington, DC: Taylor & Francis.

Williams, E. & Barlow, R. (1998). *Anger control training. Part 3: The anger control-training guide*. Bicester: Winslow Press.

Chapter 18

In the light of experience

Ruth Wyner (editorial commentary by Michael Göpfert)

Editor's comment

We are very privileged to be able to offer this first-hand account by a person who can speak from experience of having been in prison. Ruth Wyner had never expected to go there. We hope that it will help the reader to better understand the context of forensic work, especially those who are peripheral to it. The account illustrates the potentially traumatising aspects of going to prison. Of course, this experience is not the same for everyone, and this is only one account. Editorial comments aim to link the narrative to a Cognitive Analytic Therapy (CAT) framework.

My experience of prison is one of fragmentation and disintegration of the self and a regression to less adult ways of functioning. On release, elation quickly turned into depression and despair. Why is this so? How does it feel and what does it mean for the individual? I hope to look at these issues largely from a personal perspective, having been imprisoned myself for 7 months in the year 2000, but also linking it to a more objective perspective I have gained during the few years that have transpired since my release.

There are various phases to a person's imprisonment. It is well known that the first week or so can cause an intense and deeply painful response, akin to the trauma of separation. The prisoner then starts to adjust to the new environment, the reality of which tends to give rise to despair. In a few months' time, there can be another change, whereby the prisoner feels that they have got control of the situation and found ways to cope. This can be empowering and a great relief. But often it is not until later that the prisoner realises what has been lost to get to that point, and how hard it is to maintain it.

First phase

I hardly slept during my first few days at Holloway Prison. I hardly ate either. The food was completely unappetising, but it was my traumatised system that refused it, reinforced by thoughts of being so useless, so worthless, so inherently bad that I did not deserve any nourishment.

I drank tea, sweet tea, though I did not usually take sugar. And I smoked, despite being a non-smoker for 10 years past. I was desperate for a fag as soon as I lost my freedom. Shamelessly, I cadged them, hoarded dog-ends (mine and other people's), and coughed at every puff. I did not care about the damage I was obviously doing to myself. The hurt to my throat and lungs seemed an appropriate reflection to the hurt I felt inside.

I had already been turned inside out by the experience of arrest, months on bail, the trial and the sentencing. After being sentenced, I had to spend the night in a police cell because it was too late to get to a prison. I felt during that night as if I'd become less than human; little more than a piece of meat. Next morning's journey to prison in the sweat-box reinforced that feeling. I had not been allowed to change my clothes or to wash properly. I felt dirty and unpleasant, and the aptly named sweat-box made me feel even more unappetising, as if I had overnight been turned into something disgusting. I worried that I smelt.

On arrival at the prison I was scared, although, like many of my fellow inmates, I was regarded as a tough cookie by people who knew me outside. The officers booking me in seemed arrogant and high-handed. I tried not to show them how I felt. The ostensible reason for my terror was that I was being locked up in an unknown environment with people I didn't know, people who could be dangerous. The situation was unpredictable. I needed to erect tough defences, and in just a day or two I became the tough con: slouching, scowling, swearing; a don't-touch-me attitude that I supposed would keep me safe.

Now I look back and see that while the terror was initiated by the situation, it had a deeper cause. The fear of the present situation locked into the fear I held inside, the fear of the infant when it found itself in an unsafe and unknown environment. Prison might seem containing to an outsider, and indeed it does contain its inmates physically, but, psychologically, it feels uncontained: a strange, incomprehensible place where pain is the norm and fear all part of that. A place where you are powerless, and where what happens to you is of little import. A place where you become nothing; you are just a cipher in the all-encompassing bureaucracy which, in itself, seemed confusing, especially when viewed through the whirl of a new prisoner's fragmenting emotions. All the fixed points that made up one's life had been lost, to be replaced by an incomprehensible chaos.

The real terror was the feeling of losing one's selfhood. It was as if everything that marked you out as a person, as the individual that you were, had been left outside the prison gates: your home (if you had one – a third of prisoners do not), your job (also if you had one) and (for every prisoner) your family, friends, possessions, and the city, town or village where you live. Now, I was no longer a person with a place in the world: I was a number. The prison officers seemed fierce, the environment harsh, and I did not know who among my fellow inmates I could believe or trust. I feared that prison would destroy me completely.

As well as the physical responses of not being able to sleep, eat, relax or even concentrate enough to read a book, and the constant yearning I had to get outside, there were the tears. A fellow prisoner told me that I shouldn't worry because everyone felt as I did when first imprisoned. She described the tears as coming in waves, which was true: that is what they did. It felt visceral, as if the tears were not connected to any thoughts or feelings but were just responding to the raw trauma. My mind at that point was still not thinking clearly, the emotions so confused they seemed to pass too fleetingly to catch, but the tears came, as if unbidden and without thought. Many, if not most, prisoners succumbed to bouts of them at the start of a sentence, and we all tried to hide them because they showed weakness, a weakness we were anxious to deny. It was as if by acknowledging it we would fall apart completely.

For me, the weeping was reminiscent of tears shed in childhood when I was both angry and sad at not being listened to or understood. Prison, like all large institutions, has a deeply regressive effect on its inmates, but, in prison, it is, perhaps, at its most destructive. Your day is set out for you, your choices are few. Food, drinks, accommodation are all provided by the institution, on which you have no impact. You are no longer responsible for yourself. You are being 'looked after' but in an environment that aims to punish and causes considerable pain.

Every prisoner needs to make sense of his or her experience in some way. Looking back, I now see the early days of my imprisonment in terms of the first of three stages of emotion following separation (see Bowlby, 1973). This initial stage is known as the stage of protest, and my distressed shedding of hot tears evidenced it.

Editor's comment

In this case, the loss of one's identity is accompanied by the loss of one's ordinary coping mechanisms, and therefore the sense of self is invalidated. Prison takes away all sense of autonomy and enacts, in the words of Watterson (1996), the role of 'abusive parent'. The prisoner therefore will have all the reciprocal role procedures (RRPs) (e.g. 'crushed', 'abused', 'worthless') as prison-derived roles that CAT therapists are used to from their work with child-hood abuse. Of course, many prisoners have also experienced abuse in their childhood histories. Gradually, this leaves a clear and distinct mark on the prisoner's way of functioning and reacting (Pryor, 2001).

Second phase

I hated the prison officers and, like almost all of my fellow inmates, would do anything to get one over on them. Fighting the 'screws' was like fighting the hollow feelings of hopelessness that continually threatened to overtake me, and sometimes did. I was full of despair (Bowlby's second stage of loss).

I have always enjoyed collaborating with colleagues and, as a manager, I think I could listen with understanding to staff complaints. But when it came to the prison officers, I had no sympathy. These people were my jailors, and they were committing the unthinkable by ensuring that I stayed safely locked up in the appalling surroundings and deprived regime of prison.

In prison as I experienced it, the relationship between prison officers and inmates was mainly an adversarial one: it was 'us and them'. The prison officer had all the power, the prisoner had none. This was how it felt to the prisoner, and these feelings were reinforced at every turn: morning roll-check and unlock, distribution of breakfast, movement to education or work, all carefully logged and controlled by prison staff; then more roll-checks, and yet more at the end of the relatively short morning session, on to lunch and lock-up, and then a repeat in the afternoon. The routine was grim and boring, offered little satisfaction and, at every turn, controlled by the prison officers.

The officers, for their part, struggled to contain a tide of urgent emotion that constantly threatened to break its banks. No doubt in fantasy, they feared the worst from the prisoners and did their best to prevent it. They also had to work hard to defend themselves against their own emotions, ones that arose from treating their fellow human beings as they did; at causing them pain. They depersonalised the prisoner. When entering prison, I was told that the officers treated the inmates as scum. In time, I could see that this was true. Later, I understood why they had to. How else could they operate?

Some of the officers that I came across appeared to get satisfaction from being overbearing and, sometimes, sadistic. I thought the male officers sometimes quite enjoyed having the power they did over us women. Others developed a jolly banter that saw them through. While annoying to certain inmates, because of the way it made light of their predicament, others found it a helpful relief.

If an inmate wanted to make a request or complaint, it would be done, in writing, by submitting a form at the required time. An answer might come in days or weeks. Refusals could be followed up by appeals to senior officers and, ultimately, to the governor. To the prisoner, it could feel as though your voice had been submerged beneath piles of paper; your request or complaint eaten up by the bureaucracy. Everything about you became depersonalised by the system itself; it was as if nothing about you really mattered any more.

Editor's comment

This is an experience of, sometimes intensely, polarised role enactments in prison that leave no room for anything else and can be totally all-encompassing in the way they work; in short: a traumatic one. Depending on the person's vulnerability and the length of exposure, this may have a significant effect on a prisoner's further personal development. Since Keilson's seminal study on 'Sequential traumatization in children' (1979/92), we know that the context,

environment or family in which a person experiences this trauma, can signifi-
cantly add to it, and itself become part of the traumatic sequence, much as in
RRPs, in the case of incest, the rejecting and disbelieving other parent, faced
with disclosure by the child, may figure as a distinctive but significantly trau-
matic component of the overall experience that determines the developmental
outcome. In a similar way, prison and the quality of environment it provides will
determine the outcome of such experiences. In fact, much will depend on the
quality of other personal relationships that are available to the prisoner to help
modify some of these potentially annihilating polarised experiences.

The best way to maintain your personhood in prison, and to avoid being overwhelmed by such depressive thoughts, was to fight. The problem was that assertive behaviour, let alone aggression, was definitely not appreciated by the powers that be. It was easy to be labelled a troublemaker and a great deal harder to lose that label. Prisoners could, as punishment, be given days or weeks in segregation, spending all their time in a bare cell with hardly a half-hour for daily outside exercise.

So prisoners learnt how far they could go and tried to stay within that limit. It was a difficult line: nothing was ever totally clear in prison. Uncertainty was in itself a way of keeping people under control.

Editor's comment

In prison, like in an abuse situation, the fear/hope of all involved will be that the
unbearable situation is not containable any more. Therefore, emotions are kept
under tight control by the (abusive) power because they are dangerous if
genuine. The uncertainty is part of the power game enacted in prison, where
everything is ostensibly controlled by the institution. That is certainly also the
expectation of those in charge of prisons and of the general public. So the
reciprocal role here is one of 'parental' total control against an unruly 'child'
who tries to preserve some sense of self through limited fighting (autonomy).
The re-enactment of such patterns is a not uncommon experience with ex-
prisoners in group situations such as therapeutic communities, and the case
described in Chapter 9 partially demonstrates this.

Along with the pressure of the environment, most prisoners had pressures from outside: their families (especially children if there were any), financial problems, worries about accommodation and, for many if not the majority, the cravings caused by addiction to drugs or drink. The detoxification offered by prisons was generally experienced as inadequate, and rarely was enough done to work properly with the psychological issues.

As a result, prisoners felt their fight to be useless, their position hopeless, and the waves of tears were replaced by waves of the deepest depression. When I was in prison, I imagined that the place was inhabited by a spirit of despair that alighted on individuals haphazardly and chose when to withdraw from them: after days, weeks, months or years. My fantasy was not without foundation. Prisoners' overall lack of control of their lives extended to their emotions. Like the tears, it was as if the most awful depression came upon us without either warning or any particular reason. Perhaps it found its own way of creeping unnoticed past the wall of defence the prisoner tried to erect and maintain, never entirely effectively.

The despair is perceived to be what society, and the prison staff, most want, but if you don't fight, you are lost. I have on several occasions been surprised by feisty prisoners attempting suicide. I had thought that they were coping well. The spirit of despair had managed to sneak in, taking them by surprise, with potentially dreadful consequences. They would assure me that, at the time, they had really meant it. They had wanted to die.

As for me, the crying was much less frequent now and was of a different order, as if I was grieving the loss of my freedom and, most especially, the loss of contact with my home and family. I still had a constant urge to be outside, but a new symptom of my incarceration had come upon me: I could recall, in absolute detail, memories of my house, the street where I lived, the city where I lived, every city I'd visited, my parents' house, my sisters', my pets, old friends and new ones, all the events of my life. These memories flooded in as if the paucity of my surroundings gave them the space. For a while, they haunted me. Then they disappeared.

Third phase

After a few months of being in prison, I reached a point that I described to myself as a plateau. My mood was much steadier, though inevitably still quite low, and I felt a little more in control of my life, despite still being subject to the dreary prison routines. I had learnt to manage prison.

The learning had a variety of components. The main one was to take life at a slower pace. Nothing happened quickly in prison, and there was endless queuing. We had to queue for our meals, queue for medication, queue to be checked out before going to work or education, queue to get in for a visit if we had one. Then there was the waiting: waiting to go back to the unit at the end of a work or education session, waiting to use the phones, waiting to see our visitors once we'd been checked in, waiting for an appointment with the doctor or the dentist (I had to wait 6 months for a dental check, even though I was having trouble with my teeth). One thing you have in prison is time.

I also learnt to manage the lock-ups: how to stay calm and find things to do to get through them. Light reading was now possible. I would write letters, and even penned a couple of articles and poems. If I felt sleepy, I'd take a snooze, and I became very proud of my acquired ability to sleep through the constant noise in prison of radios blaring out along the corridors, often tuned to different channels, and the disruption of other inmates fooling about.

Prison is a noisy place; the long blank corridors and paucity of furniture meant that sounds bounced and echoed through the buildings. Prisoners often used noise and sometimes childish activity to blot out their difficult feelings. The officers regularly shouted through the units, calling for particular inmates or announcing the start of activities, such as movement to gym or the chapel.

It didn't bother me. I had erected a tough defence. The other inmates and officers no longer scared me. I knew how to handle them all. Although I still longed to get out and back to the world, prison no longer held any fear. I knew how to survive it.

In the process, I had cut myself off from much of my sensitivity. I had become a hardened con and, although I still tried to support my fellow inmates, I no longer felt so much concern for them, for myself, or for the world in general. In fact, I soon felt quite disconnected from the things going on around me. I went through my days, accepted the routines and took less and less interest in life. It was a more manageable state, but not a very healthy one.

One day, sitting alone in my cell, I had a kind of waking dream where my dead father and brother came to see me inside. It was a comfort, to have them close, urging me to take care of myself, but on reflection it seems somewhat unhinged, in that I felt such strong contact with these dead people rather than the alive ones around me.

This experience reminds me of Bowlby's third and final phase of separation: that of detachment.

Editor's comment

This is akin to the dissociation in response to serious abuse that many children develop as a coping mechanism. It is the precondition of the further psychological damage that can now take place as a result of the splitting off of the experience so that it can be endured without risk to the remaining 'self', ultimately resulting in the development of restricted role repertoires and consequently a limited capacity to live life.

The smoking as a symptom, the picking up of cigarette ends as mentioned earlier, could then be seen as the first sign of self-harming tendencies in response, a self–self role enactment as the only means of control and sense of self.

Regression versus rehabilitation

The environment of prison caused me to regress. I had little responsibility. The major decisions in life were not in my hands: where and how to live, food, shelter, work. Choices of when and what to eat (choosing meals from a menu with two or three choices is hardly empowering) and choices about work or

education were severely limited, as were choices about possessions and pur-
chases, all of which got completely embroiled in the prison's bureaucracy. I
felt 'parented' by the establishment, or 'looked after', as stated in the prison
service's mission statement. I felt responsible only for cooperating with the
systems imposed, which I experienced as grim and tedious. I felt that these
systems and the overarching bureaucracy attacked my individuality and
depersonalised and objectified my existence.

Given the regressive nature of prison, and the pain and frustration of
prison life as described above, it is paradoxical that prison should also be
attempting to rehabilitate people so that they become more responsible for
themselves and less likely to fall into practices that lead to crime on release. In
fact, I experienced prison as a kind of double bind: to be treated as a child
and, simultaneously, to be urged to take more responsibility for one's life. It is
not surprising that, in most cases, rehabilitation work done in prison is
scorned by the inmates and does not seem to work. Like others, I cooperated
to the extent that I could get out of my cell as often as possible and gain
brownie points for my parole. Some prisoners do make real efforts to improve
their basic education. But the fact is that the majority go on to reoffend.

I felt that current practices were damaging for us prisoners and for prison
officers alike. I was appalled that society should be content with this. We have
good knowledge about how groups and communities work, and about milieu
therapies. While in prison, I saw, on the rare occasions when it happened, the
most unlikely prisoners respond positively when offered a responsible role
and a chance to affect their environment. This gave me hope that it might
be possible to develop environments and regimes that, in themselves, are
rehabilitative. This would benefit both the prisoner and society as a whole.

References

Bowlby, J. (1969). *Attachment and loss (Volume 1: Attachment)*. London: Hogarth.
Bowlby, J. (1973). *Attachment and loss (Volume 2: Separation)*. New York: Basic
    Books.
Keilson, H. (1979). *Die sequentielle Traumatisierung von Kindern*. Stuttgart: Enke.
Keilson, H. (1992). *Sequential traumatization in children*. Jerusalem: Hebrew University
    Magnes Press.
Pryor, S. (2001). *The responsible prisoner: An exploration of the extent to which
    imprisonment removes responsibility unnecessarily and an invitation to change*.
    London: Prison Service.
Watterson, K. (1996). *Women in prison*. Boston, MA: Northeastern University Press.

Chapter 19

Final thoughts

The way forward for Cognitive Analytic Therapy in forensic settings

Philip H. Pollock

Cognitive Analytic Therapy (CAT) as a new form of forensic psychotherapy

CAT has suffused many clinical areas since its inception. Its application to forensic settings is yet another extension of its development as a therapy model. The aim of the present work was to illustrate its use across a range of settings, offence types and clinical disorders. Although the evidence base is scant for CAT as a form of forensic psychotherapy, the descriptions of the model and therapy here were intended to provide a novel, perhaps even innovative, illustration of a different form of psychotherapy for offenders. Case studies are, of course, anecdotal reflections of clinical practice, but they do display some of the intricacies of therapy. It is hoped that CAT for offenders will become a possible option for the 'evolving species' of forensic psychotherapists (Adshead, 1991).

Psychotherapists' preferences for a theory, model or form of therapy are influenced by many factors. We are not advocating that CAT for offenders should be perceived as in competition with other psychotherapies in forensic settings or that CAT should be granted a market segment. Those who worship in the church of a particular psychotherapy are often narrow in their thinking and blinkered by their loyalty and allegiance. The authors of the present work argue that CAT is here offered as a therapeutic option with its deficiencies and attributes. On a case-by-case analysis, it is proposed that CAT is a fresh way of thinking about and intervening with offenders and their contexts. The objective is to promote CAT as a theory and method that can, perhaps, join the league of forensic psychotherapies and improve clinicians' choices for effective intervention and conceptualisation of criminals and their offences. Of course, the reformulation process in CAT permits the clinician to incorporate other modalities (e.g. imagery rescripting and reprocessing, eye movement desensitization and reprocessing, anger management, trauma work, art and music therapy, etc.) within the therapy without losing sight of the overarching model of the offender's personality, offence and target problems. Examples of such integrations of different therapies or techniques have been reported by Pollock (2001), showing that the conceptual 'mental model' derived from the client is not compromised when applying CAT reformulation.

The evidence base for CAT with offenders

The debate about 'what works' (McGuire, 1995) in psychological therapies for offenders and the impetus to collect an 'evidence base' of efficacy and effectiveness within the criminal justice system are of primary importance because of the human cost of failure in forensic settings. It is acknowledged that the outcomes for CAT are anecdotal and limited at this juncture. Efforts are under way to address the lack of anchoring data to guide choices about CAT as a forensic psychotherapy. Two particular studies are worthy of mention. Firstly, a treatment-based project is being undertaken that investigates the use of CAT within the sex offender treatment programmes of prisons. The project uses individual CAT reformulations for each sex offender and a group SDR, in addition to examining the offender-to-victim RRPs, to trace the dialogical sequences within the offences and also to focus on the offence-dominant RRPs that denote peak risk potentials for the offenders. Repertory grid evaluation is employed as a specific outcome measure.

Secondly, a group of rage-type homicide perpetrators ($n=19$) have been treated by individual CAT with a battery of CAT-specific and other psychometric measures, and positive changes resulted (Pollock, 2004, unpublished). These studies are likely to inform future therapeutic endeavours and herald the beginning of the accumulation of the evidence base for CAT with offenders.

A valid form of forensic psychotherapy?

Examples have been offered here of CAT for a diversity of contexts, offence types and clinical disorders. It was argued that a 'valid' forensic psychotherapy should exhibit a number of attributes, and review of the material in this book would indicate that CAT shows a range of particular strengths which promote its utility and worth as a model of psychotherapy for offenders. Firstly, the explicit focus on the link between the offender's personality and idiosyncratic actions during the crime is a core part of CAT. In terms of the underlying model of new learning and change in CAT, the thrust of therapy is to make clear, precise acknowledgement of the link between the unique functioning of the offender and his/her actions and to facilitate the offender's assuming responsibility for and ownership of the crimes. One of the objectives of CAT is to scaffold the offender's acquisition of the psychological tools to promote self-knowledge, insight and the ability to self-reflect, developing a mental model of the connection between both personality and crime. The examination of the offender's internal world, the meaning of the offence and its predicable recurrence are overt features of the therapy.

Furthermore, devising a formulation of the relational components of the crime is a central task, encouraging a focus on the offender-to-victim dyads and specifying the origins, manifestations and motivations of such relating. The offender's personality is not reduced to its pathological parts within CAT, and healthy capacities are acknowledged in a way that diagnosis of disorder fails to recognise. The risk potential is understood as a dynamic, fluctuating factor which is analysed within the reformulation to aid prediction and to promote self-awareness, self-monitoring and improved self-regulation. The offender-to-victim relationship is assigned primary significance when creating a mental model of the offender's internal world and its expression through crime.

The issue of enhancing the offender's active assumption of responsibility and ownership is directly endorsed from the commencement of therapy. Within CAT, the context of the offender's existence and experience is understood and used to develop non-collusive, therapeutic responses from other parties (such as nursing or prison staff). Advice to decision makers can be articulated through CAT models and reformulations, which provide a focused approach to reporting within-therapy outcomes and changes in target problems. The expected patterns of new thinking, feeling, acting and relating in the 'real world' are identified, and constructive solutions sought within a collaborative relationship between therapist and offender. In terms of positive attributes compared against the set criteria, we can vouch that CAT shows many of the components of a valid forensic psychotherapy.

The way forward for CAT

An accumulation of evidence of the effectiveness of CAT and its expansion into other areas of forensic work is required. CAT is conducive to the three core principles (the risk, needs and responsivity principles) of the 'what works' for offenders debate (McGuire, 1995). CAT can be applied to any type and any seriousness of offence, conceptualising risk potential in a particular way. In terms of criminogenic needs, CAT directly focuses on the dynamic risk factors, and targets these needs for change. In some ways, the use of reformulation, dialogical sequence analysis, identification of the dominant offence position and RRPs is similar to functional analytic approaches to understanding crime (e.g. Jackson, Glass & Hope, 1987), in that pathways to the offence are noted and addressed. Furthermore, CAT can be adapted to provide an idiosyncratic model of each offender's personality and crime without assuming that, because a particular offence has occurred, a 'sophisticated idiosyncratic assessment' cannot be completed in accordance with the responsivity principle. It is hoped that further applications of CAT in forensic settings will support or negate its value as part of this debate.

References

Adshead, G. (1991). The forensic psychotherapist: Dying breed or evolving species? *Psychiatric Bulletin, 15*, 410–412.

Jackson, H. F., Glass, C. & Hope, S. (1987). A functional analysis of recidivistic arson. *British Journal of Clinical Psychology, 26*, 175–185.

McGuire, J. (Ed.) (1995). *What works: Reducing reoffending.* Chichester: Wiley.

Pollock, P. H. (2001). *Cognitive Analytic Therapy for adult survivors of childhood abuse: Case conceptualisation and treatment.* Chichester: Wiley.

Pollock, P. H. (2004). Cognitive Analytic Therapy for rage-type homicide (unpublished).

Chapter 20

An invited critique of Cognitive Analytic Therapy for offenders

James McGuire

This book provides a potentially rich source of ideas and practical illustrations for those clinicians who wish to apply Cognitive Analytic Therapy (CAT) in their work with individuals who have broken the law. As a hybrid or integrative form of therapy, CAT is generally employed with the more complex forms of personal distress and criminal conduct. The cases considered in these pages are far removed from the ordinary or 'volume' crimes that constitute the bulk of the official statistics. The vignettes presented in various chapters consist for the most part of offences of homicide, rape, child abuse, arson, stalking, and other serious and serial crimes generally involving extreme violence and causing or threatening enormous harm. These patterns are typically compounded by other behaviours including self-injury, substance abuse, victim mutilation, and even cannibalism. Furthermore, perpetrators often meet diagnostic criteria for one or other, and sometimes several, of the psychiatric categories of personality disorder. Some chapters consider the wider implications of the CAT framework for the way mental health or criminal justice services are conceptualised and delivered, in both institutions and the community. The editors are highly experienced and knowledgeable practitioners, and it would be difficult to think of anyone better able to act in their role in relation to a book on this topic.

The invitation to write a brief critique has presented a challenging task, as my own theoretical and clinical outlook has very different roots from those underpinning the use of CAT. Yet, the types of individuals discussed in this book are probably at or beyond the limits of any of our currently available conceptual models. It would be foolhardy, therefore, not to consider the prospective value of a method that appears to derive primarily if not exclusively from clinical work with this very demanding client population.

On the positive side, it appears to me that, as depicted here, CAT constitutes a bold and innovative step in combining and synthesising ideas from psychodynamic, cognitive and personal-construct models of therapy. Some chapters exemplify usage of yet other treatment modalities, such as attachment theory or imagery reprocessing work, within the same framework. Since the 1940s, many attempts have been made to integrate therapies with supposedly incompatible theoretical bases. Their degree of success has varied, and more often than not such efforts have failed, at least in the sense that the results had little impact on widespread practice. But if the level of interest shown by practising clinicians, and growing popularity, are valid measures of progress, CAT could be said to enjoy steadily increasing credibility.

Nevertheless, and ungrateful though it might be as a response to the editors' invitation to critique *CAT for offenders*, it would be dishonest of me not to express some reservations about the scope and utility of the material offered in this volume. There are several grounds for doing so, and perhaps they would be best condensed into a few key concerns and posed as questions for those who seek expansion of the applicability of CAT.

First, there are crucial theoretical issues to be addressed. They derive from the problem known in the philosophy of science as the 'underdetermination of theory' (Klee, 1997). The explanations for action that are offered within CAT result in the construction of immensely elaborate series of hypothetical mechanisms, often only tenuously linked to the clinical data that have been collected. The available data are often compatible with more than one theoretical position, and there are no firm grounds for choosing between them.

Below the rather abstract altitudes of epistemology and theory construction, essentially the same problem arises on an everyday clinical level. Imagine you are referred a person with a cluster of long-standing, deep-seated problems, including a history of frequent antisocial acts. There could be many explanations and accounts – alternative 'case formulations' – all apparently plausible. Again, how does the clinician choose between them? It is possible to depict someone's behaviour as a contest between good and evil. Many media reports and (by implication) lay theories draw on such concepts, but assertions of that kind are neither provable nor disprovable on the basis of evidence. My own very strong inclination, indeed conviction, is to rely upon those models and processes that are best connected to theoretical constructs that in turn have been subject to extensive, methodical testing and also account for a wide array of other psychosocial phenomena (McGuire, 2004).

Second, it is a valid criticism that, until recently, cognitive and allied therapies neglected the relational elements of therapeutic work. The solution within CAT is to incorporate a psychoanalytic model for doing this, focused on the processes of transference and counter-transference (Freud, 1933). It seems both unfortunate and redundant to draw on psychodynamic thinking to achieve this. Is it not strange that nearly a century after its initial conception, Fried, Crits-Cristoph & Luborsky (1992) reported the 'first empirical demonstration' of this cornerstone of psychoanalytic thinking? Yet, their study simply showed an association between certain aspects of clients' relationships with their therapists and with other people, a pattern that could exist for many reasons. As evidence that the clinician or, for that matter, the prison, takes the place of the parent in a therapeutic encounter, this is far from convincing. Furthermore, there are numerous aspects of the working alliance that are probably more important to therapy process and outcome than transference (Norcross, 2002). Overall, the empirical basis of psycho-analytic ideas and methods remains highly questionable; despite their pervasive cultural influence, they are deeply flawed in many respects (see, for example: Farrell, 1981; Macmillan, 1997; Crews, 1998; Gellner, 2003).

A third problem is the extent to which actions are seen as manifestations of pathology. The disciplines that some criminologists call the 'psy-sciences' (Groombridge, 2001) are often portrayed as taking almost any kind of behaviour that departs from social conventions or norms and applying an illness label to it. Simultaneously, it is held that they neglect or even wholly ignore situational, environmental, and socio-political factors. From the standpoint of Foucault and his adherents, their main objective has been represented (in my view, slanderously) as that of 'disciplining the population'. Even accepting that the types of offences and offenders we encounter in this book are highly unusual, could the extended usage of CAT add to a perception, already difficult to overcome, that psychology is indeed largely about 'pathologising'? The suggestion in the closing chapter that 'CAT can be applied to any type and any seriousness of offence' could lead to further alienation between the disciplines of criminology and psychology, at a time when there were signs of a new cordiality and rapprochement (Hollin, 2002). Is it not vitally important to make connections between the taken-for-granted and the bizarre in human behaviour, and develop a theoretical framework capable of encompassing both?

Finally, though, it is currently claimed that there is an emerging consensus that all psychological therapies are broadly equivalent in their outcomes (Wampold, 2001). Even if there is also evidence that some approaches have demonstrably greater efficacy in specific clinical areas, no single therapy 'brand name' emerges as outright winner (the so-called 'dodo bird verdict'). Alongside this, there are suggestions that the key to facilitating clinical improvement is to be convinced of the validity of your approach, and that the only feature that consistently differentiates therapists in their effectiveness, surpassing experience and training, is interpersonal skill (Lambert & Ogles, 2004). If these conclusions are sustained and consolidated by further research, future progress will essentially entail the development of therapeutic models capable of accounting for rarer and more intricate types of clinical problem. Models that designate the possibility of individuals entering differentiated 'self-states' could be one aspect of this. To the extent that this is reflected in the formulations provided in the present book, it is a welcome and valuable innovation.

References

Crews, F. (Ed.) (1998). *Unauthorized Freud: Doubters confront a legend*. Harmondsworth: Penguin Books.

Farrell, B. A. (1981). *The standing of psychoanalysis*. Oxford: Oxford University Press.

Freud, S. (1933). *New introductory lectures on psychoanalysis*. London: Hogarth Press and Institute of Psychoanalysis.

Fried, D., Crits-Cristoph, P. & Luborsky, L. (1992). The first empirical demonstration of transference in psychotherapy. *Journal of Nervous and Mental Disease, 180*, 326–331.

Gellner, E. (2003). *The psychoanalytic movement: The cunning of unreason*. Oxford: Blackwell.

Groombridge, N. (2001). Pathology. Entry in E. McLaughlin & J. Muncie (Eds), *The Sage dictionary of criminology*. London: Sage.

Hollin, C. R. (2002). Criminological psychology. In M. Maguire, R. Morgan & R. Reiner (Eds), *The Oxford handbook of criminology* (3rd edn). Oxford: Oxford University Press.

Klee, R. (1997). *Introduction to the philosophy of science: Cutting nature at its seams*. New York: Oxford University Press.

Lambert, M. J. & Ogles, B. M. (2004). The efficacy and effectiveness of psychotherapy. In M. J. Lambert (Ed.), *Bergin and Garfield's handbook of psychotherapy and behavior change* (5th edn). New York: Wiley.

Macmillan, M. (1997). *Freud evaluated: The completed arc*. Cambridge, MA: MIT Press.

McGuire, J. (2004). *Understanding psychology and crime: Perspectives on theory and action*. Maidenhead: McGraw-Hill Education/Open University Press.

Norcross, J. C. (Ed.) (2002). *Psychotherapy relationships that work*. New York: Oxford University Press.

Wampold, B. E. (2001). *The great psychotherapy debate: Models, methods, and findings*. Mahwah, NJ: Lawrence Erlbaum Associates.

Appendix I

Self-States Grid and Psychotherapy File

Self-States Grid

(Reproduced from Golynkina, K. & Ryle, A. (1999). The identification and characteristics of the partially dissociated states of patients with borderline personality disorder. *British Journal of Medical Psychology*, 72, 429–445. Reproduced with permission from the *British Journal of Medical Psychology* © The British Psychological Society.)

Rate each state	5 = applies strongly	4 = applies	3 =+/-	2 = does not apply	1 = does not apply at all

Patient's Name:	Therapist's Name:	Date/ Session number:

STATES									
Descriptions	**A**	**B**	**C**	**D**	**E**	**F**	**G**	**H**	**I**
Overwhelmed by feelings									
I feel weak									
I feel happy									
I feel angry									
I feel sad									
I feel guilty									
I feel out of control									

I feel unreal										
Others seem critical										
Others envy me										
Others attack me										
Others admire me										
Others care for me										
I trust others										
I depend on others										
I control others										
I want to hurt others										
Cut-off from feelings										

When completing the test I was in the following state of mind:

Names of different states:

A:	D:	G:
B:	E:	H:
C:	F:	I:

Psychotherapy File

(Reproduced from Pollock, P. H. (1990). The Psychotherapy File. In A. Ryle (Ed.), *Cognitive analytic therapy*. Chichester: Wiley. © John Wiley & Sons Limited. Reproduced with permission.)

An aid to understanding ourselves better

We have all had just one life and what has happened to us, and the sense we made of this, colours the way we see ourselves and others. How we see things is for us how things are, and how we go about our lives seems 'obvious and right'. Sometimes, however, our familiar ways of understanding and acting can be the source of our problems. In order to solve our difficulties, we may need to learn to recognise how what we do makes things worse. We can then work out new ways of thinking and acting.

These pages are intended to suggest ways of thinking about what you do; recognising your particular patterns is the first step in learning to gain more control and happiness in your life.

Keeping a diary of your moods and behaviour

Symptoms, bad moods, unwanted thoughts or behaviours that come and go can be better understood and controlled if you learn to notice when they happen and what starts them off.

If you have a particular symptom or problem of this sort, start keeping a diary. The diary should be focused on a particular mood, symptom or behaviour, and should be kept every day if possible. Try to record this sequence:

1 how you were feeling about yourself and others and the world before the problem came on
2 any external event, or any thought or image in your mind that was going on when the trouble started, or what seemed to start it off
3 once the trouble started, the thoughts, images or feelings you experienced.

By noticing and writing down in this way what you do and think at these times, you will learn to recognise and eventually have more control over how you act and think at the time. It is often the case that bad feelings like resentment, depression or physical symptoms are the result of ways of thinking and acting that are unhelpful. Keeping a diary in this way gives you the chance to learn better ways of dealing with things.

It is helpful to keep a daily record for 1–2 weeks, and then to discuss what you have recorded with your therapist or counsellor.

Patterns that do not work, but are hard to break

There are certain ways of thinking and acting that do not achieve what we want, but which are hard to change. Read through the lists on the following pages and mark how far you think they apply to you.

Applies strongly ++	Applies +	Does not apply 0

Traps

Traps are things we cannot escape from. Certain kinds of thinking and acting result in a 'vicious circle' when, however hard we try, things seem to get worse instead of better. Trying to deal with feeling bad about ourselves, we think and act in ways that tend to confirm our badness.

Examples of traps

	++	+	0
1. *Fear of hurting others* Feeling fearful of hurting others* we keep our feelings inside, or put our own needs aside. This tends to allow other people to ignore or abuse us in various ways, which then leads to our feeling, or being childishly angry. When we see ourselves behaving like this, it confirms our belief that we shouldn't be aggressive and reinforces our avoidance of standing up for our rights. * People often get trapped in this way because they mix up aggression and assertion. Mostly, being assertive – asking for our rights – is perfectly acceptable. People who do not respect our rights as human beings must either be stood up to or avoided.			
2. *Depressed thinking* Feeling depressed, we are sure we will manage a task or social situation badly. Being depressed, we are probably not as effective as we could be, and the depression leads us to exaggerate how badly we handled things. This makes us feel more depressed about ourselves.			
3. *Trying to please* Feeling uncertain about ourselves and anxious not to upset others, we try to please people by doing what they seem to want. As a result: (1) we end up being taken advantage of by others, which makes us angry, depressed or guilty, from which our uncertainty about ourselves is confirmed; or (2) sometimes we feel out of control because of the need to please, and start hiding away, putting things off, letting people down, which makes other people angry with us and increases our uncertainty.			

	++	+	0

4. *Avoidance*

    We feel ineffective and anxious about certain
    situations, such as crowded streets, open spaces,
    social gatherings. We try to go back into these
    situations, but feel even more anxiety. Avoiding
    them makes us feel better, so we stop trying.
    However, constantly avoiding situations limits our
    lives and we come to feel increasingly ineffective
    and anxious.

5. *Social isolation*

    Feeling underconfident about ourselves and
    anxious not to upset others, we worry that others
    will find us boring or stupid, so we don't look at
    people or respond to friendliness. People then see
    us as unfriendly, so we become more isolated,
    from which we are convinced we are boring and
    stupid – and become more underconfident.

6. *Low self-esteem*

    Feeling worthless, we feel that we cannot get what
    we want because (1) we will be punished, (2)
    others will reject or abandon us, or (3) anything
    good we get is bound to go away or turn sour.
    Sometimes it feels as if we must punish ourselves
    for being weak. From this, we feel that everything
    is hopeless, so we give up trying to do anything,
    and that confirms and increases our sense of
    worthlessness.

Dilemmas (false choices and narrow options)

We often act as we do, even when we are not completely happy with it, because
the only other ways we can imagine seem as bad or even worse. Sometimes
we assume connections that are not necessarily the case – as in 'If I do x, then
y will follow'. These false choices can be described as either/or or if/then
dilemmas. We often don't realise that we see things like this, but we act as if
these were the only possible choices.

Do you act as if any of the following false choices rule your life? Recognising them is the first step to changing them.

Choices about myself

1.	Either I keep feelings bottled up or I risk being rejected, hurting others or making a mess.	++	+	0
2.	Either I feel I spoil myself and am greedy or I deny myself things, punish myself and feel miserable.	++	+	0
3.	If I try to be perfect, I feel depressed and angry; if I don't try to be perfect, I feel guilty, angry and dissatisfied.	++	+	0
4.	If I must, then I won't; it is as if, when faced with a task, I must either gloomily submit or passively resist. Other people's wishes, or even my own, feel too demanding, so I put things off, avoid them.	++	+	0
5.	If I must not, then I will; it is as if the only proof of my existence is my resistance. Other people's rules, or even my own, feel too restricting, so I break rules and do things which are harmful to me.	++	+	0
6.	If other people aren't expecting me to do things for them or look after them, then I feel anxious, lonely and out of control.	++	+	0
7.	If I get what I want, I feel childish and guilty; if I don't get what I want, I feel frustrated, angry and depressed.	++	+	0
8.	Either I keep things (feelings, plans) in perfect order, or I fear a terrible mess.	++	+	0

Choices about how I relate to others

1.	Either I'm involved with someone and likely to get hurt or I don't get involved and stay in charge, but remain lonely.	++	+	0
2.	Either I stick up for myself and nobody likes me, or I give in and get put upon by others and feel cross and hurt.	++	+	0
3.	Either I'm a brute or a martyr (secretly blaming the other).	++	+	0
4.	a. With others, either I'm safely wrapped up in bliss or in combat. b. If in combat, then I'm either a bully or a victim.	++	+	0
5.	Either I look down on other people, or I feel they look down on me.	++	+	0

	++	+	0
6. a. Either I'm sustained by the admiration of others whom I admire, or I feel exposed. b. If exposed, then I feel either contemptuous of others or contemptible.	++	+	0
7. Either I'm involved with others and feel engulfed, taken over or smothered, or I stay safe and uninvolved but feel lonely and isolated.	++	+	0
8. When I'm involved with someone whom I care about, then either I have to give in or they have to give in.	++	+	0
9. When I'm involved with someone whom I depend on, then either I have to give in or they have to give in.	++	+	0
10. a. As a woman, either I have to do what others want or stand up for my rights and get rejected. b. As a man, either I can't have any feelings or I am an emotional mess.	++	+	0

Snags

Snags are what is happening when we say, 'I want to have a better life, or I want to change my behaviour but . . .' Sometimes this comes from how we or our families thought about us when we were young; for example, 'she was always the good child', or 'in our family we never . . .' Sometimes the snags come from the important people in our lives not wanting us to change, not being able to cope with what our changing means to them. Often the resistance is more indirect, as when a parent, husband or wife becomes ill or depressed when we begin to get better.

In other cases, we seem to 'arrange' to avoid pleasure or success, or, if they come, we have to pay in some way, be it by depression, or by spoiling things. Often this is because, as children, we came to feel guilty if things went well for us, or felt that we were envied for good luck or success. Sometimes we have come to feel responsible, unreasonably, for things that went wrong in the family, although we may not be aware that this is so. It is helpful to learn to recognise how this sort of pattern is stopping you from getting on with your life, for only then can you learn to accept your right to a better life and begin to claim it.

You may get quite depressed when you begin to realise how often you stop your life from being happier and more fulfilled. It is important to remember that the cause is not stupidity or bad nature, but rather that:

1. We do these things because this is the way we learned to manage best when we were younger.
2. We don't have to keep on doing them now we are learning to recognise them.

3. By changing our behaviour, we can not only learn to control our own behaviour, but also to change the way other people behave to us.
4. Although it may seem that others (such as our parents or our partners) resist the changes we want for ourselves, we often underestimate them; if we are firm about our right to change, those who care for us will usually accept the change.

Do you recognise that you feel limited in your life

	++	+	0
1. for fear of the response of others? For example, I must sabotage success (a) as if it deprives others, (b) as if others may envy me, or (c) as if there are not enough good things to go around.	++	+	0
2. by something inside yourself? For example, I must sabotage good things as if I don't deserve them.	++	+	0

Difficult and unstable states of mind

Some people find it difficult to keep control over their behaviour and experience because things feel very difficult and different at times. Indicate which, if any, of the following apply to you:

	++	+	0
1. How I feel about myself and others can be unstable; I can switch from one state of mind to a completely different one.	++	+	0
2. Some states may be accompanied by intense, extreme and uncontrollable emotions.	++	+	0
3. Others may be accompanied by emotional blankness, feeling unreal, or feeling muddled.	++	+	0
4. Some states are accompanied by my feeling intensely guilty or angry with myself, wanting to hurt myself.	++	+	0
5. Or I may feel that others can't be trusted, are going to let me down, or hurt me.	++	+	0
6. Or I may be unreasonably angry with or hurtful to others.	++	+	0
7. Sometimes the only way I can cope with some confusing feelings is to blank them off and feel emotionally distant from others.	++	+	0

Continue overleaf if you want to:

Different states

We all experience changes in how we feel about ourselves and the world. But for some people these changes are extreme, and sometimes sudden and confusing. In such cases, there are often a number of states that recur, and learning to recognise them and shifts between them can be very helpful. Below are a number of descriptions of such stages. Identify those that you experience by ringing the number. *You can delete or add words to the descriptions*, and there is space to add any not listed.

1. zombie – cut-off from feelings, cut-off from others, disconnected
2. feeling bad but soldiering on, coping
3. out-of-control rage
4. extraspecial; looking down on others
5. in control of self, of life, of other people
6. cheated by life, by others; untrusting
7. provoking, teasing, seducing, winding-up others
8. clinging, fearing abandonment
9. frenetically active; too busy to think or feel
10. agitated, confused, anxious
11. feeling perfectly cared for, blissfully close to another
12. misunderstood, rejected, abandoned
13. contemptuously dismissive of myself
14. vulnerable, needy, passively helpless, waiting for rescue
15. envious; wanting to harm others, put them down, pull them down
16. protective, respecting myself and others
17. hurting myself and others
18. resentfully submitting to demands
19. hurt, humiliated by others
20. secure in myself, able to be close to others
21. intensely critical of self, of others
22. frightened of others

Appendix 2

Personality Structure Questionnaire (PSQ)

(Reproduced from Pollock, P. H. (Ed.) (2001). *Cognitive analytic therapy for adult survivors of childhood abuse.* Chichester: Wiley. © John Wiley & Sons Limited. Reproduced with permission.)

For each statement on the opposite page, please shade one of the circles for the comment that best describes you usually, using the 1 to 5 scale.

	1 Very true	2 True	3 May or may not be true	4 True	5 Very true	
1. My sense of myself is always the same.	○	○	○	○	○	How I act and feel is constantly changing.
2. The various people in my life see me in much the same way.	○	○	○	○	○	The various people in my life have different views of who I really am.
3. I have a stable and unchanging sense of myself.	○	○	○	○	○	I am so different at different times that I wonder who I really am.
4. I have no sense of opposed sides to my nature.	○	○	○	○	○	I feel I am split between two (or more) ways of being, sharply differentiated from each other.
5. My mood and sense of self seldom change suddenly.	○	○	○	○	○	My mood can change abruptly in ways which make me feel unreal or out of control.
6. My mood changes are always understandable.	○	○	○	○	○	I am often confused by my mood changes, which seem either unprovoked or quite out of scale with what provoked them.
7. I never lose control.	○	○	○	○	○	I get into states in which I lose control and do harm to myself and/or others.
8. I never regret what I have said or done.	○	○	○	○	○	I get into states in which I do and say things which I later deeply regret.

Appendix 3
States Description Procedure (SDP)

Initials or name: Date:

The purpose of this procedure

Your replies to the Personality Structure Questionnaire indicate that you (more than most people) experience an unstable sense of yourself because you switch between contrasting states of mind or states of being. Switching between such states involves more than a change of mood; for example, in one state, one's feelings may be overwhelming, but in another state they may be blanked off, and one's sense of oneself and other people may differ markedly between states, with the result that one behaves in inconstant and inappropriate ways. Some states are unpleasant or harmful, and switches between states are often abrupt and confusing to oneself and others.

The procedure described here offers a way of thinking more clearly about your states and state switches. Going through it (either on your own or, preferably, with your therapist, psychologist, counsellor, nurse or other health professional) can help you become conscious of your patterns. Describing and making a diagram of your states can give you more control over distressing or harmful ones, and can help you develop a more connected and consistent sense of yourself.

The first part gives general descriptions of common states which can help you recognise and describe your own. The second part helps you give a more detailed account of each of your states – you will need a separate sheet for each state.

States description procedure (SDP)

Part 1. Recognising your states from general descriptions

The commonly used names and key features of a number of frequently experienced states are described below. They are identified by the letters A to J.

Select those which more or less match your own states.
Not all of the listed features will apply to your experiences.

1. *Cross out* those features that do not apply and *add others if necessary*.
2. You may prefer to give your states a different name.
3. Then write the identifying letters of the states you recognise as ones you experience from time to time – people usually identify from two to five such states.
4. If you experience a recurrent, clearly recognisable state that is not described here, add this to the list under K, L, etc.

(A) OK STATE

I feel:

Emotionally secure
Mostly content
Satisfied with myself
In control of my life
I can look after myself

People in my life:

Seem friendly
Seem concerned
Seem sympathetic
Seem respecting

(B) VICTIM, ABUSED STATE

I feel:

Powerless
Weak
Guilty
Worthless
Cheated
Damaged
Like hurting myself
Like neglecting myself
Self-blaming
Striving to please or perform

People in my life:

Threaten me
Bully me
Hurt me physically
Hurt me emotionally
Control me
Provoke me
Abandon or neglect me
Look down on me
Criticise me

(C) SOLDIERING ON STATE, COPING

I feel:

Hopeless
I must submit
I feel resentful
I must do what is expected

People in my life:

Make demands
Ignore my needs
Are disappointed in me

(D) RAGE STATE, CRAZY

I feel:

Out of control
Dangerous
Like harming myself
Wanting to hurt/destroy others

People in my life:

Do not care about me
Seem like threatening abusers

(E) REVENGEFUL STATE

I feel:

Enraged
Self-righteous
Violent
Envious

People in my life:

Threaten me
Control me
Neglect me
Attack me

(F) ZOMBIE STATE, BLANK

I feel:

Emotionally numb
Indifferent to others
Indifferent to pain
'On automatic'
Unreal

People in my life:

Seem indifferent
Seem threatening
Seem abandoning

(G) BULLYING STATE

I feel:

I want to hurt others
Without pity
Guilty
Contemptuous
Like hurting or punishing myself

People in my life:

Fear me
Attack me
Ignore me
Reject me

(H) HIGH STATE, SPEEDY

I feel:

Efficient
Energetic
Competent
Happy
Strong
Quick
Accurate
Speedy
Unstable
Over the top

People in my life:

Envy me
Admire me
Are tired by me
Give in to me

(I) CLOUD-CUCKOO-LAND STATE, BLISSED OUT

I feel:

Blissfully close to others
Cared for
Safe
Protected
Suffocated

People in my life:

Care for me
Adore me
Protect me
Meet all my needs

(J) DISMISSING STATE, CONTEMPTUOUS

I feel:

Better than others
Special
Deserving admiration
Suspicious of emotion
Intolerant of weakness in myself
Empty of feeling
Cruel
Dismissive of others

People in my life:

Important people admire me
Weak people give in to me

You can add other states here and label them K, L, etc

Part 2. Describing the states in more detail

NOTE: You will need a copy of this page for each of your states. Underline the correct description for each item.

Write here the letter/name identifying the state described on this page

STATE . . .

*Frequency

Over the past 100 days, I estimate I have experienced this state on:

1 day   2–10 days   11–20 days   21–40 days   41–70 days   71+ days

*Duration

This state usually lasts for:

| Minutes only | Less than 1 hour | Several hours | All day | 2 or more days | A week or more |

*How it feels emotionally

In this state I feel: Humiliated   Out of control   Anxious   Angry
   Blank   Despairing   Excited   Powerful Efficient

*How it feels physically

In this   Energetic   Slowed   Exhausted   Headache   Other
state I feel: Unreal   down   Outside   As if I
Physical   Strangely   myself   am in
symptoms   detached   a film

*This state usually starts

Abruptly   Over a few minutes   Gradually

*This state usually comes on

For no apparent reason   In response to what   In response to what
                             somebody says or does   somebody does not
                                                          do or say

This state usually ends

Abruptly   Over a few minutes   Gradually

This state usually ends

For no apparent reason   In response to what   In response to what
somebody says or does   somebody does not
do or say

This state is likely to come on when

I am tired   I have drunk alcohol   I have taken other drugs   other
(specify)

I can get out of this state by

Drinking   Taking drugs   Hurting   Talking to a   other
myself   close friend   (specify)

I find being in this state

Very   Distressing   Boring   Despairing   Indifferent
distressing   Pleasant

Index

DATE DUE

GAYLORD   PRINTED IN U.S.A.